4th Edition

MANAGING and COORDINATING NURSING CARE

MANAGING and COORDINATING NURSING CARE

Illustrations by
Cathy Miller

Janice Rider Ellis, PhD, RN
Professor and Director of
    Nursing Education
Shoreline Community College
Seattle, Washington

Celia Love Hartley, MN, RN
Curriculum Consultant
Camano Island, Washington

And

Professor Emerita
College of the Desert
Palm Desert, California

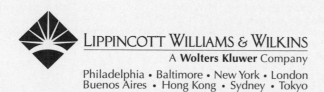

LIPPINCOTT WILLIAMS & WILKINS
A **Wolters Kluwer** Company

Philadelphia • Baltimore • New York • London
Buenos Aires • Hong Kong • Sydney • Tokyo

Senior Acquisitions Editor: Quincy McDonald
Managing Editor: Helen Kogut
Editorial Assistant: Marie Rim
Senior Production Editor: Debra Schiff
Director of Nursing Production: Helen Ewan
Managing Editor /Production: Erika Kors
Art Director: Brett MacNaughton
Interior Design: Melissa Olson
Cover Design: Melissa Walter
Senior Manufacturing Manager: William Alberti
Compositor: Graphic World Publishing Services
Printer: RRD-Crawfordsville

4th Edition

9 8 7 6 5 4

Library of Congress Cataloging-in-Publication Data

Ellis, Janice Rider.
  Managing and coordinating nursing care / Janice Rider Ellis, Celia Love Hartley ; illustrations by Cathy Miller.—4th ed.
      p. ; cm.
  Includes bibliographical references and index.
  ISBN 13: 978-0-7817-4106-4
  ISBN 10: 0-7817-4106-8
  1. Nursing services—Administration. 2. Nursing—Planning. I. Hartley, Celia Love. II. Title.
  [DNLM: 1. Nursing—organization & administration. 2. Nurse's Role. 3. Patient Care Planning—organization & administration. WY 105 E47m 2005]
RT89.E43 2005
362.17′3′068—dc22

2004004868

Reviewers

Preface

This book is written with the belief that every nurse can expect to have a leadership role in nursing and that all nurses are managers. Although leadership and management have distinct components, they also overlap in some of their applications. Because of the conviction that all nurses participate in these roles, we recognize the need for students at all levels of nursing education to develop core skills of management and leadership that will enable them to meet the challenges they face in their workplace. This textbook is written for those students. It presents content that will help the new graduate apply principles of leadership to the management and coordination of care for groups of patients, to better understand and manage the health care environment and its resources, and to supervise the care delivered by those with less education or experience. In addition, the text brings to the student content related to information technology in health care; describing the many ways in which it is being used in care delivery and offering suggestions regarding its application. An important aspect of this is a review of evidence-based practice that finds its foundation in nursing research. Just as all nurses have a leadership and management role, they also have a role to play in nursing research.

ORGANIZATION OF THE TEXT

This textbook is organized into three units. Although the content of each chapter can stand alone, a greater sense of the whole can be seen if the reader begins with Chapter 1 and progresses through the text to Chapter 14.

Unit 1

Unit 1 takes the student on a journey that explores the many aspects of working within organizations. The development of leadership behavior and management skills provides a foundation for individuals to look at themselves, their own perceptions of what the management role entails, and how they will develop their own management styles. Understanding the structure and function of organizations is critical to the implementation of management skills. The managing of resources increases in importance as pressure to contain costs grows in the health care system. The nurse's role in managing both supplies and personnel cannot be overemphasized. Similarly, discussion of the nurse's role in supporting quality care stresses the shared responsibility of all nurses for evaluating nursing care and nursing care delivery within the health care team. In this context, the processes of quality assurance, total quality management, and continuous quality improvement are explained.

Unit 2

Unit 2 focuses on the many roles of the nurse and provides many helpful guidelines for implementing these roles. "The Nurse as Communicator, Teacher, Motivator, and Team Builder" includes a discussion of professionalism as well as the role in building teams and empowering others. "The Nurse as Decision Maker and Delegator" provides guidelines for these activities as well as suggestions for effective assignment of responsibilities and prioritization of care. "The Nurse as Supervisor and Evaluator" describes the responsibilities encountered when directing the work of others and provides suggestions for giving meaningful feedback, accurate evaluation, and describes the steps to be followed in progressive discipline. "The Nurse as Change Agent and Advocate" pursues the challenges of overcoming the resistance to change, implementing change, and assuring its acceptance. As an advocate in the system, the nurse needs skills in determining who needs an advocate and in determining the best way to be an advocate for the client or for other staff. "The Nurse as Conflict Manager, Negotiator, and Mediator" provides essential understandings of these roles and makes suggestions for building skills in these areas. Content related to the collective bargaining process as it applies to nursing is included.

Unit 3

Unit 3 is directed toward the evolving issues in nursing practice. The unit begins with a discussion of activities that will help in advancing a career, including career mapping, seeking employment, preparing for interviews, and moving to new positions. "Attaining and Maintaining Competence," with emphasis on cultural competence, interpersonal competence, and technical competence, provides key information about the importance of competent practice and how it might be measured in health care organizations. The challenges of today's workplace are described and discussed, with a focus on the problem employee. Suggestions and guidelines for working with a wide variety of personalities are included. The importance of nursing informatics in today's health environment and the increasing emphasis on evidence-based practice are emphasized. Students are provided information to allow them to understand the basic terms used in research, various types of research that are employed in nursing, and the importance

of their role in collecting data for research. The book concludes with a look into the future. A brief discussion of the evolution of nursing education leads to an exploration of differentiated practice. The goals of the National Advisory Council on Nurse Education and Practice (NACNEP), entrepreneurial roles for nurses, and nursing classifications as a language for nursing are also described.

SPECIAL FEATURES

In this edition, we have identified a number of pedagogies that we believe will enhance student learning.

- **Learning Outcomes.** Each chapter begins with a list of learning outcomes to assist students in planning and evaluating their study.
- **Key Terms.** Key terms are listed at the opening of each chapter and are highlighted as they occur in the chapter text to alert students to terminology that is used in the management context.
- **Examples.** Examples of concepts being discussed are integrated throughout each chapter to assist the student to understand the application in health care.
- **Critical Thinking Exercises.** Critical thinking exercises that provide students opportunities to apply for themselves the concepts being discussed occur throughout each chapter.
- **Cultural and Legal/Ethical Icons.**   Icons pointing out cultural concepts and legal/ethical considerations occur throughout each chapter.
- **Key Concepts.** Key points are summarized at the conclusion of each chapter.
- **Illustrations.** Illustrations throughout the text are designed to highlight important points and help students to visualize concepts. Their humor helps lighten what students often find to be difficult content.

We hope that you will find this textbook a useful and beneficial aid as you progress to your role as a professional nurse. As we have done with all previous editions, we welcome and appreciate your feedback and suggestions. Through this kind of professional interchange we are able to more effectively meet the needs of tomorrow's students.

Janice Rider Ellis, PhD, RN
Celia Love Hartley, MN, RN

Acknowledgments

As with all projects such as writing a textbook, there are many individuals who have contributed significantly to this work. First, we thank those individuals who took the time and effort to conscientiously review the previous edition and send their suggestions to us for consideration. Their names are listed in the reviewers section.

We also thank the faculty members who have used this text in the past and who have shared with us their ideas for an improved text. We invite this continued activity.

We welcome and thank Cathy Miller for her creative artistic interpretation of the concepts presented in each chapter. Her chapter openers are a new feature with this edition.

We express appreciation to the people at Lippincott Williams & Wilkins who have assisted in the production and publication of this text. We want to give special recognition to Helen Kogut, with whom we have worked in other capacities in the past, but who provided expert assistance as managing editor on this edition.

We owe much to our respective parents, Lillian and Evert Rider and Warren and Ella Love, who instilled in us a belief in our potential and a commitment to lifelong learning. And finally, we thank our respective husbands, Ivan and Gordon, who continue to provide support with humor and caring and to, as one of them stated, "Hold the lamp" while we work to meet deadlines.

Janice Rider Ellis, PhD, RN
Celia Love Hartley, MN, RN

Contents

1

WORKING WITHIN ORGANIZATIONS

To best prepare for your role as a registered nurse with responsibility for managing and coordinating patient care, you need to develop an understanding of what this role encompasses and of the setting in which you will practice. Unit 1 provides general background knowledge about roles and leadership behaviors that are critical to functioning as a manager. What kind of manager do you want to be? How do you find a leadership style for yourself that is effective for patient care while still capturing those qualities that bring out the best in you? Because most nurses function as employees within organizations or agencies that deliver health care services, you will need to understand how organizations are structured and how they function if you are to work effectively within the organization. As you study organizations, you will soon recognize that some individuals exercise significant power within the organization. The different types of power, how it is acquired, and how it can best be used are also a part of the unit. Your ability to manage resources responsibly is also a critical element in becoming a manager. It is critical that you possess a beginning understanding of health care financing, the budget process, and the nurse's role in cost containment if you are to manage wisely. You also need to have a good comprehension of the basis for assuring the quality of care, including knowledge of the standards by which quality care is measured as well as the processes for determining the quality of care. Unit 1, therefore, lays the foundation on which you will begin to build your ability to function knowledgeably as a nurse manager, a coordinator of care, and a leader in the nursing community.

Developing Leadership Behavior and Management Skills

Learning Outcomes ■ ■ ■ ■

After completing this chapter, you should be able to:

1. Discuss the differences between leadership and management activities.
2. Apply leadership theories to nursing leadership and management activities.
3. Analyze the three basic types of management, identifying the characteristics and disadvantages of each and providing an example of a situation in which each would be used appropriately.
4. Define power, and analyze the seven forms of power, describing the differences among them.
5. Discuss the concept of empowerment as employed in management roles.
6. Discuss the role of followers and the characteristics of effective and ineffective followers.
7. Identify activities that can help develop your leadership style and develop a plan to build your own leadership style.
8. Analyze other factors that influence leadership style.
9. Describe methods of assessing your effectiveness as a leader.

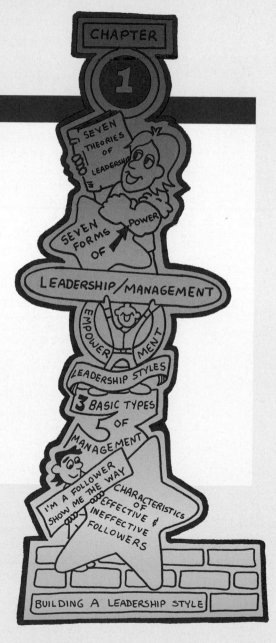

3

Key Terms   ■   ■   ■   ■   ■

authority

authoritarian or autocratic
  leadership

behavioral theory

coercive power

connection power

contingency theory of
  leadership

democratic leadership

empowerment

expert power

Great Man theory

informational power

laissez-faire leadership

leadership

leadership style

legitimate power

management

multicratic style

participative

permissive leadership

power

process theories

punishment power

referent power

relational model of
  leadership

reward power

servant leadership theory

situational theory of
  leadership

social change model of
  leadership

Theory X

Theory Y

Theory Z

trait or attribute theory

transformational
  leadership theory

EXAMPLE   *A Difference in Leadership*

Clancy Memorial Hospital is a 450-bed community hospital in a midsized urban city. Because of high census, the hospital operates two medical units, 2-East and 2-West, that provide similar services to clients. The staffing on the units is the same with regard to the number of staff employed and their educational preparation. The number of beds on each unit is identical. Nurses with equal educational preparation and experience manage the units. Yet, 2-West is a unit with a high level of esprit de corps in which a strong sense of team collaboration exists, low absenteeism occurs, and the unit consistently receives high ratings for quality of care as measured by client questionnaires. On the other hand, 2-East experiences a fair amount of dissension among staff, has a relatively high rate of absenteeism, and receives only mediocre ratings of quality of care by clients. What would cause the difference in these two units that are outwardly so similar? What are the factors that create such disparate patient evaluations? Why do staff members work together in harmony on one unit and not on the other? What style of leadership characterizes each unit manager? Could the leadership make that much difference?

As a novice, observing an experienced individual functioning skillfully in a leadership role, it would be easy to believe that leadership skills are innate within the individual or that the response the leader gets from others occurs by virtue of being appointed to the position. But leadership and management behaviors, like the other clinical skills you have acquired, are learned. It is also important to understand that all nurses occupy roles as leaders and managers, whether they are identified as such by title or position within the organization. In the present health care environment, the ability to function in a leadership role was never more important. Nurses working directly with patients need well-developed leadership skills to direct a team that will assess needs and provide care to a group of patients. Your ability to provide leadership to others will have a direct impact on how well the unit functions. Your skill in managing will have a direct influence on the quality of care your patients receive.

It is also important that you realize that you will be both a leader and a follower. At the same time that the staff nurse is serving as a leader and manager in delivering care to patients, the staff nurse also has an important responsibility as a follower. Staff nurses receive guidance from supervisors, charge nurses, patient care coordinators, or other leaders formally designated by the institution as managers. Although supervision is provided, each nurse employs management activities in carrying out professional responsibilities. You need to understand and be comfortable with the roles of both leader and follower if you are to function effectively as a manager in your own sphere of responsibility.

■ CONTRASTING LEADERSHIP AND MANAGEMENT

Leadership and *management* are two terms that are frequently used rather interchangeably. However, for our purposes, we want to distinguish between the two, although the difference may seem slight.

Leadership may be viewed as the process of guiding, teaching, motivating, and directing the activities of others toward attaining goals. It involves having the ability to influence others. Leadership often involves moving into a position because of special abilities, skills, or attributes and may be formal or informal within the organization (see Chapter 2).

Thus defined, leadership is not a new term to you; it is one you have heard and read about throughout your life. John van Maurik (2001) states that in 1996 alone, 187 books and articles were published with the word *leadership* in their title. Undoubtedly, you have looked at the leadership of international figures or of individuals who influenced history through their ability to inspire or motivate others. Names such as Abraham Lincoln, Franklin D. Roosevelt, Winston Churchill, Mohandas Gandhi, Martin Luther King, Margaret Thatcher, and Billy Graham may come quickly to mind. And you also might think of others, such as Hitler, who was able to rouse large numbers of people to action but whose leadership had an adverse effect on society and was responsible, in part, for the deaths of millions of people. Regarding leadership, Cronin (1995, p. 27) writes, "Leadership can be exercised in the service of noble, liberating, enriching ends, but it can also serve to manipulate, mislead and repress."

Management, on the other hand, involves the coordination and integration of resources through the activities of planning, organizing, directing, and controlling in order to accomplish specific goals and objectives within an organization. Management positions tend to be ones to which an individual is appointed. Typically, a manager has responsibility and accountability for tasks that must be accomplished, and

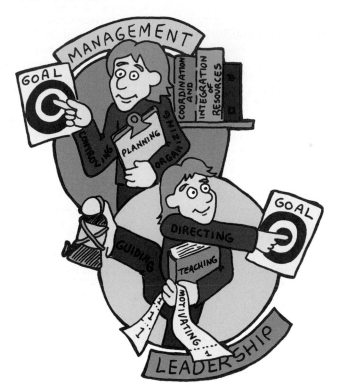

Leadership and management are terms frequently used interchangeably.

to fulfill those responsibilities plans, hires, coordinates, directs, organizes, evaluates, and budgets. If an individual functions poorly in the management role, the tendency within organizations is to replace that person with someone who can carry out the responsibilities in a more effective manner.

Ideally, a good manager should also possess leadership ability, but this does not always occur. On the other hand, a good leader may not possess management skills. However, both can be learned and improved by experience and the desire to increase your abilities and skills in both areas. Nurses must understand leadership and management as an important part of their responsibilities and must prepare themselves to participate at all levels.

In all nursing settings, the importance of leadership and management skills is equally great. Nurses in community settings, nursing homes, and hospitals require both clinical competency and the ability to lead and manage others in order to deliver effective nursing care.

This chapter provides an overview of the various theories concerning the development of leadership. It also explores the role of followers and examines the ways in which leaders and followers interact. An application of leadership to the management role is discussed. Some strategies for evaluating your own leadership style and those of managers you might choose as role models are examined. Finally, some suggestions are made to new graduates on how to begin to develop a responsive management style and how to work collaboratively with both leaders and followers.

■ LEADERSHIP THEORIES

The ways in which individuals influence and direct the activities of others has been a subject of interest for many years. As early as 1830, Hegel reportedly wrote the first book about leadership, focusing primarily on how it related to the political process (Bass, 1995). By the mid-twentieth century, researchers became interested in factors that resulted in greater or lesser productivity among workers and began to look at the role of the manager and leadership skills. As a result, a number of theories of leadership evolved. Some of the major theories are summarized in Table 1-1. We will not discuss all the theories in detail, but we will provide a general overview of the theories most commonly referenced and discuss the application of each to nursing. Theories can make a contribution to the analysis of leadership in any given situation and can also assist in the creation of environments in which nursing leadership skills can be learned and practiced. You will notice, as you review these theories, that they often build one on another, with each theorist expanding on ideas previously set forth and often reflecting the general attitude of the times. It is also quite possible for the thoughts expressed in an early theory to reemerge in the much later writings of another theorist. Although the organization is somewhat arbitrary and others may place the theories in different categories, we look at theories under four major headings, none of which should be considered mutually exclusive or totally time bound.

Great Man and Trait Theories

The Great Man theory and the trait theories of leadership were among the earliest. Evolving from Aristotelian philosophy, which contends that some people are born to lead and others are born to be led, the **Great Man theory** set forth the premise that certain people are born to be leaders, having inherited a set of innate characteristics that endow them with the unique ability to lead others. This theory grew because the ability to lead others was often seen within royal and prominent families. Others were not allowed to become leaders, a fact that also helps explain its demise. Currently, most people do not accept the idea that an individual is born to lead.

The **trait or attribute theory** evolved from the Great Man theory of leadership when social and economic barriers no longer prevented members of the general public from occupying leadership roles. Behavioral scientists began to identify the common traits of great leaders throughout the ages. These traits frequently included assertiveness, ambition, charisma, creativity, decisiveness, enthusiasm, intelligence, initiative, integrity, persistence, physical characteristics (especially above-average height), sense of self, technical mastery, verbal ability, and similar skills. In 1948, Stogdill reviewed more than 120 such studies of traits, looking for a reliable and coherent pattern and concluded that no such pattern existed.

The trait theory approach to leadership lost appeal because it failed to look at the situation in which action was occurring, neglected the role of the follower, and did not consider the importance of the group situation. Leaders in one situation may function as followers in another. In addition, leaders who are effective in some circumstances calling for sociability, popularity, and dependability are ineffective in others that require prompt and decisive actions. This said, the idea continues to fascinate many.

TABLE 1-1	MAJOR RESEARCHERS IN LEADERSHIP AND THEIR THEORIES OR POSITIONS		
Time Developed	**Theorist**	**Theory Name or Approach**	**General Concept**
1830	G. F. Hegel	Some of the first writing about leadership	Believed that leaders must first serve as followers to best understand their followers. This understanding was a paramount requirement of effective leadership.
1841	Thomas Carlyle	Great Man	Believed the leader to be a person endowed with unique qualities and characteristics needed to lead others.
1924	Max Weber	Charismatic leadership	Believed that leaders emerge in a time of crisis owing to their inherent charisma.
1940	C. Bird	Trait	Compiled a list of 79 traits of leaders. Natural born leaders possess certain physical traits and personality characteristics that establish them in the leadership role.
1951	K. Lewin	Behaviorist	Looked at the ability to lead in relationship to leadership style, comparing leaders who made unilateral decisions with those who involved followers in decision making.
1958	R. Tannenbaum and W. H. Schmidt	Humanistic	Looked at the range of leadership styles open to a manager, expressed as a continuum ranging from manager-centered leadership to subordinate-centered leadership.
1957, 1962, 1964	C. Argyris	Humanistic— maturity– immaturity	Perceived a conflict between the organization and the individual, believing that the organization will be most effective when leadership provides means for followers to make a creative contribution.
1960, 1966	Douglas McGregor	Humanistic- Theory X and Theory Y	Looked at the way different leaders view followers—titled Theory X and Theory Y. **Theory X** assumes that people are passive and resistant to organizational needs and need to be directed and motivated. **Theory Y** assumes people desire responsibility, are motivated, work hard, and are cooperative.
1967	Likert	Humanistic	Suggested leadership is a relative process in which leaders must consider expectations, values, and interpersonal skills of those with whom they interact.
1964, 1978	Robert R. Blake and Jane S. Mouton	Humanistic— managerial grid	Identified five management styles, placed on a grid that combines concern for production and concern for people and is related to the maturity of subordinates.
1965	Abraham Maslow	Self-actualization	Stressed importance of leaders developing the self-esteem and psychological health of subordinates so that subordinates could become what they have the capacity to achieve.

continued

TABLE 1-1	MAJOR RESEARCHERS IN LEADERSHIP AND THEIR THEORIES OR POSITIONS *continued*		
Time Developed	**Theorist**	**Theory Name or Approach**	**General Concept**
1967	F. E. Fiedler	Contingency approach	Suggested that no one leadership style is effective in all situations. The best style is contingent on the situation.
1971	Robert J. House	Path–goal	A leader's effectiveness is determined by the ability to minimize obstructions to goals, establish outcomes, and reward followers for high production.
1971	G. A. Yukl	Multiple-linkage model	Proposed that the leader's initiation of structure aided subordinates' ability to cope; consideration for subordinates' welfare enhances worker satisfaction.
1977	P. Hersey and K. H. Blanchard	Situational approach	Developed model to predict which leadership style would be most effective in situations, based on followers' maturity.
1977	Robert Greenleaf	Servant leadership	Suggested that successful leaders influence others as a result of dedicating their lives to serving others.
1978	J. M. Burns	Transactional	Examined leadership as related to striking a bargain in which there is a mutual exchange between leaders and followers.
1981	W. G. Ouchi	**Theory Z**	Expanded McGregor's Theory Y to support democratic leadership, which includes consensus decision making, job security, quality circles, and strong bonds between superiors and subordinates.
1994	Heinrich von Pierer	Transformational leadership	Placed emphasis on the collective purpose and mutual growth of leaders and followers. Places more responsibility on leader for vision and relationship building.
1994	Peter Senge	Visionary leadership	Viewed the role of the leader as that of being a strategic visionary. Advocated "learning" organizations in which the leader was a designer, steward, and teacher who built a shared vision.
1994	Ronald A. Heifetz	Ethical leadership	Examined the ethical questions that surround the area of leadership and turned to the leader as an educator.
2001	C. E. Johnson	Ethical leadership	Looked at the questionable aspects of leadership, the character and disposition of leaders, and ethical standards and strategies.

Based on information gathered from Bass, B. M. (1990). *Bass & Stogdill's Handbook of Leadership: Theory, Research, and Managerial Applications,* (3rd ed.). New York: The Free Press.

Critical Thinking Exercise

Identify the traits, attributes, or characteristics that you believe should be exhibited by nursing leaders. Compare your list of traits with those of a classmate. How many were similar? How many were different? Which of the traits will you want to build into your own leadership style? Explain why you view each as important.

Behavioral Theories

Behavioral theories, at times also referred to as the humanist approach, emerged during the 1940s and 1950s and led to studies of the 1960s. They were so named because they looked at the behaviors in which leaders engaged. Early researchers most identified with this approach are Chester Barnard and Herbert Simon. These theories went a step further in analyzing organizational effectiveness by examining the contribution of social relations and formal structure in interaction. Barnard, who was very influential in introducing the need to look at behavioral, intuitive, and emotional aspects of leadership, looked at both the formal and informal structures that exist in any organization and identified additional components, such as the cooperative system, that must be a part of any organizational assessment. He suggested that authority is delegated upward and is granted by one's subordinates.

Herbert Simon described the organization as an exchange system in which employees produced work for specific inducements as long as they perceived the inducements as more substantial than the effort required. Simon felt that there were no ideal solutions to management problems, but that some could be seen as more satisfactory than others. This principle of "satisficing," or arriving at mutually satisfying solutions, meant that effective decisions could be reached in which the participants saw the results as individually beneficial.

A number of studies evolved that looked at the attitude that prevailed between the task (or production or structure) to be accomplished and the relationship (or employee or consideration) focus. Workers could no longer be considered simply as cogs in a machine; their attitudes, their concerns, and their relationships were as important to effective operation as their abilities to perform a task. One of the best-known studies based on this approach was conducted at the Hawthorne Works of the Western Electric Company. These studies repeatedly demonstrated that when management gave special attention to workers, productivity would most likely increase, regardless of the working conditions. The importance of interpersonal relations between supervisors and subordinates and the role of social conditions in organizational effectiveness took on new significance.

McGregor (1960), Argyris (1964), and Maslow (1970) expanded on these theories. Other studies included the Ohio State leadership studies, the Michigan leadership studies, and group dynamics studies. Blake and Mouton (1964) developed a managerial grid based on concern for task and concern for relationships. This grid placed the leader on a bipolar grid that looked at the leader as task oriented, who is concerned with getting work done; and relationship oriented, who is concerned with interpersonal relationships and needs of group members. Leaders who were uninvolved, did little planning, and showed little concern for team members earned the lowest ratings. The most effective leadership approach was identified as one involving both a high-task and a high-relationship orientation, in which the leader promotes open communication, sets goals, intervenes in conflicts, and involves team members in decision making.

Critical Thinking Exercise

Spend a few minutes recalling the leadership approach used by several of the clinical managers on the units to which you have been assigned. In what ways did these managers demonstrate a behaviorist approach to leadership? What degree of consideration was provided to the nursing staff? In what ways was that consideration demonstrated? How did the staff react? What might have made the situation even better?

Situational and Contingency Theories

As a reaction to the early trait theories, another school of thought developed that focused on the context or the situation in which the leader functions, which thus became known as the **situational theory of relationship** and the **contingency theory of relationship.** These were based largely on the premise that the leadership style that would prove successful in one set of circumstances may not be effective in another. For example, in a crisis a strong and assertive leader might be needed but would not be wanted in another situation.

At the beginning of the twentieth century, Follett (1918) began to view organizations as systems composed of contingencies and published books setting forth her ideas. Her theories, which received little credit until much later, suggested that the situation should determine the approach to be followed. Situational theories examined such things as hierarchical structure of the organization, atmosphere of the organization, and characteristics of the leadership role and the follower role. They remain popular today.

Hersey and Blanchard (1995, p. 207) believed that "the leader must remain sensitive to the follower's level of readiness" and looked at leadership as having four basic styles: telling, selling, participating, and delegating. The readiness of the group determined which style would be most effective in a given situation; the leader's behavior must change appropriately in order to maintain the performance of followers.

Situational theories helped explain how leaders effective in one instance might be ineffective in others, but they tended to ignore the role of individual characteristics or that individuals can vary in their approaches to situations.

Fiedler (1967) believed that leadership style alone was not enough to explain leadership effectiveness. In the 1960s, he developed the contingency theory approach in which he described three components of any situation that must be included in an examination of leader effectiveness: (i) the nature of the leader–member relationship, (ii) the structure of the task to be performed and (iii) the authority or power the leader had to act as determined by job description and organizational support. Fiedler went on to describe eight situations, referred to as situational favorableness, ranging from favorable to unfavorable, that impact the type of leadership that results in the most effective outcomes.

A number of contingency-based theories followed. Vroom and Yetton (1973) suggested the normative decision theory, identifying a range of decision-making styles.

House (1971) looked at the successful leader as one who shows followers the rewards that can be earned by meeting the goal and illustrates the paths by which rewards can be obtained. His theory was named the path–goal theory and looked at supervision more than decision making. Currently, most contemporary theories reflect a contingency perspective. No single style of leadership is appropriate to all situations.

In nursing, we find that the situation impacts the type of leadership that is effective. A nurse providing leadership to a team employed in an emergency department may use approaches entirely different from those used by the manager of a rehabilitation unit. Trauma conditions require different direction and action than do situations that are more predictable and in which time is not of higher essence.

Critical Thinking Exercise

Explore the various situations nurses encounter in the health care environment. How do these situations vary with regard to the criticality, time available for decision making, opportunity for input from those involved in the situation, and structure of the environment in which it occurs? How might that affect the type of leadership demanded in that situation? How might it affect the way that subordinates respond?

Process Theories

The studies we have discussed might all be regarded as leader oriented in that they tend to look at the leaders' actions and attitude. More recently, we have witnessed a trend to what could be referred to as **process theories,** so named because they look at leadership as it relates to group interaction. In 1965, Hollander looked at how far valued members of a group were allowed to deviate from group norms or to act idiosyncratically. Thus, valued members of the group are allowed to exchange their competence and loyalty for group-mediated rewards, ranging from physical rewards such as money to less tangible rewards such as honor or influence. The individual's achieved value (status) allows new ideas and new ways of doing things to be introduced to the group (Chemers, 1995).

The **transformational leadership theory** developed by Burns (1978) is often reflected in nursing literature and practice. Essentially, a transformational leader may be defined as a leader who motivates followers to perform at their full potential by influencing changes in perceptions and by providing a sense of direction to the group. The group is encouraged to set aside personal interests for the good of the group. Group members are empowered and motivated and provide input to decision making, and leaders and followers raise one another to higher levels of performance.

Other process theories include the **relational model of leadership** described by Komives et al. (1998), in which leadership is viewed as a relational process designed to accomplish a common goal to benefit all. As with transformational leadership, the leader is empowering and process oriented, moving the group toward the goal. Greenleaf (1995) developed the **servant leadership theory,** in which he pictured successful leaders as being able to influence others as a result of dedicating their lives to serving others. The **social change model of leadership** (Higher Education Research

Institute, 1996) is developed around the process by which individuals and groups work toward a common goal and improve the quality of life for all by promoting basic values.

Recent research on leadership has looked at behavior across cultures. For example, in Western industrialized nations, directive and task-oriented leadership behaviors are usually differentiated from those that are more considerate or interpersonally oriented. Chemers (1995, p. 97) reports that research in developing nations indicates that "the leaders who have the highest group performance and the most satisfied subordinates are those who combine directive task styles with interpersonal warmth and consideration." Chemers concludes that the culture, through the processes of socialization, helps shape the needs, values, and personalities of both leaders and followers. Another cultural difference noted is that Western democracies place more emphasis on individualism whereas the rest of the world possesses group-oriented values.

In summary, each theory of leadership makes a contribution to our understanding of this complex role. Clearly, many variables contribute to effective leadership, including personal attributes, characteristics of the group, resources, cohesiveness of the group, relationships of the leader to the group, and ability. Over the years, the continuum of leader behavior has tended to shift from a task-oriented to a relationship-oriented focus. Effective leaders are those who acknowledge the importance of both task-oriented and relationship-oriented actions and seek to provide structure and support for subordinates. As you move into positions of leadership in nursing, the challenge to you will be finding an approach to directing the activities of others in a manner that will recognize and give credence to the relationship considerations in a health care environment that has never before been more highly task oriented.

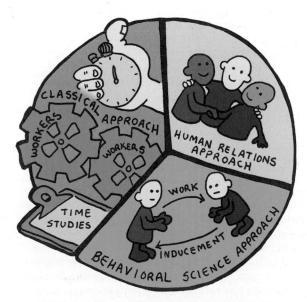

Many variables contribute to effective leadership.

■ WOMEN AND LEADERSHIP

Historically, women have been viewed as less effective in leadership positions than men. Some suggest that the lower prestige and desirability of nursing as a profession is related to the fact that it is primarily female oriented. Bass (1990) reports a number of studies on women and leadership. By and large, the studies have found that stereotypes have identified women as less competent, less aggressive, less task oriented, more dependent, and more emotional than males. He also noted that women were found to be more effective communicators and more attentive to upward communications from their subordinates and more relations oriented than their male counterparts. Bass (1990, p. 737) concluded that the role of women in leadership is changing so rapidly that earlier research may need to be discounted, but encourages continued consideration be directed "to the underlying dynamics and dimensions of importance to success and effectiveness of women leaders."

  ## ■ LEADERSHIP AND CULTURES

Culture has a strong influence on leadership. In Western countries, the rugged individualist who courageously takes charge and leads others to victory is honored and admired. In some Eastern cultures, this rugged individualist might be thought of as offensive. Over the years, each culture has selected its leaders from among its own, using the standards of that group. In the United States, which each year becomes more and more diverse, it is important that no one be excluded from leadership positions because of race or culture; in fact, it is against the law.

Despite legal mandates, affirmative action, civil rights regulations, and social pressure, the number of minorities in major leadership roles in businesses and government is limited. Although the situation is much improved over what it was a decade ago, greater representation by minorities in leadership roles is being encouraged. Such changes will occur only as a result of a national effort involving both public and private sectors. Educational institutions will play a significant role in this effort as they develop programs that will assist members of minority and ethnic groups to master the skills that will prepare them for leadership roles.

■ TYPES OF LEADERSHIP STYLES

Your effectiveness as a manager may be greatly influenced by your **leadership style,** the pattern of behavior you exhibit when attempting to influence and direct the activities of others. All nurses need to examine their leadership style and develop it appropriately.

Individual characteristics constitute one important variable that determines the type of manager a nurse might be. How does the leader view subordinates and are they basically ego centered or other centered? Correspondingly, the characteristics of the followers will also influence the style of leadership employed. Another factor affecting style is the type of institutional organization or the situation in which the nurse functions. In Chapter 2, you will become acquainted with various types of organizations. The degree to which authority is centralized or dispersed and the way in which communication and consultation occur have great influence on management style. In addition, the nurse manager can choose to focus on the tasks to be done, on the motivation and satisfaction of the subordinates, or on a combination of approaches. Within the constraints of leadership style and organizational structure, three basic leadership styles can be described: authoritarian, democratic, and laissez-faire. Each type of leadership style can be appropriate when used in the right situation. A fourth style, referred to as the multicratic style, has evolved from the application of the other three.

Authoritarian or Autocratic Leadership

The **authoritarian** or **autocratic leadership** style is characterized by strong control by the manager over the workgroup and also may be referred to as the directive approach. The activities of the group are primarily directive, with activities determined by the leader and dictated to the followers, with no input from the followers on decisions. Communication flows downward and emphasis is on accomplishing the task. Managers who exercise this style of leadership are characteristically found in bureaucratic organizations that reinforce the centrality of authority and reliance on formal rules, such as seen in the military. Their authority is generally derived from position power that is tied to their official job title within the organization. Chemers (1995) states that this directive style, in which the leader tells followers what to do, is most likely to work when the leader knows what the followers should be doing and the followers are inclined to do what they are told.

Disadvantages of this type of leadership style are clear. When subordinates feel that they are not listened to or supported, they are less likely to have a personal stake in the achievement of management goals. In addition, this style of leadership can create hostility and dependency among followers. An advantage of this style of leadership is that decisions can be made expeditiously without the lengthy time required for consultation to arrive at a collaboratively agreed-on course of action.

An authoritarian leadership style is appropriate when there is a need for immediate action and the manager is the individual with the best understanding of the situation. An example of this type of leadership might occur in an emergency department setting.

EXAMPLE *Authoritarian Leadership*

Janice Brown is in charge of the emergency department, working with a receptionist, an EMT, and the ER physician Dr. Black. In the waiting room at 9:00 p.m. is a mother with a young child who is complaining of an earache, a teenager who cut his hand hitting a window, and just arriving is an older gentleman who is in obvious distress. His face is pale and his skin is clammy, but he dismisses his discomfort as indigestion. The EMT begins to take the bleeding teenager back to a treatment room. The mother of the young child protests that she was there first. The receptionist announces that it is time for her supper break and prepares to leave for the cafeteria.

Because of her position as leader of the group and because of her greater knowledge of the possible ramifications of each patient's presenting symptoms, Nurse Brown takes charge of the situation in an authoritarian style. She instructs the EMT to take the older gentleman into the cardiac assessment room and instructs the receptionist to call Dr. Black first and then to call the cardiopulmonary technician and the laboratory technician. She gives the teenager a temporary dressing for his wound and tells him and the other waiting patients that someone will be with them as soon as possible. Then she prepares to start an IV, draw blood samples, and attach ECG leads on the older gentleman. Later, when all patients have been cared for, she thanks the staff members for their prompt response and shares with them the knowledge about some of the early indications of a myocardial infarction.

This situation is one in which an authoritarian leader functions best. The leader is in the best position to make judgments and decisions. There is not time to explain to subordinates why things must be accomplished, and there is not time to allow for discussion of alternative approaches. Because of the authority vested in the charge nurse, her instructions will be followed.

Authoritarian leaders will continue to have the full support of their subordinates only if they are able to involve them in the organization's overall goals and processes. Given the nature of the emergency department, this may have to be done at times other than when decisions are actually being made. By recognizing the contribution of subordinates and by assisting them in increasing their own skills and knowledge, managers help ensure that their authority is maintained and that their orders will be effectively followed in the future.

Democratic or Participative Leadership Style

The individual exercising a **democratic leadership** style, in contrast to the authoritarian leader, focuses on involving subordinates in decision making. This style of leadership may also be referred to as **participative.** Democratic leaders see themselves as coworkers, rather than as superiors, and stress the importance of communication, consensus, and teamwork. Although the leader may hold a position of higher authority, this authority is not exercised in a coercive manner, and the leader leads by providing information, suggesting direction, and being supportive of coworkers. Human relationships are important, and communications flow both up and down. Generally, the democratic leader functions best in an organization in which power is less centralized and there is less reliance on formal rules and policies.

Disadvantages of this style of leadership are that decision making can become a lengthy process. In addition, if coworkers are not confident about their own abilities to participate in planning and decision making, they may feel that the manager is not doing his or her job and is foisting difficult decisions off onto others who are not being paid to manage. Further, if decisions of the group cannot be implemented, coworkers may feel that the time and effort invested have been wasted.

Advantages of the democratic style are that coworkers who are consulted and who have input into decisions are more motivated to support such decisions. Involving subordinates in data gathering, analysis, planning, implementation, and evaluation of tasks ensures the widest possible scope and may provide information to which the manager alone would not have had access.

Democratic leadership is appropriate when the task or decision at hand is not one that requires urgent action, when subordinates can be expected to make meaningful contributions, and when their input can be taken into account. An example of democratic management might occur on a medical-surgical floor.

EXAMPLE *Democratic Leadership*

John Smith is working with a newly graduated nurse, an experienced LPN, and a nursing assistant. Together they have the responsibility for medical patients in one wing of Hastings Hospital. Nurse Smith has confidence in his subordinates because he has worked with them for some time. He knows that they make keen observations and often bring him important information about their patients. He also knows that they function within their assigned roles and are careful not to exceed their authority.

As they report for duty, Nurse Smith and his subordinates receive the report on their group of patients. Following the report, they meet to formulate a plan to deliver care. Nurse Smith requests their input, particularly on patients they might have cared for previously. LPN Jones indicates that one patient has to be watched particularly closely because of a tendency to climb over the bed rails. Nursing Assistant White suggests that another patient might be a particularly interesting assignment for the new graduate nurse, because the patient has a condition that is rarely seen at this hospital. The four coworkers design a plan for jointly caring for the assigned patients, with the team manager, Nurse Smith, providing information, encouragement, and direction as it is needed.

Laissez-faire Leadership

Also called **permissive leadership, laissez-faire leadership** provides the least structure and control and is also referred to as the delegating approach. Little or no direction is provided: coworkers develop their own goals, make their own decisions, and take responsibility for their own management. Managers concentrate on providing maximum support and freedom for coworkers, and decision making is dispersed throughout the group.

Disadvantages of this style in most health care settings are numerous. Generally, it is not possible to let each coworker arrive at an individual approach to decisions about patients. Because of the multidisciplinary nature of patient care, there usually must be more centralized decision making and agreement in following generally accepted policies and procedures.

Advantages of this style of leadership include providing maximum freedom for individuals and, presumably, increased motivation of subordinates to perform at high levels because of this independence. An example of laissez-faire leadership might occur in an inpatient psychiatric unit.

In circumstances in which a laissez-faire approach to leadership is inappropriately attempted, a leadership vacuum may occur. In these instances, it is not uncommon for an informal leader to arise who will give direction to the group. Coworkers recognize an implicit authority or degree of expertise in the informal leader. This may temporarily allow the group to continue to function while the informal leader provides the necessary direction and assistance.

EXAMPLE *Laissez-faire Leadership*

Nancy Stevens is one of four registered nurses who provide care to established patients on an inpatient psychiatric unit. The supervising nurse, recognizing the competence and accountability of the four RNs, allows them individually to structure and deliver care for the patients for whom they are responsible, as long as they adhere to general schedules for meals, group meetings, and medication administration. Each nurse develops a plan of care in conjunction with the individual patient and shares the patient's progress with other members of the staff at regularly scheduled case conference meetings at which the psychiatrist, the social services worker, and other professionals also present information.

Multicratic Leadership

Each of the three management styles may be used effectively, depending on the situation involved. One of the skills of leadership is identifying which style of leadership a particular situation requires. This so-called **multicratic style** combines the best of all styles, mediated by the requirements of the situation at hand. The multicratic leader provides a maximum of structure when the situation requires it, a maximum of group participation when needed, and support and encouragement for subordinates in all instances. For the new graduate, learning which is the best approach for a particular situation requires study and practice, just as with other nursing skills. Looking at this leadership style, it is not difficult to identify the various theories of leadership that could be applied. For example, situational theories support using the structure demanded by the situation. Encouraging group participation would be advocated in process theories. Supporting subordinates would be a part of the behaviorist theories.

■ POWER AND THE LEADERSHIP ROLE

The term **power** evokes many different feelings, such as fear, mistrust, control over others, and domination. It also has a wide variety of synonyms, such as force, strength, potency, stamina, vigor, control, and command. Thus, power has many different meanings.

Defining Power

Among the definitions of power one finds in a dictionary is "the ability to do, act or produce; the ability to control others; authority; sway; influence" (Neufeldt, 1996,

p. 1058). We tend to be in awe of the power of an individual who is able to accomplish significant tasks. We also notice that power can be defined as the ability to influence others either through persuasion or coercion. However, the concept of power should not be thought of as synonymous with leadership.

Our first experiences with power occur in the family unit as parents exercise control over children. Children are conditioned to follow the directives of their parents (and later their teachers), either through persuasion or punishment. These experiences may have been positive or negative, depending on the family structure and whether the parents relied more on persuasion or coercion. As we move into adulthood, we tend to transfer this concept of power to the workplace.

Individuals view power differently. Because women often have been culturally socialized to view power as dominance versus submission, they may hold more ambivalent or negative feelings toward power than do their male counterparts. However, as with women and leadership mentioned earlier in this chapter, this view appears to be changing. To fully develop your potential as a leader and manager, it is critical that you possess an understanding of power and its use.

Power is not a static phenomenon; it can change and shift, increase or decrease. Bass (1990) points out that differences in power in a group, organization, or society influence the kind of leadership that can be effective. When there are great differences in power among individuals or groups, a more directive leadership is likely; when the differences in power are small, a more participative leadership is likely.

Within an individual, power may vary from one time to another or from one situation to another. For example, the unit manager may have a great deal of power when it comes to the operation of a particular unit but very little in meetings chaired by the hospital administrator.

Types of Power

French and Raven (1959) identified five types of power based on the source: legitimate, referent, reward, coercive, and expert. These five types can be seen in many different settings.

(margin note: Cooperation)

(1) **Legitimate power,** often termed **authority,** is most frequently thought of as the power granted by an official position. Whoever holds the position has the same amount of authority, which may include making decisions on behalf of the organization, acquiring or controlling information, having access to people of higher status or power, and controlling the human and material resources of the organization. Most often, the individual holding legitimate power is given a title to indicate the authority that has been delegated, such as unit manager, vice president of patient care services, or administrator.

(margin note: Charisma)

(2) **Referent power** refers to the potential influence one has because of the strength of the relationship between the leader and followers. For example, when people admire leaders and see them as someone to model, leaders are said to have referent power. The individual has power based on the desire of followers to identify with leaders, or what leaders symbolize, and to be accepted by them. An expert and established staff nurse may possess referent power with the new graduate who wishes to emulate the skill and behavior demonstrated by the more experienced nurse. Referent power also exists because others tend to perceive the individual as powerful, as in the case of political figures. The term *charisma* has been used to describe this type of referent power and is sometimes referred to separately as another basis of power (Heineken & McCloskey, 1985). Charisma is the power that attracts one person to

another and relates to the way leaders act, talk, walk; the organizations to which they belong; and personal associations. Such behavior communicates the message "I am confident, sure of myself, and in charge," and tends to encourage others to ascribe power to the individual. The manner in which one dresses has also been associated with referent power and has resulted in people speaking of "power dressing" or wearing a "power suit." This concept evolved from the work of Molloy (1988), who examined the responses of people to various forms of dress. He concluded that most people associate certain types of clothing with power. The majority of powerful people in business choose to dress conservatively and avoid extremes of fashion.

Reward power is achieved by having the potential to influence others because of one's control over desired resources. These may include the power to give raises, bonuses, and promotions; select individuals for special projects or assignments; or distribute valued resources. In addition, an individual in a management position has a wealth of rewards that can be provided to employees, including praise, commendation, respect, and support. All persons have the ability to control rewards in any given environment. A client controls the rewards associated with positive feedback for the care you provide. You control the rewards of praise and recognition given to coworkers.

Coercive power, also referred to as **punishment power,** is the opposite of reward power. It ranges from negative sanctions to verbal threats of punishments and is based on the fear of punishment if the manager's expectations are not met. It implies the ability to impose penalties for noncompliance. The manager can control through the fear of loss of job or of punishment, such as undesirable assignments or shifts. Although we tend to view coercive power negatively, some situations may require coercion.

Legal aspects are frequently associated with coercive power. An individual who drives 75 miles per hour in a 50 mile-per-hour zone is subject to fine imposed by regulations. The law exercises coercive power to maintain safety for citizens. Similarly, the activities that nurses may perform are spelled out in the nurse practice acts of each state. A nurse who is discovered abusing drugs faces the threat of loss of license, position, and salary. The safety of clients must be the first consideration.

Expert power is gained through the possession of special knowledge, wisdom, sound judgment, good decisions, skill, or ability. Experts wield power and are able to accomplish their purposes because others recognize their abilities and turn to them for guidance. Typically, this type of power is limited to a specialized area. For example, persons with expertise in nuclear physics would not be powerful in a critical care unit unless they also possessed expertise in critical care. As nursing becomes ever-more specialized, we see an increase in expert power among professionals.

Various writers have identified additional sources of power. Heineken and McCloskey (1985) added **informational power** to the list. Informational power exists when individuals have information that others must have to accomplish particular goals. Examples would be when an individual has information regarding a budget, income, important upcoming events, or similar critical information. Information power may also be found in the person who has access to many different communication channels within an organization. Information is an integral part of some positions, and such jobs are powerful ones.

Connection power may be described as power based on having connections (or associations) with others who are powerful (Raven & Kruglanski, 1970). One often sees politicians exercising connection power when being seen with a powerful political figure may infer a higher personal status. Connection power may also involve working with others to accomplish a common goal. You can readily see how nurses could use this form of power to great advantage. Nursing is the single largest health care occupation. The force of all nurses working together could be phenomenal.

Influence and Influence Tactics

Just as there are various forms of power, there exist a number of influence tactics. In organizations, power, influence, and influence tactics are related to your ability to provide direction to others or to bring about change. It is useful to distinguish among these terms that are often used somewhat interchangeably. Hughes et al. (1995) define power as the capacity to produce effects on others. Influence is defined as the change in a target agent's attitudes, values, beliefs, or behaviors as a result of influence tactics. Influence tactics are defined as the actual behaviors an individual uses to change another person's attitudes, beliefs, values, or behaviors. In simpler language, they may be viewed as ways to persuade others to change their attitudes, beliefs, values, or ways in which they act. The tactics described by Hughes et al. (1995) are listed and explained in Table 1-2.

Influence tactics have been a part of our culture for years. They may be found in a myriad of situations, including advertising campaigns, public elections, contract negotiations, and even marriage relationships. Influence tactics have gained enough attention for researchers to develop taxonomies of behaviors.

Many of the tactics we use to influence others are good. Among positive tactics we think of things such as mutual respect, openness, trust, and mutual benefit. However, other tactics can be far less ethical. When we attempt to get others to act in a particular manner by creating obligations, through pressure tactics, or other coercive behaviors, it may be viewed by some as unethical. For example, attempting to persuade another individual to adopt a new behavior or to cease an old one

TABLE 1-2	INFLUENCE TACTICS
Type of Influence	**Description of Behavior**
Rational persuasion	The use of logical arguments or factual evidence to influence others
Inspirational appeals	A request or proposal designed to arouse enthusiasm or emotions in those to whom it is directed
Consultation	The process of asking others to participate in planning an activity or action
Ingratiation	The situation that occurs when one attempts to place another in a good mood before making a request
Personal appeals	Asking another to do a favor out of friendship
Exchange	The process of influencing through the exchange of favors
Coalition tactics	Occur when one seeks the aid or support of others in order to influence another
Pressure tactics	The use of threats or persistent reminders to influence another
Legitimizing tactics	Occur when one makes requests based on his/her position or authority

(such as smoking) can be interpreted as interfering with that individual's right to autonomy. Increasing attention is being directed toward the ethics of management behaviors.

Critical Thinking Exercise

Review the content presented in Table 1-2. Identify a situation in which each of the nine influence tactics might be used appropriately. Identify a situation in which it would be inappropriate to use each of the influence tactics. Do you believe that all nine are ethical? Explain your response. Would some be ethical in some situations and not in others? Explain your rationale.

■ EMPOWERMENT

Much has been written about empowerment in the last decade, whether referring to empowerment of staff or patients. The role of the manager in empowering subordinates forms the basis of many new approaches to management.

Defining Empowerment

Empowerment may be viewed as the process by which a leader shares power with others or enables them to act. It is the basis of transformational leadership, discussed earlier, in which the leader shares the vision of what is to be accomplished, delegates a great deal of authority for decision making, and allows employees to share in the satisfaction derived from goal achievement. It results in employees having a strong sense of self, which encourages the motivation to excel. John van Maurik (2001) views this as giving subordinates a mixture of three factors when assigning them a task:

Direction: Sufficient instructions to give confidence
Challenge: An element of stretch that will bring out creativity and satisfaction on completion
Autonomy/support: Confidence that there is further help and direction available if needed

Thus, empowerment involves changing the way in which individuals view themselves and their abilities. It means helping them realize that they have the skills needed to cope successfully with given situations, people, and events.

In many instances, empowerment requires a change in the organization's structure and the locus of decision making, which will be discussed in depth in Chapter 2. The opposite of empowerment is powerlessness, in which the individual feels demotivated, unable or incapable of accomplishing desired activities, and frustrated with the work environment. Powerlessness leads to dependent behavior.

Empowering Others

Because our approaches to leadership are moving toward involving others in decision making, the ability to empower others is a required skill for all good managers. What steps and actions should be taken to help a subordinate develop new skills and to feel enabled?

First, empowerment is best facilitated in an organization that supports such activity. It is difficult for a supervisor to empower subordinates when the individual is not empowered. Fortunately, most hospital units operate in some type of transformational leadership that involves individuals other than the manager in decision making and supports democratic leadership. When this is the case, we can move forward

Empowerment can begin with modeling the personal behaviors that will encourage others to be active participants. This requires that we be patient with others, that we communicate belief and trust in others, that open channels of communication be created, and that a sense of openness be established. It entails a demonstration of basic respect for others. We need to nurture an organizational climate that sends a message of acceptance, support, and collaboration. Once an environment exists that will allow the empowerment of others, we need to allow time for them to grow.

Encouraging others to make choices for themselves and to have input in decisions is a good beginning point. In other words, we delegate the power to make decisions to subordinates, thus fostering greater initiative and responsibility for tasks. For example, rather than directing the nursing assistant to bathe Mr. Jones, then Mrs. Archer, and finally Mrs. Katz, permit the nursing assistant to decide which is the best way to proceed. In this way you can help the nursing assistant build self-confidence in his or her own ability, a hallmark of empowerment.

You can also empower others by developing the habit of asking questions rather than giving directions. When we ask productive questions we stimulate others to think through issues or situations for themselves, to seek answers, and to problem-solve the situation. Such thoughtful questions that probe for answers should focus on concepts and strategies rather than on facts or figures.

When things go well, share your pleasure and pride with the subordinate, and, when appropriate, share the successes of individuals with the group. Allow them to experience the good feelings that accompany knowing that their work was done well and appreciated. This helps build confidence and self-esteem, the critical elements of feeling empowered. If things go poorly, you should focus on improving the situation rather than dealing with the errors of the individual. For example, if the nursing assistant is unable to complete the care of assigned patients in a timely manner, assist her or him to complete the work. At a later time, sit down with the individual and review how the assistant planned the care. Offer helpful suggestions to improve the situation and give recognition to the improvement when it occurs. Be supportive and encouraging. This is an especially crucial behavior during times when an individual is feeling stress and anxiety.

Encourage those working on your team to make suggestions about team problems or concerns. One of the characteristics of teams as we see them in today's health care environment is the diversity reflected in their makeup. Creativity is often greater in heterogeneous groups. We may discover hidden talents in a team member in the process. Constructing a work environment that encourages others to make suggestions and contribute ideas can capture this creativity. Again, good ideas need to be recognized and credited to the individual who provided them. This should be

TABLE 1-3	EMPOWERING STATEMENTS VERSUS STATEMENTS THAT MAKE ONE FEEL POWERLESS	
Empowering Statements		**Statements Encouraging Powerlessness**
What ideas do you have regarding the problem?		Here is what you should do.
What are your strategies for working with this client?		Just follow these steps and everything will be fine.
In looking at the outcomes, what do you think worked best?		Did you learn anything from what you just did?
How can I be of help to you?		I would tell you if I thought things were not going well.
How do you feel about how things went?		You must feel a lot better about that.
Next time, would you do anything differently?		Next time it would be a good idea to . . .
What things seem to be getting in your way?		Your problem is that you do not . . .
What other data do you need?		This is all that is really important.
What were your goals when you began?		Do you have any idea of where you are going?
You are really improving; that was a wonderful job.		Well, that's a lot better than the last time.

done publicly if possible; however, often it is appropriate to recognize the efforts of others through a note or short letter thanking them for their contributions and praising the accomplishment. All recognition and praise must be provided in a sincere manner and not to excess. In an effort to begin to empower others, we do not want to praise others for things they have not accomplished. Insincerity is quickly recognized in most instances. Table 1-3 provides examples of statements that help people feel empowered versus those that make people feel powerless.

If you have existed in work situations in which little empowerment occurred, initially you might not feel comfortable empowering others. However, like so many of the leadership skills we will discuss in this book, these skills can be learned. Display 1-1 summarizes the actions that can be taken to empower others.

EXAMPLE   *An Empowered Work Force*

At Clancy Memorial Hospital, Mary Loftus was Unit Manager on 2-West. The staff members respected Mary and admired her leadership ability. Mary involved others in decisions regarding patient care. They established unit goals as a group and she frequently asked for staff input regarding unit decisions. The staff felt consulted and valuable. Mary encouraged staff members to participate in hospital in-service programs and established work schedules to allow this to occur. She was patient and understanding, particularly with new employees or when something went wrong. Mary frequently praised members for care that was done especially well. It was not uncommon for staff from other units to request transfers to 2-West.

DISPLAY 1-1	**Actions to Empower Others**

PERSONAL BEHAVIORS
- Practice patience and understanding
- Model behaviors you wish to see in others
- Communicate clearly and kindly
- Develop a willingness to accept change
- Engage in self-awareness and self-evaluation

ONE-ON-ONE ACTIVITY
- Demonstrate respect for individuals
- Be patient and understanding
- Encourage openness and honesty
- Promote active participation
- Allow time for growth
- Recognize and give credit for accomplishments

WITH A GROUP
- Promote group participation and interaction
- Identify and clarify common visions and goals
- Establish group values
- Establish open channels of communication
- Foster a climate of respect, acceptance, collaboration, and cooperation
- Promote the sharing of information among group members
- Recognize accomplishments of others
- Celebrate accomplishments

■ THE RECIPROCAL ROLE

There are two parties to any leadership situation. The general would be of no importance if there were no army to command. Similarly, the role of the company president would be insignificant without the employees in the organization. Frequently, followers are incorrectly viewed as merely passive recipients of management strategies who carry out directives or who fail to do so. However, the effectiveness of an organization can be determined on the basis of how well followers follow. Certainly, we often find ourselves occupying two roles—one of leader, another as follower. When we have subordinates, we also have bosses. For example, the clinical supervisor of a medical unit who is responsible for subordinates on the unit reports to a vice president for patient services. The importance of recognizing this interchanging of roles in today's health care setting is great. Registered nurses who are expected to manage the care of patients at the bedside and to lead subordinates who support them in this process are also expected to be competent followers of nurse specialists, supervisors, and administrators.

We all begin our careers in a follower-type position. Some individuals choose to stay in follower roles and serve as team players who gain satisfaction from helping accomplish the goals of the organization in that role. This is the basis of the clinical ladder we will discuss in Chapter 14.

Role of the Follower

In reality, both the role of the leader and the role of the follower have responsibilities and expectations, and each individual is an active agent within the relationship. But what distinguishes an effective follower from and ineffective one? Kelley (1995, p. 195) states, "What distinguishes an effective from an ineffective follower is enthusiastic, intelligent and self-reliant participation—without star billing—in the pursuit of an organizational goal." He further lists four qualities of followers: "1) They manage themselves well; 2) They are committed to the organization and to a purpose, principle, or person outside themselves; 3) They build their competence and focus their efforts for maximum impact; and 4) They are courageous, honest, and credible" (Kelley, 1995, p. 196). Certainly, a follower possessing these qualities would function well in an organization that embraces a transformational form of leadership that counts on shared decision making.

Being a Good Follower

As a new graduate, there are several ways to ensure that you assume an effective follower role:

1. *Invest yourself.* You decided to accept your new position because you saw the opportunity to accomplish your own goals and objectives. Perhaps the organization specializes in caring for a particular type of patient with whom you are interested in working. Perhaps the institution has a reputation for delivering excellent nursing care. Whatever your motivation, you must begin to see how your own goals fit into the goals of the larger organization, whether this is viewed as the nursing service or the organization as a whole. To the degree that they are congruent, you will feel more of an investment in your role as follower. If you discover that there is a fundamental conflict between organizational goals and your personal goals, it may be necessary for you to reevaluate your decision to work there, because such conflict may substantially compromise your ability to be an effective follower or leader. (See Chapter 4 for a further discussion of goal setting.)

   Another part of being an effective follower is maintaining your competence. Look for opportunities to expand your skills through continuing education and workshops and seminars related to your area of practice. Set high standards for yourself. Recognize your strengths and the areas needing improvement. Seek to improve the latter without being pushed to do so.

2. *Clearly identify your responsibilities as a follower.* What is expected of you? What does your job description involve? To whom do you report? How is your performance evaluated and by whom? You only will be able to fulfill your role if you know specifically what it is. As a new graduate, you will be using your orientation time to learn your new role. Usual resources will include your job description; the procedure manual for the unit on which you will be working;

and policies dealing with institutional functioning, including evaluation and training of workers. During the orientation process, make certain you identify the resource person to whom you can go for continued clarification and assistance during the period following the orientation.

3. *Clearly identify your expectations of the leader.* Ensure that you understand the leader's role and relationship to you. Just as you must be cognizant of your own responsibilities, you need to understand what realistically to expect from your leader in relation to you and other members of the group. Holding unrealistic expectations of the leader may compromise your ability to perform your own role effectively and may make it difficult to establish an appropriate relationship with this person.

4. *Support your leader and your group.* Once you are committed to jointly held goals and have a clear understanding of your role as follower and the manager's role as leader, work toward the effective functioning of your group. This may sound self-evident, but unfortunately it is not uncommon for nurses to feel that their only obligation is to patients directly in their charge. Learning to work productively with others to achieve patient care goals is a much more effective way of ensuring that goals for all patients are met.

5. *Provide stimulation for your leader and your group.* One of the most important services followers can provide is to stimulate discussion, provide a fresh look at problems, and propose other potential solutions. Obviously, this is most effective when carried out in a constructive manner and with the support of the leader and group. Effective followers are not merely compliant subordinates, but rather are coworkers who see a personal responsibility in maintaining the best possible work environment. Establish yourself as an independent, critical thinker whose judgment can be trusted.

6. *Follow channels of communication and responsibility.* As a new graduate, you should be oriented to the organizational structure, including channels of authority and routes of communication. Although you may be tempted to take questions or problems to the most sympathetic coworker or leader, it is important to follow established channels. This course of action ensures that the leader who is responsible for overall operation of the area is aware of the concern, and it also serves to hold the leader responsible for a constructive response. The only time it is appropriate to approach someone further up the chain of authority is when you do not receive a response from your immediate supervisor; generally, it is best to inform the immediate leader of your intent to contact this person. This helps ensure that leaders are accountable for responsibilities assigned to them and for assuming authority appropriate to that position. Followers as well as managers have responsibility for ensuring that the organization operates effectively.

■ DEVELOPING YOUR LEADERSHIP ABILITY

It can be safely said that no one sets out to do a poor job. Yet, clear-cut differences can be observed between how two different individuals might go about accomplishing a task or in providing direction and guidance to others. As you work at developing your own leadership style and techniques, the following may help accomplish that goal:

1. *Increase your personal competence and knowledge.* Everyone expects that you will perform tasks well. If you are going to be recognized as a leader, your knowledge and skills will have to be exceptional. Subscribe to at least one nursing journal and read it thoroughly each month. Attend meetings, workshops, and in-service sessions, even if it requires doing so on your own time. Volunteer for new assignments or committees. Accept responsibility for researching a particular aspect of patient care to share with your colleagues. Initially, you may wish to seek out a role model or ask someone you admire to serve as your mentor. Aligning yourself with an individual recognized within the organization is an excellent way to begin building power.

2. *Develop and maintain flexibility.* Persons who expect to provide leadership to others must develop a reputation for flexibility and maneuverability. Getting locked into one position, one way of viewing issues, or one method of approaching concerns compromises and obstructs the ability to change and make progress. Possessing a broad vision of the entire organization is critical to its function, and being able to see how your unit fits into that picture is important. Be willing to compromise and negotiate. Allow yourself to be vulnerable and learn to laugh with others. Accept willingly your share of weekend work or night shift rotations. Develop the reputation of being a team player and get to know the team and what is important to it.

3. *Develop self-confidence, decisiveness, and integrity in decision making.* Know who you are and the things that you stand for. Share this with others. If you do not believe in yourself and your ability, no one else will believe in you either. Become visible within the organization by offering to serve on committees or work groups. Develop keen skills in listening, observing, and communicating. Encourage others to question your beliefs and approaches. These skills will give you access to important information that can be used to shape your future. Make others feel important, respected, and valued as part of the organization. Learn to accept graciously compliments for work that is well done. Let others know when you have received a special commendation or award, not in a boastful manner but rather in one that reflects a sense of self-worth and accomplishment. On the other hand, be willing to admit and accept responsibility for mistakes. Accept feedback from others and don't become defensive when faced with a negative comment.

4. *Walk, talk, and look poised and confident.* Be well groomed with clothes that are clean and pressed and hair that is maintained in a professionally acceptable style. Avoid loud and gaudy jewelry and makeup. Be assertive and articulate. Use basic good manners that include saying "please" and "thank you." How you look and act will influence others' perception of you.

5. *Develop and maintain alliances.* This involves communicating and networking with others who share similar goals and ambitions. Focus beyond yourself and listen, support, provide feedback, and coach. Share your knowledge with friends, value professionalism, and give credit to others when their achievements deserve recognition. Help others feel safe and valued.

6. *Develop your personal physical resources.* Health provides the energy and enthusiasm for activity. To successfully provide leadership to others, you need sufficient time to unwind, relax, rest, and have fun. This will provide time and

energy for necessary reflection on work activities. It is important to have outside interests and relationships that will supply reinforcement when the organization makes heavy demands on one's energy. Healthy living includes a healthy diet, exercise, rest, and relaxation. The leadership style you choose to develop will be influenced to some extent by your personal philosophy, roles with which you are comfortable, your values, and your personality and attitude. Develop self-awareness and belief in yourself. You must think positively about yourself before you will be able to provide leadership to others. These are internal factors. Also, factors in the work situation will have an even stronger influence on the approach you use.

Critical Thinking Exercise

Jim Morton, RN, is working as a staff nurse on an oncology unit at University Hospital. He is anxious to move into a position involving greater leadership roles and responsibility. What steps or actions should he take to achieve this personal goal? Which should be started immediately? What actions might be most effective? Why? What might he do if 1 year later he has not been offered any new roles?

■ OTHER FACTORS INFLUENCING YOUR LEADERSHIP STYLE

The size of the group for whom you are responsible will influence your approach. Larger groups require greater coordination. Typically, large groups also require more task orientation than do smaller associations.

The abilities, educational preparation, and maturity of the group will also influence your leadership style. If all the persons you direct have similar educational preparation that involves a number of years of study, you will choose to exercise a different approach than if the group is composed of individuals with varying educational and experience backgrounds, most of which are far less than your preparation for the positions. Is the group committed to the task to be done or does it view it as just a job? Is the group capable of making sound decisions?

The structure of the organization will greatly influence leadership styles. A hierarchical organization will provide less freedom, autonomy, and feedback than a more decentralized organization committed to shared governance. (Organizational structure will be discussed in detail in the Chapter 2.) In organizations in which there is less bureaucracy, employees feel more freedom to express new ideas and approaches and to make changes. Along with this, you will want to consider the traditions and values that have been operating in the organization. What leadership style is supported by the organization? What type would not be effective? What are the formal and informal power structures within the organization? What limitations do they impose or what opportunities do they offer? What is the culture of the organization?

The task to be accomplished will also influence leadership style. How long will it take? Is it short term or long term? What resources are needed? Does the nature of the task provide time for input from others or is it such that immediate action must be taken without delay?

The degree of stress in the situation or environment will also play a role in determining the leadership styles used. Situations that experience continued high levels of stress reduce the ability of all individuals, both the leaders and the followers, to think and creatively problem-solve. This is especially true if the stress is between the various individuals employed in the work situation or if it is between the leader and the group to be led.

■ ASSESSING YOUR OWN EFFECTIVENESS AS A LEADER

Each person develops an individual leadership style. The following self-assessment will help you explore ways to make your leadership style most effective.

Self-Assessment

You already have developed a style of working with both leaders and followers. Begin to analyze the ways in which you interact with others, including fellow students, instructors, nursing staff, and patients. Do you find that you are more comfortable in situations in which you are told precisely what is expected? In this case, as a follower you may feel more comfortable in a bureaucratic organizational structure in which the leader uses an authoritarian management style. When you relate to other students in groups, do you feel more comfortable when members all have a voice in the operation of the group? Do you feel that members of the group ought to be unfettered by constraints? If so, you may feel more comfortable with a democratic or permissive management style. Obviously, your preferences will depend to some extent on the situation in question, but developing an awareness of your comfort level with the various styles of management will provide important background data for you.

Environmental Assessment

Just as important as a knowledge of self is a knowledge of the work environment. Assess the nature of the unit and the hospital in which you will be working. Based on what you know of the relative advantages and disadvantages of different leadership styles in different work environments, begin to identify those that might be most productive in this setting. For example, is the agency in which you work developing shared governance structures? If so, staff nurses will be expected to contribute directly to making decisions not only about patient care but also about the overall operation of the agency itself. Does the agency have councils or committees on which nurses have membership? If so, these provide a valuable opportunity to influence policies and decisions that affect patient care. Does the agency have a strategic plan for development? Thomas (1993) points out that such a model can communicate long-range goals and provide staff an opportunity to contribute. Does the agency encourage individual initiative and innovation? Benefits can accrue to the organization and to individuals if both entrepreneurs (those outside the organization who assume the risks of a new endeavor) and intrepreneurs (those inside the organization who assume the risks of a new endeavor) are supported (Manion, 1994). If the agency for which you work is traditional in terms of its organization, with most decisions made at the upper levels of management, there may be many changes to be anticipated as health care reforms are introduced on both state and national levels. Being aware of changes in law and regulation may help you take advantage of new opportunities to be a part of important decisions affecting management at all levels. Does the agency for which you work operate any units using a differentiated practice model? If so, is the differentiation made by education or experience? Does it matter to you?

Identifying Role Models

You have most likely observed nurses who are particularly effective as leaders and followers. Begin to look more closely at their operating styles. How do they interact with subordinates and superiors? How do they involve coworkers in activities with joint responsibilities? What communication strategies do they use? What bases of power do they access? Frequently, effective managers are quite willing to talk about their approach to followers and can provide very helpful suggestions to new nurses. Practice using the leadership skills worksheet in Display 1-2 to examine the management style of nurses you might wish to emulate. You can also use the worksheet to analyze your own management style as it develops. An effective management style makes use of the skills and techniques discussed in subsequent chapters. It includes setting goals and objectives, understanding and using power, managing resources, making decisions, managing time, developing motivation, teaching staff, using feedback, managing conflict, and serving as an effective advocate.

Trying Out Leadership Styles

All the observation, data gathering, and assessment of leadership styles are ineffective if not put into action. After you have assessed yourself, assessed your environment, and identified a management style you feel you would like to emulate, practice using it in your work.

If this means a change from your current operating style, it is usually helpful to inform subordinates or coworkers that you are trying something different and to enlist their assistance. If you are moving to a more democratic structure, it may be important to make clear to subordinates exactly what their responsibilities will be under the new system. For example, if you, as the registered nurse, were accustomed to assigning subordinates responsibilities without consulting them, and you wish to begin incorporating their input, you would let them know that you expect such input, plan to use it in making assignments, and value their participation.

As a new nurse, you may find the leadership skills worksheet (Display 1-2) helpful in beginning to explore your own approach to management. You may use it to evaluate the leadership skills of nurses you observe and to keep track of strategies you decide to try out.

Evaluating Effectiveness

Just as with any other nursing intervention, evaluation of the effectiveness of your leadership style is important, particularly during the formative period or periods of change. Identify specifically the characteristics of your leadership style on which you

DISPLAY 1-2   **Leadership Skills Worksheet**

Identify a nurse whose leadership style you would like to emulate. Observe the manner in which this person interacts with team members, supervisors, and other members of the health care team. Identify whether this individual is using an authoritarian, democratic, or laissez-faire approach in the following situations. Note skills and techniques you might like to consider in developing your own leadership style.

Description of Situation _____

Leadership Skill	Management Approach	Effectiveness
Setting goals—Sharing vision		
Developing motivation		
Decision making		
Empowering others		
Teaching staff		
Using feedback		
Managing time		
Managing resources		
Advocating		
Managing conflict		
Using research		

Note: _____

_____

want feedback. Do you want to know whether communications are effective? Whether decision making is expeditious? Whether subordinates feel consulted and valued? Requesting specific information on these aspects of your leadership style will assist you to make ongoing adjustments and to develop a style of leadership that is effective for you and the group.

Fawcett and Carino (1989), in their discussion of hallmarks of success in nursing practice, identify changes in nursing care delivery systems as an important emerging hallmark. They point to the development of case management approaches and of other approaches growing out of primary nursing structures as evidence of substantive progress in nursing practice. In these approaches, management, whether practiced by the supervising nurse or the nurse at the bedside, is crucial. Further, the use of conceptual models to guide nursing practice—another important hallmark of nursing success—implies a coordinating, directing role that can only be expected to increase as nursing assumes its full responsibility in the delivery of patient care.

As changes occur in our health care system, accompanying changes will occur in organizational structures. Nurse executives will need to be involved with their organization's strategic plan and the marketing strategies that have been identified. Management approaches and relationships between leaders and followers will also undergo change. Staff nurses will be an essential part of evaluating current structures and practices and helping develop new structures for the future. Emphasis on patient satisfaction and evaluation will result in modifications in the delivery system (Nield et al., 1998). Relationships within organizations may take on new perspectives that will require greater facilitative roles among leaders (Crowell, 1998).

The present health care environment is dominated by three major trends: consumerism, competition, and change (Stahl, 1998). Keeping abreast of developments on both national and state levels will be increasingly important.

■ KEY CONCEPTS

- Leadership is the process of guiding, teaching, motivating, and directing the activities of others toward attaining goals.
- Management involves the coordination and integration of resources through planning, organizing, directing, and controlling in order to accomplish specific goals.
- There are many theories about leadership, including the Great Man theory, the trait theory, situational theories, the contingency theory, the path–goal theory, and tri-dimensional theories. Each makes a contribution to our understanding of how effective leadership involves characteristics of leaders, followers, and the situation in which they function.
- Effective leaders vary their style with the demands of the situation, providing both structure and support to subordinates.
- Transformational leadership models are products of the 1990s that place emphasis on mutual growth and deemphasize the role of the leader.
- Three different leadership styles are authoritarian leadership, democratic leadership, and laissez-faire leadership. Each has advantages and disadvantages and may be used productively in differing situations by those adopting a multicratic style.
- Power is an important aspect of leadership and management. Different individuals view it variously.
- At least seven different types of power have been identified in literature, each of which might be characterized by individuals in power positions.
- Empowerment may be viewed as a process by which a leader shares power with others or enables others to act. It forms the basis of transformational leadership.
- There are a number of activities the leader can embrace that will facilitate the empowerment of others.
- A number of suggestions for developing your own leadership style exist. These include developing your personal physical resources, increasing your personal competence and knowledge, developing and maintaining flexibility, developing self-confidence and decisiveness, and developing and maintaining alliances.

- Nurses function as both leaders and followers. An effective follower takes an active role in the relationship with the leader.
- The leadership style may be influenced by a variety of factors, including the size of the group, the abilities of the group, the structure of the organization, the task to be accomplished, and the degree of stress in the situation or environment.
- Developing your own effective management style begins with an assessment of your own leadership and followership characteristics. Assessment of the work environment, identification of good role models, experimentation with different styles, and evaluation of their effectiveness are part of the ongoing process of developing a good management style.
- All registered nurses, regardless of position, must be prepared to function as leaders and managers. Although management ability may not come as comfortably as psychomotor-skill competency in a particular clinical setting, nurses must be prepared to function as leaders, because they are responsible for coordinating and managing care of patients, delegating tasks to subordinates, and supervising the subordinates' activity.
- As you begin your career in nursing, you must exercise the same diligence and commitment in learning leadership and management skills as you expect to do in other professional areas.

REFERENCES

Argyris, C. (1964). *Integrating the Individual and the Organization.* New York: John Wiley and Sons.

Bass, B. M. (1990). *Bass & Stogdill's Handbook of Leadership: Theory, Research, and Managerial Applications* (3rd ed.). New York: The Free Press.

Bass, B. M. (1995) Concepts of leadership: the beginnings. In: Wren, J. T. (Ed.), *The Leader's Companion: Insights on Leadership through the Ages* (pp. 49–52). New York: The Free Press.

Blake, R. R., & Mouton, J. S. (1964). *The Managerial Grid.* Houston: Gulf.

Burns, J. M. (1978). *Leadership.* New York: Harper & Row.

Carlyle, T. (1902). *On Heroes, Hero Worship, and the Heroic in History.* New York: Ginn & Co.

Chemers, M. M. (1995). Contemporary leadership theory. In: Wren, J. T. (Ed.), *The Leader's Companion: Insights on Leadership through the Ages* (pp. 83–99). New York: The Free Press.

Cronin, T. E. (1995) Thinking and learning about leadership. In: Wren, J. T. (Ed.), *The Leader's Companion: Insights on Leadership through the Ages* (pp. 27–32). New York: The Free Press

Crowell, D. M. (1998). Organizations are relationships: a new view of management. *Nursing Management, 29*(5), 28–29.

Fawcett, J., & Carino, C. (1989). Hallmarks of success in nursing practice. *Advances in Nursing Science, 11*(4), 1–8.

Fiedler, F. E. (1967). *A Theory of Leadership Effectiveness.* New York: McGraw-Hill.

Follett, M. P. (1918). *The New State.* Gloucester, MA: Peter Smith.

Follett, M. P. (1926). The giving of orders. In: Metcalf, H. C. (Ed.), *Scientific Foundations of Business Administration.* Baltimore: Williams & Wilkins.

French, J., & Raven, B. (1959). The basis of social power. In: Cartwright, D., & Lander, A. (Eds.), *Studies in Social Power* (pp. 150–167). Ann Arbor, Michigan: Institute for Social Research.

Greenleaf, R. K. (1995). Servant leadership. In: Wren, J. T. (Ed.), *Leader's Companion: Insights on Leadership through the Ages* (pp. 18–23). New York: The Free Press.

Heineken, J., & McCloskey, J. (1985). Teaching power concepts. *Journal of Nursing Education, 24*(1), 40–42.

Hersey, P., & Blanchard, K. H. (1995). Situational leadership. In: Wren, J. T. (Ed.), *Leader's Companion: Insights on Leadership through the Ages* (pp. 207–211). New York: The Free Press.

Higher Education Research Institute. (1996) *A Social Change Model of Leadership: Guidebook III.* College Park, MD: National Clearinghouse for Leadership Programs.

House, R. J. (1971). A path-goal theory of leadership effectiveness. *Administrative Science Quarterly, 16,* 321–338.

Hughes, R. L., Ginnett, R. C., & Curphy, G. J. (1995). Power, influence, and influence tactics. In: Wren, J. T. (Ed.), *Leader's Companion: Insights on Leadership through the Ages* (pp. 339–351). New York: The Free Press.

Kelley, R. E. (1995). In praise of followers. In: Wren, J. T. (Ed.), *Leader's Companion: Insights on Leadership through the Ages* (pp. 193–204). New York: The Free Press.

Komives, S. R., Lucas, N., & McMahon, T. R. (1998). *Exploring Leadership: For College Students Who Want to Make a Difference.* San Francisco: Jossey-Bass.

Manion, J. (1994). The nurse intrepreneur: how to innovate from within. *American Journal of Nursing, 94*(1), 38–42.

Maslow, A. (1970). *Motivation and Personality* (2nd ed.). New York: Harper & Row.

McGregor, D. (1960). *The Human Side of Enterprise.* New York: Harper & Row.

Molloy, J. (1988). *The New Dress for Success.* New York: Warner Books.

Neufeldt, V. (Ed.) (1996). *Webster's New World College Dictionary* (3rd ed.). New York: MacMillian.

Nield, M., Ecoff, L., Miller, L. A. et al. (1998). Evaluation: closing the loop. *Nursing Management, 29*(5), 34–35.

Raven, B. H., & Kruglanski, A. W. (1970). Conflict and power. In: Swingle, P. (Ed.), *The Structure of Conflict.* New York: Academic Press.

Stahl, D. A. (1998). Reengineering: the key to survival and growth under PPS. *Nursing Management, 29*(3), 14–17.

Taylor, F. W. (1911). *The Principles of Scientific Management.* New York: Harper & Row.

Thomas, A. M. (1993). Strategic planning: a practical approach. *Nursing Management, 24*(2), 34–38.

van Maurik, J. (2001). *Writers on Leadership.* London: Penguin Books Ltd.

Vroom, V. H., & Yetton, P. W. (1973). *Leadership and Decision-making.* Pittsburgh: University of Pittsburgh Press.

Wolf, G. A., Boland, S., & Aukerman, M. (1994). A transformational model for the practice of professional nursing. Part II. *Journal of Nursing Administration, 24*(5), 38–46.

2

Understanding and Working in Organizations

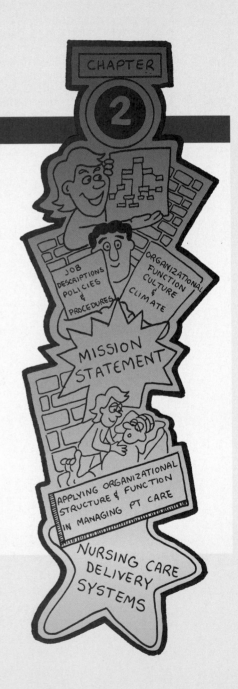

After completing this chapter, you should be able to:

1. Discuss the structure and relationships of an organization by using an organizational chart; include type of structure, span of control, chains of command, channels of communication, and lines of authority and accountability.

2. Analyze the effect of job descriptions, policies, and procedures on organizational function, culture, and climate.

3. Discuss the purpose of an organizational mission statement and a statement of philosophy and describe factors that result in these statements being different.

4. Analyze factors that affect organizational effectiveness and give the reason each is important.

5. Analyze the various nursing care delivery systems describing the situation in which each would be employed most appropriately.

6. Characterize ways in which the informal organization affects organizational function.

7. Analyze the various actions you could take to affect the culture and climate in an organization.

8. Describe specific situations in which you may need to apply knowledge of organizational structure and function in managing and coordinating patient care.

Key Terms ■ ■ ■ ■ ■

acceptance theory
accountability
adhocracy
authority
bureaucracy
case management
case method
centralized
chain of command
channels of
   communication
communication
   relationships
cross-functional
flat or decentralized
   organization
functional method

informal organization
informal structure
job descriptions
lines of authority
matrix structure
mission statement
modular care
organization
organizational chart
organizational climate
organizational culture
organizational
   effectiveness
organizational function
organizational hierarchy
organizational structure

partnership models
philosophy
policy
policy manuals
primary nursing
procedures
project structure
protocols
shared governance
span of control
standards of care
standards of nursing
   practice
tall organization
team nursing
total patient care

Y ou are surrounded by organizations everywhere, and, in one way or another, spend most of your life in one. The school in which you are enrolled, the business for which you work, the church you attend, and your recreational club are all organizations. An **organization** may be defined as a formally constituted group of people who have identified tasks and who work together to achieve a specific purpose defined by the organization. In other words, organizations are composed of individuals and operate within systems (Baker & Branch, 2002). All organizations have purpose and structure. In the last 30 years, social scientists have devoted considerable time and effort to studying organizations and how they work. Much of the study is directed toward either organizational form and structure or organizational functions and activities.

EXAMPLE *A Need to Understand Organizational Structure*

Ellen Morrell, a recent graduate, accepted her first nursing position as a registered nurse on a medical unit of a 350-bed community hospital. After 3 months of employment, Ellen became aware that most of the staff would be happier with their work if they could be assured of every other weekend off. She outlined some plans that would make this a possibility for all unit staff who preferred such a rotation.

> Enthusiastic about her ideas and her plan, she dropped by the office of the assistant director of nursing to see whether the plan could be implemented. The assistant director acknowledged that the ideas looked good but directed Ellen to discuss them with the unit manager. Believing that she was being rerouted to the unit manager because of her inexperience and because the assistant director didn't want to bother with her plan, Ellen became discouraged and discontinued all efforts to share her ideas.

Ellen's situation provides an example of the importance of understanding organizational structure, the chain of command within an organization, and the responsibilities assigned to each individual. In the facility described previously, the responsibility for developing the work schedule rests with the unit manager. In addition, seeking input from the assistant director, to whom the unit manager reported, was improper use of the organizational structure. Without this basic knowledge, Ellen found herself handicapped in accomplishing her goals.

There are a number of questions you will have that, when answered, will provide an understanding of how the organization in which you are employed is structured. You need to ask: To whom do I report? To whom can I delegate? To whom do I go with a problem or concern? How do I report errors? Who will evaluate me? Am I responsible for evaluating someone else? These and many other questions are answered by understanding the organization's structure and function.

■ UNDERSTANDING ORGANIZATIONAL STRUCTURE AND FUNCTION

When we use the term **organizational structure,** we are talking about the way in which a group is formed, its chains of command, its lines of communication, and the process by which decision making occurs. In other words, the structure of an organization outlines the formal working relationships and identifies who is accountable and responsible for the various jobs that make the organization viable. This implies that jobs and responsibilities are systematically arranged through departments or work divisions, with workers having variously defined roles. The organization is hierarchically arranged, with people employed in the defined roles within the organization having different levels of power (or authority) and rank from what others have. The concept of organizational structure is credited to Max Weber, a German social scientist, who wrote during the 1920s and is known as the father of organizational theory. He placed high value on **bureaucracy** (the administration of institutions through departments or subdivisions managed by sets of officials who followed an inflexible routine) and its importance in the operation of an organization (Gardner, 1995). Referred to as a closed, rational system that focuses on internal interactions and places emphasis on organizational order and control, this form of organization dominated both governmental and corporate life throughout the twentieth century (Baker & Branch, 2002). However, it does not take into consideration the complexity of multifaceted health care organizations of the twenty-first century. Today we find many large-scale organizations, including health care facilities, dispersing leadership and management functions throughout the system.

Kotter (1995, p. 118) states, "A central feature of modern organizations is interdependence, where no one has complete autonomy, where most employees are tied to many others by their work, technology, management systems, and hierarchy." This is certainly true in today's health care facilities, in which transdisciplinary teams come together in an environment filled with highly technical equipment to seek the most positive outcomes for clients from very diverse backgrounds.

The structure of any organization is designed to allow it to accomplish its purposes in an efficient and effective way. No organization can continue to exist if it does not make enough money to meet expenses and to improve and develop, a factor that is significantly impacting health care delivery. In addition, structure establishes the authority and responsibility within the organization and serves to establish a method by which the organization will respond to events and situations.

Ideally, organizational function parallels organizational structure, but sometimes that is not the case. **Organizational function** is the way interactions actually occur within the organization. Organizational function is often complex and may be related to characteristics of the employees as well as to the planned structure of the organization itself. Although important to the way in which the organization works, organizational function is more informally arranged.

■ TYPES OF ORGANIZATIONAL STRUCTURE

Organizational structures commonly fall into three main patterns: tall (centralized), flat (decentralized), and matrix. In addition, two other approaches that affect structure and organizational operation are mentioned: adhocracy and shared government. These patterns or approaches also occur in combinations. Each pattern tends to have different effects on organizational function. To work comfortably and effectively within an organization, you will want to determine its major structural pattern and how the pattern affects the manner in which that organization functions. Currently, many health care organizations are restructuring, that is, changing their structure, in order to operate in a manner that is more responsive to the changing world of health care reform.

Tall or Centralized Structure

A **tall organization** is so named because a chart of its relationships appears tall and narrow (Fig. 2-1). It is also called **centralized,** because most of the decision-making authority and power is held by a few persons in central positions that typically are found at the top of the chart. For example, in an acute care hospital, the nursing position would be that of the chief nursing officer who would have two or three assistants. In a tall organization, each person who has some authority is responsible for only a few subordinates. Tall organizations have many levels, and communication must travel through these levels.

One advantage of a tall organization is the ability of an individual to be an expert in the narrow area over which he or she is responsible, such as intravenous (IV) therapy or ostomy care. A tall organization may also use fewer skilled individuals,

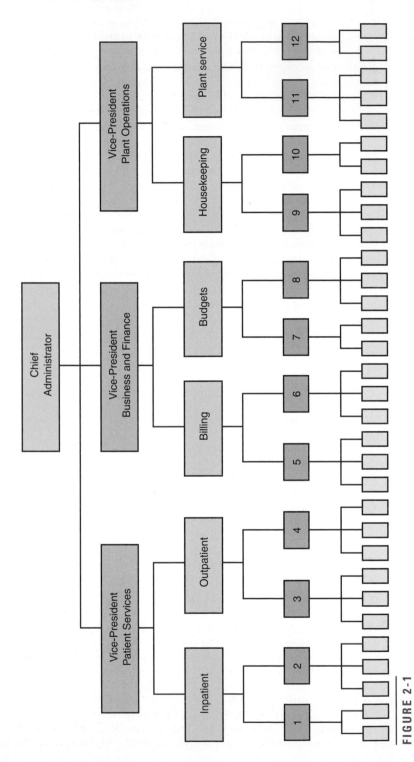

FIGURE 2-1

A tall organizational structure, with positions designated in boxes at higher levels and departments designated in boxes at the lower levels.

because the more skilled individuals are placed in positions in which they supervise others who carry out standardized procedures. Because the supervisor has fewer people to supervise, close supervision is possible. People at the top of the organization may be spared unnecessary communication if supervisory individuals in intermediate levels screen the communications. Those at the top of a centralized organization have a great deal of control over actions and are the primary decision makers.

These advantages also can become disadvantages. The most skilled individuals may end up doing nothing but supervising, whereas those less capable do the actual tasks. Those who are very closely supervised may feel stifled and in extreme cases even mistrusted. Communication is difficult because it must pass through many layers, and the person with the authority for decision making may be quite far removed from the actual situation. For the same reason, implementation of a decision may be excessively delayed. Some communications never reach the individual who might be able to make a decision for change when that is needed.

Hospitals were traditionally very tall, centralized organizations. A nursing unit might have been at the bottom of six or more levels of supervision. Decisions about equipment priorities, staffing patterns, and policies were made at the top levels, and nurses at the lower levels were expected to abide by these decisions. As nurses have moved toward more professional autonomy, they have found tall organizational structures restrictive and have sought a variety of ways to have a voice in decision making. Health care facilities, looking for ways to motivate nurses, are using participative management, continuing education, clinical ladders, and self-governance to accomplish these purposes (Longenecker, 1998).

Flat or Decentralized Structure

In the **flat** or **decentralized organization,** the chart of relationships shows few levels and a broad span of control (Fig. 2-2). In this type of organization, decision making is commonly spread out among many people and those closest to the situation are given wide latitude in determining appropriate actions. Close supervision is not possible when the supervisor is responsible for many people; therefore, the manager relies on individuals to make independent decisions. Individuals within a decentralized organization have an opportunity to develop their own abilities and autonomy and often see the organization as more humanistic. The result is greater job satisfaction for the majority of individuals. Many nursing settings are moving toward a more decentralized structure in which nurses directly involved in care have greater autonomy in decision making. Providing nurses with more autonomy and a greater involvement in decision making has been recommended as a strategy to keep good nurses in nursing.

One of the strengths of the decentralized organization is the simplification of communication patterns, which flow easily from lower levels to higher levels in a direct manner. With fewer levels through which messages must pass, there is less chance of the communication becoming lost or distorted as it moves within the organization. Another asset is the speed with which the organization can respond to problems or new opportunities, because decisions do not have to be referred upward through the hierarchy but can be made by those in the situation.

Disadvantages also exist in the decentralized pattern. For example, the individual in charge may have so many individuals with whom to relate that the various parts of the organization do not work together as effectively as desired. In addition,

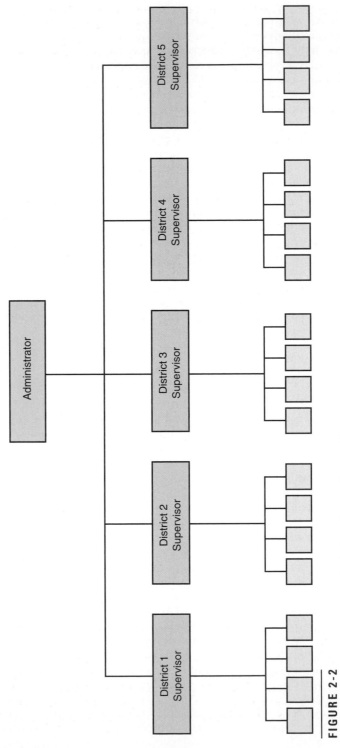

FIGURE 2-2
A flat organization with few levels and a broad span of control for managers.

managers may find that they cannot process all the communication that arrives, or if communication is limited, the manager may lack critical information to make decisions at that higher level. Managers in a flat organization may lack expertise in the wide variety of operations for which they are responsible and thus make inappropriate decisions. A greater need exists for ongoing education of individuals within the organization to enable them to make good decisions and appropriately to share decision making, and this may be costly. If individuals within the organization are not competent, their inappropriate decisions and actions may do great harm before their lack of ability is identified.

Many health care organizations are moving toward more decentralized models for nursing service. Although these models take a variety of forms, greater decision-making authority by individual nurses is common to them. Nurses are sharing in governance through committee structures, primary care for clients, and case management (shared governance is discussed later). In some settings, a nursing unit may not have a traditional manager. Instead, administrative responsibilities may be placed with a supervisor, and the nurses in some sort of democratic forum carry out decision making within the unit itself. Many nurses find this shared governance a positive setting in which to practice, because they believe it affords maximum potential for professional growth.

One aspect of restructuring in health care that is of concern to many nurses is the addition of more layers of unlicensed personnel at the bottom of the organization. These unlicensed individuals often lack any formal educational background; therefore, their abilities vary widely. As nursing roles change from providing direct care to supervising unlicensed assistive personnel, many different skills are demanded of nurses.

Matrix Structure

Recent years have seen changes in the structure of health care facilities as those organizations try to apply principles of business that gained popularity in the 1970s to health care. This has resulted in the organization of areas around product lines and service lines, with the product lines focusing on the end product of health care and the service lines representing the tasks required to accomplish the delivery of the product. Matrix structures are most often found in very large, multifaceted organizations. These may be seen as autonomous units within a hospital established to offer a special type of service, such as women's centers or sports medicine centers. All the resources needed to offer complete care in the chosen area are brought together under one administrator. For women's care, this might include obstetricians and gynecologists, weight loss specialists, psychologists and psychiatrists, plastic surgeons, and specialists providing breast care services. The goal is to attract more patients who will appreciate having all the services available in one area and involves a team approach.

Another example of this type of matrix organization is a corporation that owns many nursing homes. It may employ a nurse who is an expert in gerontological nursing and in the reimbursement process for long-term care to serve as a project manager. The nurse may have responsibility for establishing policies and procedures to maximize reimbursement for all the nursing homes in the group and may organize teams to assist with the work. Members of the team may continue to work part of their time in their base or original department and part of their time with the project team (Fig. 2-3).

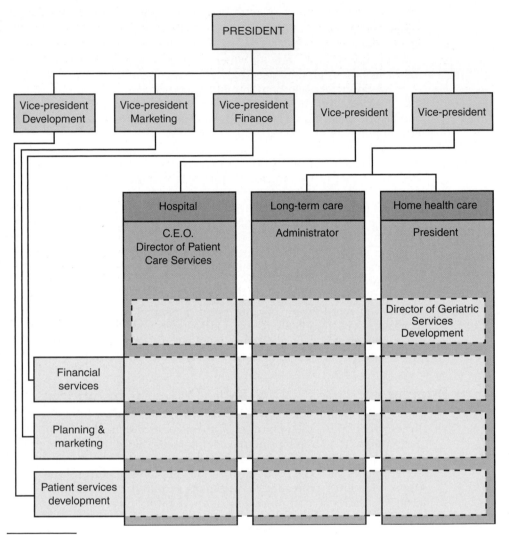

FIGURE 2-3
A matrix organization with some departments connected by dotted lines representing communication relationships.

Ford and Randolph (1992) discuss the difficulty that continues to exist in defining a matrix organization despite more than 30 years of use in work settings. They suggest that matrix management often is whatever a company defines it to be and state that project management has likewise come to mean a variety of things. Typically, a **matrix structure** will have an underlying structure that is either tall or flat and is thought of as the functional structure. A second structure, referred to as the **project structure,** overlies the first, creating two directions for **lines of authority,** accountability, and communication or a multiple command system. These structures may also be referred to as **cross-functional.** Functional managers (or line managers) have the responsibility of maintaining adequate staffing, developing or acquiring skills needed to support the project, maintaining standards, overseeing the assignments of personnel to projects, and providing for evaluation and career development of personnel. The project manager directs the project team that develops project standards and management practices and oversees their application to the various projects (Levine, 2000). The project manager also has the authority to see that these policies are carried out. However, the project manager's position in the organization is in addition to the basic lines of authority and accountability. This overlying structure represents a special relationship of individuals that is not part of the regular chain of command.

Such dual responsibility and accountability constitute both the advantage and disadvantage of the matrix structure. However, most of these concerns can be avoided with a good orientation and leadership (Levine, 2000).

A team approach to projects or problems brings together wide expertise and often generates more creative solutions as a result of the flexible use of human resources. The team members learn more about one another's concerns, and this involvement may also improve their usual working relationships, functional integration, and skill development. Advantages are derived from creation of horizontal communication linkages that solve information processing problems. Communication is improved by the close contact with all organizational groups, which is required of managers to assure project success (Ford & Randolph, 1992).

Matrix organizations are not without their problems, which can result in areas of leadership conflict, poor communication, lack of understanding of roles and expectations, costs created by dual authority, and concerns regarding personal evaluation. Dual-reporting relationships may also be a concern. Individuals within the organization may report to at least two managers, the nursing manager and the project director. This can lead to confusion, conflict, and ambiguity: a price individuals may have to pay for working in a matrix (Ford & Randolph, 1992). A team member who will be evaluated by both the team leader and the base department manager may feel a conflict and find it frustrating to be asked to do more than is realistic within the time allotted.

Time allocation between working for the team and working for the base department may become an issue. This is particularly true if the base department must operate with a shortage of personnel while the project person participates in the team. Frequent meetings can be very time consuming.

Persons working in a matrix organization need good interpersonal skills and training because they will be working in a collegial rather than a hierarchical relationship. Power balance between the two structures may become a concern.

Adhocracy Structure

Although not found frequently in health care organizations at the present time, recent literature on organizational structure describes an **adhocracy** structure. The National Aeronautics and Space Administration (NASA) used this type of organizational structure to accomplish its goals. Frequently, a bureaucracy- and an adhocracy-type structure coexist within the same organization. This type of structure uses teams of specialists who are organized to complete a particular project or task. (This explains the basis for the name, which is formed from the term *ad hoc*.) Typically, these groups are referred to as a project team or task force. Composed primarily of highly specialized professionals, the work is delegated by a director to members of the project team who provide particular expertise. Members of the team may come from a variety of disciplines or areas of expertise. Teams serve as think tanks, are creative, flexible, and fluid. The role of the leader is to create the process for effective problem solving and is based on the belief that the best thinking comes from team effort. The leader blocks out time for meetings, coaches the team, encourages it to think broadly, and ensures that it has necessary resources (Waterman, 1990). Teams of this nature work especially well when trying to implement change. In the health care arena, it might be seen in hospice organizations, community health, or nurse centers. We briefly mention it here, because as health care becomes increasingly specialized, it seems realistic that this model will soon be employed in the health care environment.

Shared Governance

Shared governance represents a professional practice model in which the nursing staff and the nursing management are both involved in making decisions as opposed to having the decisions made at an administrative level only. Shared governance is a relatively new concept in organizational structure that developed in the mid-1980s as a substitute for a more bureaucratic approach to management.

No single model for shared governance exists. It may take any one of a number of approaches, including a councilar model in which committees and councils have defined authority and functions, a congressional model that involves an elected representative system, or an administrative model consisting of committees or forums in which people communicate and share ideas (Porter-O'Grady, 1987). Through committees and councils, staff has an active role in management. As a consequence, it gains autonomy, greater control over the work environment, and greater job satisfaction. Decisions are made closer to the site of action, often resulting in improved patient care.

A nursing executive board often serves as a coordinating and approval body to which the councils report. In this structure, nurses are held to greater accountability within the context of peer-defined and peer-operated parameters (Porter-O-Grady, 1990).

The implementation of shared governance requires that staff nurses participate in professional development sessions that are designed to increase the nurses' understanding of decision making, team building, group dynamics, leadership, and budgeting. As one may anticipate, the time involved in shared governance is costly to organizations and its cost-effectiveness in terms of patient outcomes is being questioned. The continuance of shared governance models in the present health care system, replete with mergers, restructuring, and reorganization, may be in jeopardy. Some models of participatory governance are based in negotiated contracts. These models can only be changed through the negotiation process.

■ RELATIONSHIPS WITHIN ORGANIZATIONS

Crowell (1998) views organizations as living entities that are composed of people in relationships. She believes that these living open systems demand a different leadership—leaders who treat people and organizations as self-organizing and self-renewing and who see the work as accomplished through relationships. Therefore, when one examines an organization, it is important to identify relationships among people and departments, including who has authority or control over others and who is responsible or accountable to specific individuals in authority.

Authority and Accountability Defined

Authority refers to the official power an individual has to approve an action, to command an action, or to enforce a decision. Heifetz (1994) points out that authority is both formal and informal. Formal authority is conferred by virtue of an explicit set of expectations, such as those found in job descriptions, the manager agrees to meet. Informal authority comes from promises the manager makes that are often left implicit, such as the expectation that the individual will be trustworthy, competent, considerate, and demonstrate values and skills that are predictable. Thus, in a hospital, the unit nurse manager or the head nurse has the formal authority necessary to manage the day-to-day operations of the unit by directing the behavior of others, making decisions, and perhaps hiring staff for the unit. The manager also works at maintaining informal authority (respect, trust, admiration), because it affects the ability to influence fellow workers and create the most effective working environment.

The concept of authority is often associated with power, because it legitimizes the right of the manager or supervisor to give direction to others and expect them to comply. In bureaucratic organizations, such as hospitals, authority originates at the top of the organizational hierarchy and works its way down. The expectation that the subordinate will follow direction from a manager exists because of the belief that it is appropriate for managers to give instructions and for subordinates to comply with the instructions. If a manager leaves that position, that individual no longer has that power. (See Chapter 1 for a more detailed discussion of power.)

A second view of authority also exists—the **acceptance theory.** The acceptance theory proposes that a leader earns authority from the subordinate. It is a bottom-up approach in which the subordinate gives authority to the manager. The view employees hold regarding authority influences the practice of supervision and the manner in which it is approached (Dunn, 1998). In reality, in the best-working organizations, perhaps it is a bit of both.

EXAMPLE *Learning About the Acceptance Theory*

Leslie Goforth was excited when she was offered the position of unit manager on 7-South. As the relief manager on 4-West, she had observed the strong relationships that existed among staff on 7-South and she was eager to be part of it. However, 4 weeks after assuming the manager role, Leslie realized things had changed. She did not feel she had been granted the authority she had expected from the unit staff. As a result, her ability to influence others and provide direction was less than she had hoped. Leslie reviewed information in the management book she had purchased as a student. She realized in her review that although she had been appointed to her new position by the management, she had yet to earn the acceptance of the unit staff. She developed a plan to help accomplish that.

Accountability refers to the process of answering for what occurs in an ethical and legal sense. It represents an obligation to perform certain activities and duties. We may use this term interchangeably with *responsibility.* When we are responsible for something, it is up to us to see that the task or job is completed. As nurses move into roles in which they delegate more tasks to others, the concept of accountability has taken on more meaning. Although the tasks may be delegated, the nurse who delegates that task to others remains accountable—or legally liable—for the outcome. For example, registered nurses are responsible for the care of patients to whom they are assigned. If they assign the task of taking the blood pressure to the nursing assistant, the registered nurse is still responsible and accountable for assuring that the readings were correct and that they are appropriately documented. (See Chapter 6 for a detailed discussion on delegation.) If the care is not completed according to established standards, it is the nurse who remains liable and whose license to practice may be jeopardized.

The structure of an organization helps designate the authority and accountability of all persons working within that body. It indicates who gives instructions to whom and who must answer for the actions that follow and thus influences individuals within the organization. The charge nurse on a shift will have different authority and accountability from those of the unit manager and therefore would need to respond in a different way.

In turn, individuals may have an effect on the organization of which they are a part. A very experienced charge nurse may have greater authority than an individual who is new to such a position, which may be a reflection of the acceptance theory of authority and the authority accrued through the informal system. The more experienced charge nurse is viewed by his or her subordinates as competent and knowledgeable regarding his or her leadership role. Thus, there is always interaction between the individual and the structure of the organization.

Problems arise in organizations when people are asked to be responsible for certain outcomes but are not provided with the authority with which to accomplish the goals. Organizations are healthier when the structure and function are well described, authority is appropriately provided to match responsibilities, and this information is known to all involved. Let's look at some of the ways organizations provide these needed descriptions.

Chain of Command

A chain of command exists in all organizations. The **chain of command** identifies the path of authority and accountability from one individual with top administrative authority to the individuals at the very base of the organization. It is also referred to as **organizational hierarchy.** Thus, in hospitals we usually see that the nursing administrator gives directions to and evaluates the performance of the assistant administrator, who in turn gives direction to and evaluates the performance of the nursing manager, and so forth. Each of these people is considered to be on a different level or layer. When we are looking at this process from the base of the organization to the top (that is, in reverse), we frequently use the language "reports to," which indicates that the nurse manager is accountable for his or her activities to the nursing administrator. As a registered nurse, you will likely have the responsibility of giving direction to and overseeing the activities of the practical (vocational) nurse and the nursing assistant, and they, in turn, report to you.

Channels of Communication

Channels of communication may be defined as the patterns of message giving within an organization, and they typically correspond to the chain of command. Formal communications are not supposed to skip or loop any levels; the staff nurse is expected to take concerns to the unit manager and not to the supervisor of the unit manager. (See the example at the beginning of the chapter). Referred to as looping the system, in a bureaucratic organization it is generally considered improper and inappropriate to skip or bypass any of the levels in the communication system. If the staff nurse does not feel that there was a satisfactory response at the level of the unit manager, there is usually some method for the staff nurse to communicate those concerns to the next higher level. Jumping levels in this way usually requires that the individual first exhaust all usual avenues of communication.

Not all communication follows these formal pathways. They are designed for communications that deal with conducting the business of the organization. Some organizations adhere closely to the formal lines of communication; others, especially those that involve subordinates in decision making, encourage communication outside those lines if the desired action would be accomplished more efficiently. Effective function often requires that a manager communicate directly with individuals at many different positions in the organization. When managers on the same level in different departments build bridges of communication from one to another rather than rely on formal communication going up through one department and down through another, problem solving and accomplishing tasks is facilitated.

Critical Thinking Exercise

You have been working the night shift at Community Hospital for 9 months after spending 4 months in orientation on the day shift. A clinical manager who reports to a medical-surgical supervisor manages the unit on which you are assigned. The supervisor had a major role in your initial orientation and stressed the fact that her door was always open if a problem occurred. You have been aware of the fact that nurses on a unit that is adjoining yours take turns sleeping during the night shift. You often see patients' lights on and are concerned that proper care is not being provided. One morning as you are leaving the hospital, you meet the supervisor in the parking lot. She is congenial and asks you how things are going. Should you tell her about what you have observed on the adjoining unit? Would that be using appropriate channels? What are your alternatives? What would be the best way to approach this problem? Explain the rationale for the alternative you would choose.

Span of Control

Organizations operate by identifying who has authority and responsibility for directing others. The number of individuals a person is responsible for managing is called that person's **span of control.** With a narrow span of control, the individual will be responsible for only a few people and perhaps one or two task areas. For example, in a smaller community hospital the responsibilities of the manager of IV therapy might be limited to administration of all IV solutions given in the facility and the manager may have a team of fewer than six persons—a narrow span of control. This individual is likely to be an expert in the area of IV therapy and might provide direct care as well as supervise others. Conversely, if given responsibility for the IV team, the emergency department, and the staffing office, this person would be considered to have a wide span of control. In this instance, the person could not possibly be a clinical expert in every area and it is unlikely to be involved in providing direct care in those departments.

The ideal size of the span of control has been the subject of much research. A number of factors influence whether the span should be broad or narrow. Factors affecting appropriate span include size of the organization, its philosophy, services provided, and availability of resources, especially human resources. These factors would also include the manager's experience and ability, the skill and experience of the employees, the task to be accomplished, and the level in the organization at which the position occurs. In hospitals, one reason often cited for a narrow span of control is the need for specialized skills and abilities in a specific clinical area. The ultimate goal is to maximize productivity and job satisfaction among employees while effectively providing services.

Job Descriptions

Position or job descriptions also help define organizational structure and function. **Job descriptions** are written statements, usually found in **policy manuals** that describe the duties and functions of the various jobs within the organization. They outline the scope of authority, responsibility, and accountability involved in each position. A formal job description never gives a complete description of everything individuals do as part of their jobs, but it should provide the broad general guidelines under which the individual will function. It should provide the basis for performance evaluation of the person working in that role (see Chapter 7). The job description for a nurse in a hospital that has a primary nursing system in place will be quite different from the job description for a nurse in one that has a team nursing system. Even within the same institution, the job description for a nurse in an outpatient clinic will be quite different from that for a nurse in critical care.

Organizational Charts

All the relationships described previously are outlined on an **organizational chart,** which is used to depict the structure of the organization. It identifies to whom various individuals within the organization report. The organizational chart is a graphic, pictorial means of portraying various roles and patterns of interaction among parts of the system. It clearly presents the formal structure of an organization, showing relationships of people or departments to one another and providing information on the size of the organization, the formal chain of command, lines of communication, and the authority for decision making.

The organizational chart is typically represented by boxes stacked in a pyramid-shaped chart. The greatest authority exists at the top of the chart (often a single box) and declines as you move toward the base of the structure (many boxes). The persons occupying jobs that are located at the top of the organizational chart are considered executives, administrators, or the management, and those closer to the base are referred to as staff or employees. Located between the two is a level generally known as middle management, a group responsible for coordinating and controlling activities of a specified group of workers. Middle management positions are typically considered administrative, although that may not always be the case.

Lines connect positions on the organizational chart. Solid connecting lines on the organizational chart represent communication relationships between individuals or departments. Vertical lines are referred to as lines of authority and accountability. Lines of authority represent the responsibility of individuals to supervise others officially and are identified by moving downward on the chart. Lines of accountability, also called reporting relationships, represent a responsibility to report to another person. (Again, refer to the example at the beginning of this chapter.) The same lines that represent authority when moving down the chart represent accountability when moving up the chart. Taken together, the vertical lines demonstrate the chain of command. In a hospital, solid lines would connect staff nurses with the unit nurse manager, because the unit nurse manager has authority over the staff nurses and the staff nurses are accountable and report to the unit nurse manager.

Horizontal solid lines indicate the communication between individuals with similar levels of authority within the organization. For example, a solid horizontal line would exist between the unit manager on a surgical unit and the unit manager on a medical unit. These individuals are required to work together to reach certain objectives within the organization, have similar responsibilities and power, but none has authority over the others. They may report to the same supervisor. These persons occupy the same level in the organizational chart.

Dotted (or broken) lines in organizational charts represent **communication relationships** rather than authority relationships. These relationships may be between managers of different divisions such as the nursing unit manager and the housekeeping supervisor. They may also be used to designate positions referred to as staff positions rather than line positions. *Line* in this case means part of the direct lines of authority and accountability. Staff positions are advisory in nature with the individuals who occupy these positions, providing information and assistance to others. The organizational authority vested in this position is limited. An example of such a position is the staff education director in a health care facility or a clinical nurse specialist whose focus is education and planning.

Parts of the organization that do not have connecting lines are considered separate units, and formal communication follows the chain of command. Therefore, the official communication between a nursing unit and the housekeeping staff might proceed from the staff nurses up the solid lines through the unit manager to the level of the chief nursing administrator, where there are communication lines between the administrator of nursing and the administrator of housekeeping. The communication could then move across from the nursing department to the housekeeping department and then down the housekeeping structure to the appropriate person.

A current trend in many health care organizations is to group all employees who must work together under one manager, regardless of the individual job description. In this system, the nurses, the nursing assistants, the housekeeping personnel, a respiratory therapist, and a laboratory technician who care for patients on one unit might all report to the nurse manager of the unit. The goal of this organizational change is to increase the ability to solve problems and accomplish goals through coordinated efforts.

Organizational charts have limitations. First, it does not show the **informal structure** of the organization. The informal structure, sometimes called the organizational grapevine, has its own leaders and communication channels. It provides the sense of belonging that is a part of most organizations and is responsible for much of the socialization of employees within an organization. Social activities outside the organization may be a part of the informal structure. There may be informal, unwritten rules and expectations regarding communication, dress, etc., which influence the operation of the organization. This structure can either assist in the goals or special endeavors of the institution or sabotage them. The leaders are often from among the long-term employees or may be in key positions, such as the secretary to the vice president for patient care services. More discussion of the informal organization follows later.

Another limitation of the organizational chart is that it is difficult to keep it current. As the individuals in various positions change, the chart gets obsolete quickly, particularly in this time of restructuring. However, the new graduate or employee can gain a great deal of information about an organization by studying its organizational chart.

Critical Thinking Exercise

Jennifer Jorgenson, RN, has been working for 3 months as the evening charge nurse in Merry Mount Nursing Home. One of the nursing assistants, Mabel Worth, who has worked there for 5 years, approaches Jennifer and states that she and the other nursing assistants are just about ready to quit because their load is getting so heavy because of the level of care required. Mabel asks that Jennifer schedule more nursing assistants to divide the workload. Jennifer knows she does not have the authority to do this. How might she use her knowledge of the structure of the organization to solve this problem? Where should she begin? What resources are at her disposal? What should she do if she is unsuccessful in securing more staff?

■ OTHER FACTORS UNIQUE TO ORGANIZATIONS

In addition to the formal aspects of organizational structure that have been discussed, several other factors help outline the operation of successful organizations or businesses.

Mission Statement

All organizations have a purpose or a reason for existing. This purpose is expressed in the form of a **mission statement,** which outlines what the organization plans to accomplish, its aims or function. This may be as short as a single clause or sentence (Display 2-1). The mission statement may also include a statement identifying the group (or constituency) to whom the services are directed. It may also specify who

---

DISPLAY 2-1 **Mission, Vision, Values, and Strategic Goals for the Swedish Medical Center**

Mission: Improve the health and well-being of each person we serve.

Vision: Demonstrate the highest-quality, best-value health care in the Pacific Northwest.

Values:
- Patient centered
- Respect, caring, and compassion
- Teamwork and partnership
- Continuous learning and improvement
- Leadership

Strategic goals:
- Best place to receive care
- Best place to work
- Best place to practice
- Best place to purchase care
- Best partner

---

sponsors the organization (Display 2-2). The mission statement of a small community hospital may indicate that its purpose is to serve the health care needs of the immediate community, provide first-line diagnosis, and care for commonly occurring illnesses. A large university hospital may have a mission statement that encompasses research, teaching, and care for rare or complex problems. These two organizations will establish different priorities for spending, choose different technologies

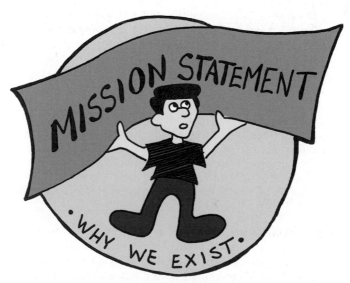

A mission statement outlines what the organization plans to accomplish.

DISPLAY 2-2	**Mission Statement and Values for the Holy Family Hospital**

MISSION STATEMENT

The Holy Family Hospital represents the vision and commitment of our founders, the Dominican Sisters of Spokane, and our sponsors, the Sisters of Providence, to meet the health care needs of the people of the North Spokane community and the Inland Northwest.

  Committed to this mission, Holy Family Hospital will:

■ Promote and uphold Christian values with patients and their families.

■ Offer a broad range of high-quality health care and health-related services regardless on one's ability to pay.

■ Encourage community outreach activities, which promote health living.

■ Provide responsible resourceful management to support the successful achievement of the goals and mission of the hospital.

■ Promote a Christian, value-based work atmosphere in which human values are honored and people are committed to caring for one another.

VALUES

Holy Family Hospital is committed to carrying on the healing ministry of Jesus in the Catholic tradition, emphasizing the values of:

■ Respect

■ Compassion

■ Competence

■ Collaboration

■ Justice

as essential to their missions, and structure their staff in different ways. Therefore, the establishment of a current and responsive mission statement is a critical element in the strategic planning of any institution because it provides the overall umbrella under which all functions of the organization take place. The small community hospital might not encourage individuals to engage in research, and the large university hospital might admit only patients who meet the criteria for research studies underway in a certain unit. When the budget is prepared, the large research hospital might include an entire department that works with research and statistics. The small hospital might decide not to include a very expensive diagnostic tool. Thus, the mission statement guides planning.

  The mission statement is often followed by a vision statement and perhaps a statement of values and a listing of strategic goals (see Display 2-1). If this is the case, the values statement may serve as the statement of philosophy for the organization.

Statement of Philosophy

The **philosophy** flows from the purpose or mission statement and provides a statement of beliefs and values that are basic to the operation of the organization, service, or unit. Most frequently, currently the philosophy is identified as a listing of values (see Displays 2-1 and 2-2). It may also include a listing of goals or objectives. Health care facilities may have an organizational philosophy and also a philosophy of nursing service. Fidellow and Hogan (1998) identify the statement of nursing's mission, vision, and philosophy as setting the standard of care that promotes a coordinated medical system, which ensures quality health care across the continuum. Thus, the philosophy, along with the mission statement, provides a benchmark against which an organization's performance can be evaluated. This implies the understanding that the philosophy will be specific and operational, a document that will help establish priorities, as opposed to being a lofty, theoretical statement to be buried somewhere in the organization's policy manual.

Policies, Protocols, Procedures, and Standards of Care

A **policy** is a designated plan or course of action to be taken in a specific situation (Ellis & Hartley, 2004). Typically, the responsibility and authority for assuring that appropriate policies are in place rest with the governing board, whether it is a board of trustees, board of governors, or a board of directors. The responsibility for implementation of the policies is delegated to the chief executive officer or administrator. The responsibility for policies specific to a department or a unit are usually delegated to the individuals or groups in the department that will be most affected by the policy. Policies developed at this level are often approved, adopted, or endorsed by the board.

Written policies usually can be found in a policy manual that is available within each department or on a computer network. Depending on the nature of the unit on which you are working, you may have greater or lesser need to refer to the policies. Special care units, such as birthing rooms and emergency departments, have more need to refer to policies than does an area in which care is more standardized. For example, an emergency department would have policies that govern the actions to be taken for the reporting on animal bites, managing the care of rape victims, or reporting gunshot wounds.

The policy for dealing with a patient suffering from a dog bite who is seen in the emergency department would provide a series of actions to be taken, such as which local authorities must be notified, who among the staff is responsible for this notification, and the time frame in which the notification must occur. Assuring accuracy with regard to reporting policies, public notification of statistics, and patient and public rights are areas of concern in such units.

There also may be **protocols** related to this same issue. A protocol is a detailed standard plan for patient care, such as a protocol relating to the general management of the patient with a dog bite. This would include the wound assessment instrument to be used, a reference to the procedure to be used for wound care, when a tetanus immunization would be included in care, discharge criteria, and teaching needed.

Procedures spell out how a particular nursing activity is to be completed, often described in a number of steps or processes. For example, you may find a procedure for flushing a heparin lock or for changing a central line. Procedures, once written, are incorporated into procedure manuals that are kept on the unit or stored in the computer.

Nurses frequently have considerable responsibility in developing and updating nursing policies, protocols, and procedures. Health care facilities will establish committees that are assigned to nursing policy and procedure review, and representatives to various committees monitor, review, and revise them to assure state-of-the-art care. Involving staff in decisions regarding nursing standards and the grassroots participation in policy formation is becoming commonplace in today's restructured health care delivery system.

Standards of care are specific, detailed plans of care for individuals with a specific health problem. A standard of care covers a broader range of concerns for the individual than does a protocol. The purpose of a standard of care is to establish the best practice and eliminate as much variation as possible. Standards of care often include aspects of medical care and various therapies as well as nursing care. They identify specific desired outcomes for each day of hospitalization and actions that are to be taken to achieve those outcomes. In some institutions, standards of care may take the form of nursing care plans or may be incorporated into care pathways, critical or clinical pathways. Designed to direct the health care team in daily care, these identify both outcomes and care activities that are expected to be appropriate for each 24-hour period of hospitalization. The standards of care become the basis for determining the level of care delivered and for quality improvement within the organization as well as for cost analysis.

Standards of Nursing Practice

Standards of nursing practice are authoritative statements that describe a common or acceptable level of professional nursing performance. Standards of practice therefore define professional practice. The American Nurses Association (1991) has developed general standards and guidelines for nursing practice that apply across the nation and are broad and general in nature. These standards are currently in their second edition and represent more than 20 areas of specialty practice. State boards of nursing also have developed standards of practice that address special areas such as child and elder abuse and advocacy. These standards apply to all nurses licensed in that state.

■ ORGANIZATIONAL EFFECTIVENESS

Organizational effectiveness refers to how well an organization accomplishes the purposes for which it exists. This is determined, in large part, by how well the organization is structured and includes all the items discussed up to this point. As health care organizations more and more frequently become the objects of public scrutiny regarding their operation strategies and costs, greater attention will be directed toward organizational effectiveness in the care arena. In 1999, the Malcolm Baldrige National Quality Award, given by the president of the United States to organizations that apply and are judged to be outstanding in seven areas, was opened to education and health care. The award program was established in 1987 to recognize U. S. organizations for their achievements in quality and performance. The seven areas specified in the evaluation are leadership, strategic planning, customer and market focus, information and analysis, human resource focus, process management, and business results. These areas continue to be major areas viewed as critical to effective organizational operation, with workshops and conferences scheduled for health care audiences for fostering improvements in health care (Frequently Asked Questions . . . , 2002).

■ STRUCTURING NURSING CARE DELIVERY SYSTEMS

At no other time in the history of nursing has there been such a wide variety of systems used for nursing care delivery. The need to control costs, the increasing professional role of the registered nurse, and the increasing emphasis on employee job satisfaction represent reasons for the multiplicity of approaches to care. Although many of the nursing actions may be delegated to another care provider, the registered nurse remains responsible for assessing the patient, identifying nursing care problems, planning and providing care, and evaluating care in all these systems. In addition, today the registered nurse may have responsibility for coordinating the care with the various individuals and agencies that provide a certain aspect of care and rehabilitation, such as physical therapy, speech therapy, rehabilitation, and home care. The following methods of care delivery may be used together in a variety of patterns.

The Case Method

The **case method** was the predominant organizational structure for nursing care delivery at the beginning of the twentieth century and should not be confused with the term *case management* used today (discussed later). Like the name implies, a nurse was hired to care for an individual patient, providing all the care needed, often living in the home with the family and assuming other household responsibilities such as cooking for the patient and family and doing light housekeeping. (Doesn't that sound a bit like the responsibilities of the home health aide today?) Nurses worked long hours and received poor wages. Advancing technology and increasing costs made this type of care delivery impractical at a time when physicians wanted patients hospitalized and many of the procedures required special equipment and service.

We currently see this form of nursing in home health nursing, although a nurse seldom has a single case and does not live in the home. In many instances, the personal care is provided by a home health aide; a registered nurse does the assessment, planning, skilled intervention, and supervision. The care may be arranged through an agency, and the individual nurse assigned to a case has a great deal of autonomy and relatively little supervision.

The Functional Method

The **functional method** of care delivery emerged around 1930 when the United States saw a tremendous growth of hospitals around the nation, and physicians preferred to have their patients hospitalized rather than cared for in the home. This method allowed for the care of greater number of patients than were previously cared for. The head nurse assigned various nursing tasks to different nurses in that unit. One nurse might take all the temperatures, change the dressings, and apply hot compresses (the treatment nurse); another might give all the medications and chart them (the medication nurse); and yet another would give all the baths (the bath nurse). Assignments varied depending on the size of the units, the number of patients and personnel, and the skill level of the personnel. The personnel all reported to the head nurse, who gave report to the next shift.

You can see that this form of care delivery, although economical and efficient, resulted in the fragmentation of care. Patients were often confused about who was caring for them and did not know to whom to address questions if they had concerns. Nursing came to be viewed as a series of tasks and technical procedures. Today, you may see this form of care delivery in use in long-term care facilities and nursing homes. The registered nurse assumes the role of manager of care providing the assessment, planning and evaluation that were missing from the functional care of the 1940s. The licensed practical nurse may be assigned to specific skilled tasks such as medication administration and treatments. Nursing assistants provide the personal care. This method is effective in situations in which there are few registered nurses and others must provide direct care.

Team Nursing

The concept of team nursing was introduced in the 1950s at a time when the nation was feeling a tremendous nurse shortage. World War II had ended and nurses returned to their homes to be wives and mothers. Also, the public was demanding a more patient-centered approach to care.

With **team nursing,** an identified team leader, who is an experienced registered nurse, was responsible for assigning care of patients to team members who typically have various levels of nursing education. Other team members could be another registered nurse, a practical nurse, a nursing assistant, and perhaps a nursing student. In addition to providing leadership to the group, the team leader might have responsibility for the administration of all the medications to patients for whom her team was responsible. The team leader gave report to the team that assumed care on the next shift.

An important part of this form of care delivery was the team conference at which all members of the team met, discussed, and planned the care of all patients assigned to the team. The team leader reported to the head nurse, who had overall responsibility for managing the unit. Typically, each unit had two or three teams, depending on the size of the unit and the number of patients. The system worked fairly well if the team leader had leadership skills and if there was always time for team conferences. If these factors were lacking, it had few advantages over the functional method.

Modular Care

Modular care is viewed by some as a variation of team nursing and gained popularity during the mid-1980s. It is dependent on structural and spatial changes in health care facilities that would enable nurses to stay close to the bedside. Patient care units were divided into modules, and the same team of care providers was consistently assigned to each module.

Total Patient Care

Total patient care, in which a registered nurse or licensed practical (vocational) nurse is assigned to all care needs of a group of four to six patients, became popular in the 1970s and 1980s. Nurses felt a greater sense of control, autonomy, and involvement in patient care. Focusing on the total patient (from which the name is derived), more emphasis was placed on the holistic approach to care rather than tasks or procedures. Total patient care became more difficult to implement when technological advances resulted in patients with far greater acuity but who remained in the hospital for shorter periods of time. The expense of this care delivery system was also a disadvantage; an individual with less education could satisfactorily complete many of the tasks performed by the RN and at a lesser cost. Total patient care is currently used in intensive care units, labor and delivery units, and other settings in which patients have very high acuity.

Primary Nursing

The use of **primary nursing** on general nursing units began in the late 1970s, peaking in the late 1980s. Primary care and total patient care are closely related and coexisted in many places. With primary care delivery, one nurse was assigned the responsibility for the care of a patient from the time the patient was admitted to the hospital until the patient was discharged. The primary nurse developed and updated the nursing care plans, performed care and patient teaching, and provided discharge planning. An associate nurse would work with the same patient on other shifts and on the primary nurse's days off. Some facilities advertised primary nursing but were really using total patient care. The nurses were responsible for care only during the time they were on duty.

Studies conducted on primary care showed that when this form of care was initiated, patients experienced fewer complications, had shorter lengths of stay, and the registered nurse did not spend time delegating and supervising. Thus, it was viewed as providing a higher quality of care to the client and allowing maximum autonomy to the nurse. Primary care has long been used in intensive care units, with certain variations on how it is implemented.

Although patients benefited from the continuity of care when used in other areas of the hospital, and nurses usually experienced a high level of job satisfaction, this form of care delivery was viewed as expensive because of the number of professional staff required to assure its implementation. This method required nurses who were knowledgeable and could work autonomously.

When decision-making skills were lacking among the new employees, the facility needed to educate staff for this role, which was another big expense to the agency. As the nursing shortage became more pronounced in the 1980s, institutional employers of nurses investigated using nurses in different ways. In the 1990s, economics became the rationale for moving away from primary nursing, and the method of care delivery again changed.

Partnership Models

At present, we see a number of **partnership models** in operation. Sometimes referred to as care pairs, patient care is provided to a group of patients by a registered nurse and either a licensed practical (vocational) nurse or, as is more often the case, an unlicensed nursing assistant. When working with an unlicensed assistant, the non-nursing tasks are assigned to this individual, whereas the registered nurse provides the professional care. The registered nurse maintains responsibility and accountability for all care delegated to the assistant. When the partnership is that of a registered nurse and a licensed practical nurse, patient care is shared with the registered nurse who is planning and directing the care.

Case Management

Case management is not an approach to the structuring of patient care in the same sense as the systems mentioned previously. However, because nurses may be involved in case management, it bears mention here. **Case management** results in the monitoring of an individual patient's health care by the case manager for the purpose of maximizing positive outcomes and containing costs. The key to the management of the case is identifying a critical pathway for care and treatment with specified time lines and protocols. The case manager typically follows the patient from the diagnostic phase through hospitalization, rehabilitation, and to home care, assuring that necessary arrangements have been made and that patient care goals will be realized. Case management goes beyond primary nursing to add responsibility for managing the patient's interaction with the entire health care system. It may not include the provision of any direct patient care.

Case management requires that nurses be well prepared for the role, both educationally and experientially. Also, they must possess good interpersonal skills. Case managers are usually employed by a particular institution and also may have additional responsibilities such as administering wellness programs.

Nurse case managers also are hired by insurance companies or managed care organizations. These external case managers facilitate the use of all care resources in a cost-effective manner. They often work to assure that the rehabilitation program is planned and ready when the patient reaches the point when that might begin. They assure that the patient is not simply marking time or waiting for the next phase of treatment.

Patients or family members hire independent case managers themselves. These case managers assess the individual, determine what services are needed, and then

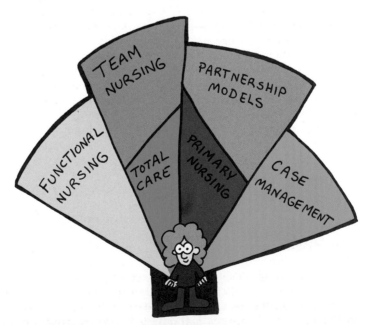

Nursing uses a wide variety of systems for nursing care delivery.

research and recommend appropriate resources. Geriatric case managers are perhaps the largest group of independent case managers. They are often hired by families to help with difficult care decisions for an elderly relative.

■ THE INFORMAL ORGANIZATION

The informal organization was mentioned previously while discussing the organizational chart. It is worthy of greater discussion. The **informal organization** is essential to the functioning of the system. It is unlike the formal organization, whose structure is highly planned and structured. The informal organization operates with great flexibility, pays little attention to boundaries, and carries the bulk of communication relating to the organization's internal politics (Gardner, 1995). It is primarily social in nature.

Informal organizations arise within the formal organization to meet the needs of the people within an organization. In a structured organization, the informal organization may provide for ease of relationships and ways to accomplish desired outcomes without using the entire formal structure. In an organization that has a loose formal structure, the informal organization may provide the additional structure that some people need to function comfortably.

Meeting Social Needs

One of the benefits provided by the informal organization is the meeting of workers' social needs. In the informal organization, a person may be viewed more as an individual and a friend than as a worker. Through informal association, an individual may find a sympathetic ear when he or she is troubled and friends with whom to rejoice when there are joys and successes in life. The informal organization may bring a sense of belonging that is not present in the formal organization.

In some employment settings, you will find people celebrating birthdays, planning holiday parties, and creating opportunities for social interaction in a variety of ways. In other employment settings, the individuals have independent social relationships that do not include people at work. Some people welcome the opportunity to socialize with those at work; others prefer to keep work life and social life completely independent.

Sometimes the social organization is closed, and new individuals remain outsiders. This may make the work environment unpleasant and create turnover among those who feel they are outsiders. If the social organization expects individuals to invest a lot of time in group activities, the person who does not want to socialize with coworkers may not fit in and therefore may seek employment elsewhere.

Accomplishing Goals

In addition to its effects on the personal lives of workers, the informal organization may contribute significantly to the success of the organization in meeting its goals. People may assist one another based on their informal relationships, even though the formal structure does not mandate this. For example, on a nursing unit, the housekeeping staff may be organizationally quite separate from the nursing staff. An informal working relationship might create cooperation that results in housekeeping people working closely with nurses to make sure that units are cleaned promptly and in coordination with admission needs. Often, these informal relationships are built over time as favors are done in both directions, and these relationships rely on both parties contributing for their existence. If one person fails to contribute, the relationship will be lost. Changes in personnel may result in the loss of effective informal relationships and thus a loss of efficiency that was not anticipated by management.

The informal organization may be detrimental to the formal organization as well as supportive of it. If the leadership of the informal organization undermines the authority of the formal leader, the result may be lessened effectiveness. Sometimes the informal organization may resist needed change and undermine efforts to achieve new ways of performing through passive-aggressive or aggressive defensive behavior. The informal organization may tolerate mediocrity and may even discourage those who would try to demonstrate excellence or ambition.

Providing Communication

One of the more important functions of the informal organization includes providing a means of communication and disseminating information that is flexible and personal. Some formal channels are inadequate for the information needs of individuals; thus, the needs are met through the informal organization.

Sometimes an organization may deliberately withhold information from those with less authority. These individuals may want and need some means of obtaining the information that is important to them. The informal organization provides the mechanism. For example, in some businesses, information regarding the budget and whether a profit is being made is a closely guarded secret. An employee who plans to ask for a raise in salary may find this information important. An informal relationship with an employee in the business office may yield the general knowledge that the business is doing well financially, thus allowing the person to negotiate for the raise from a stronger position.

Sometimes the informal organization communicates important information for job performance that the formal organization has not identified. On a nursing unit, a new nurse may need to know how nurses share the workload when unforeseen events occur. This would not be covered in a formal policy, but it is very important to effective functioning.

A danger of informal communication is that it also may disseminate rumor and inaccurate information. We have all had experiences with grapevine messages that create anxiety. It is important to be wary of messages that promote extreme views or that are detrimental to relationships and reputations. You should always check the accuracy of informal communications.

EXAMPLE *Grapevine Messages*

Maxine Teller, a licensed practical nurse on the medical unit at Southgate Hospital, arrived at work Monday morning and announced to the staff that she had been at a party Saturday night where she heard that the unit was going to be closed and the staff redistributed among other units of the hospital. The staff on hearing this was very distressed by the news and spent much time Monday morning discussing it in small groups. Patient care suffered as a result. At one o'clock, the unit manager arranged for the vice president of patient services to meet with the unit staff. She verified that the closure of the unit was an empty rumor.

Preserving Values

Another important function of the informal organization is preservation of the values of the group. For example, on one nursing unit, you may find an informal standard regarding participation in continuing education. Everyone is expected to participate in staff development programs, and group members offer whatever support is necessary to make this possible. On another unit, you might not find this same value or the corresponding actions to support continuing education efforts by colleagues.

 ## The Informal Organization and Persons from Other Cultures

Recent research suggests that it is highly probable that informal organizations are affected by national cultures. Certainly, the informal organization offers a number of benefits to groups who feel alone in the formal organization that offers little room for emotions or the sharing of personal thoughts. Through the informal organization, individuals who feel that they are in a minority can meet affiliation needs—the need to belong to a group. Belonging to a group enhances and confirms the individual's sense of identity and boosts self-esteem. It serves to reduce uncertainty and stress created by the formal organization. Because of these benefits, it is not unusual to find a large representation of individuals from different ethnic and cultural groups finding their voice in the organization through the informal structure.

Informal Leaders

Within the informal organization, varying levels of status and informal leaders may exist. These informal leaders may wield far more power than their official title or position in the organization would indicate. Some informal leaders are charismatic in their effect on others. Others may be leaders based on specific abilities and actions in job performance. Informal leadership may change based on the situation.

■ ORGANIZATIONAL CLIMATE AND CULTURE

Organizational climate refers to the perceptions employees have of an organization with regard to the prevailing feelings and values of the organization. Just as physical climate—hot versus cold, rainy versus sunny—affects your engaging in outdoors activities, the psychological climate affects your ability to carry out activities in an organization. Feelings of trust, belonging, esteem, and loyalty would be a part of the climate. The organizational climate is influenced by the **organizational culture,** which is the sum total of organizational values, formal and informal communication patterns, and historical patterns that influence how an organization operates. The culture is based on the interaction of the official policies and procedures of the organization, the behavior of supervisors, the behavior of coworkers within the informal organization, and the feedback provided within the organization. It is important that employees perceive the organizational climate as positive and that their values are compatible with those prevailing in the organizational culture.

Effect of Policies

Formal policies describe expected behaviors and limit the amount of discretion that an individual is permitted. These policies may be structured on basic philosophies of how people are motivated and respond. In Chapter 5, you will learn more about theories of motivation.

Effect of the Behavior of Managers

In addition to formal policies and procedures, the manner in which managerial personnel carry out policies and procedures also contributes to culture and climate. The personality of the manager and his or her general method of interacting with others have a major effect on the culture in any organization. For example, a study of 623 staff nurses in three Midwestern hospitals revealed that staff nurse job satisfaction clearly improves as the management style nears a participative management style (Moss & Rowles, 1997).

Although the official policy may seem restrictive when it is read, an individual manager may interpret the policy broadly, giving individuals the benefit of latitude in expectations. By word and action, the manager may say to the staff, "I trust in your commitment to patient care" and "I value your contribution." Staff members may be supported when they risk failure by trying something new, or they may be so harshly criticized for failure that they are unwilling to take risks. When the official policy supports continuing education, the immediate manager often makes the policy a reality through careful scheduling and consultation with staff. Conversely, the official policy may have little effect if the supervisor does not make the effort to adjust scheduling or otherwise support the individual in attempting to gain more education.

The manager does not have to be friends with other employees, but a concerned and friendly approach to interactions makes a difference in the general climate. Some managers unknowingly create an atmosphere of suspicion and fear through their criticism and unwillingness to tolerate less than perfection. Chapter 1 discussed the various management styles in greater detail, and Chapter 7 provides guidelines for giving feedback. As you study these chapters, reflect on the effects these management styles and guidelines would have on the climate of an organization.

The Informal Organization and Climate

The way individuals relate on a personal basis within an organization has a profound effect on the climate. When employees support one another, provide assistance as needed, and help answer questions or solve problems, a climate of cooperation and collaboration is fostered. If the informal relationships are based on trust, honesty, and working cooperatively, these feelings will permeate the organization. Conversely, if fellow employees focus on themselves and their own needs to the exclusion of the needs of others, the climate will be very different. If the accepted approach to the job is one of "me first," without concern for the effects of one's actions on others, the climate will be one of isolation and estrangement. Some organizations have a high level of competition, but this competition is accompanied by respect for others and a sense of fair play. Consequently, it creates a positive climate.

Relationships in some organizations are quite formal, with all individuals being addressed by last names and title. In other organizations, relationships are informal, with everyone being called by their first names. Neither situation is intrinsically better, but the climate each creates is different.

Changing the Organizational Culture and Climate

Organizational cultures and climates are not static; they can change. Although most changes in organizational culture and climate occur gradually as the people in the organization change and each brings a different approach to the work setting, you can change an organizational climate through deliberate action.

Why would you want to change the climate of an organization? There could be a number of reasons. You may feel that the efforts and accomplishments of the employees receive too little recognition. Or perhaps policies or processes exist that are not appropriate for the situation. Steps could be taken to provide nurses with greater autonomy or involvement in decision making. Any of these might provide a basis for wanting to change the climate.

When thinking about any kind of change, refer again to the basic nursing process you learned early in your nursing program and refer to the suggestions related to change given in Chapter 8. First, assess the current organizational climate. What is the climate of the work setting? Is this the tone that you would like to see? Clearly state to yourself the problem you see with the climate. Do others share your concern, or do you seem to be the only person who believes a change is needed? Then assess the factors that contribute to the climate in this particular setting. There will be both negative and positive factors. What actions contribute to the feeling tone? Are there policies and procedures that have an effect on the climate? Is there a particular individual within the organization who is responsible for the climate? Identify as many of the determinants of the organizational culture and climate as you can.

Once you clearly understand the situation as it is and have identified the problem, you need to set a clear goal for a new, changed culture. What exactly would you like to see in this new culture? Would you like to see a greater sense of trust? More autonomy? A stronger support for achieving excellence? Try to set your goal in a realistic way. We would all enjoy a perfect work setting, but that is not going to happen; however, we may be able to improve our work situation.

Once you know where you are and where you want to go, you can begin planning the actions that will get you to your goal. Some of the factors affecting culture may be out of your control, but you may be able to affect others directly. You may change the way you relate to others and begin noting evidence of changes you would like to see. You may involve others in the change process. If you have identified a problem, others may have identified it also. Policies and procedures may be changed through the prescribed route, which may involve the actions of committees and consultants as well as of those individuals in the specific situation.

Critical Thinking Exercise

Joan Antler is concerned about the climate that exists on the unit to which she is assigned. Recently, a new unit manager was hired to replace a much-loved manager who retired. The new manager seems unnecessarily critical of staff, provides little freedom for independent actions, but is a hard worker herself. What might Joan do to change the climate on the unit? With whom should she talk? What should be her first steps? What factors do you believe are operating in this situation? What alternatives are open to Joan?

■ KEY CONCEPTS

- The structure of an organization affects the interactions that occur with an organization. Organizational charts help you understand the structure of relationships within an organization, the lines of authority and accountability, the concepts of chain of command, the channels of communication and span of control, and the effect of the level of a person on his or her role in the organization.
- An organization's structure may be described as tall (centralized), flat (decentralized), or matrix. A new approach to structure called an adhocracy is evolving in some areas. Shared governance, developed in the mid-1980s and which gives nurses a greater voice in decision making, is being implemented in health care institutions. Each of these organizational types has strengths and weaknesses.
- The mission statement provides a statement of the purpose of an organization. The philosophy outlines the values and beliefs that guide the activities of the organization. Together they provide a benchmark for measuring the outcomes of the organization and the organizational effectiveness.
- Health care organizations are also guided by the policies, procedures, and standards of care that they endorse. Nurses are assuming ever-increasing roles in the development of hospital policies, procedures, and standards of care.
- Nursing care delivery systems may be structured to provide functional nursing, team nursing, total patient care, modular care, primary nursing, partnership models, case management, or any combination of these. The case method was an early forerunner of the various patterns of nursing care delivery.
- The informal organization meets social and communication needs of employees. In addition, it may assist with effective attainment of goals and preservation of values within the organization.
- Informal leaders arise within organizations and are able to influence others. These informal leaders may make an important contribution to the organization's functioning, but they may also be counterproductive. Other problems that may originate within the informal organization include distortions in communication, support for nonproductive behavior, and resistance to accepting new individuals within the social structure.
- The organizational culture is the sum total of values, formal and informal communications, and other factors that affect how an organization operates. The organization climate is how employees perceive the organization. These two factors may be similar or different and are not static. Many things may affect them.

■ As a beginning nurse, you can in many ways use knowledge of the structure and function of any organization in which you are employed. There may be problems you will want to help solve or a climate you wish to change. Your knowledge will be important to you in all these endeavors.

REFERENCES

American Nurses Association. (1991). *Standards of Clinical Nursing Practice*. Washington, DC: American Nurses Association.

Baker, K. A., & Branch, K. M. (2002). *Chapter 1. Concepts Underlying Organizational Effectiveness: Trends in the Organization and Management Science Literature* [Online]. Available at http://www.s.doc.gov/sc-5/benchmark/CH%201%20Trends%2006.19.02.pdf.

Crowell, D. M. (1998). Organizations are relationships: a new view of management. *Nursing Management, 29*(5), 28–29.

Dunn, R. T. (1998). *Haimann's Supervisory Management for Healthcare Organizations* (6th ed.). New York: McGraw-Hill.

Ellis, J. R., & Hartley, C. L. (2004). *Nursing in Today's World: Trends, Issues, and Management* (8th ed.). Philadelphia: JB Lippincott.

Fidellow, J. A., & Hogan, M. (1998). Strategic planning: implementing a foundation. *Nursing Management, 29*(6), 34, 36.

Frequently Asked Questions about the Malcolm Baldrige National Quality Award. (2002). *Fact Sheets from NIST* [Online]. Available at http://www.nist.gov/public_affairs/factsheet/baldfaqs.htm.

Ford, R. C., & Randolph, W. A. (1992). Cross-functional structures: a review and integration of matrix organization and project management. *Journal of Management 18*(2): 267–305.

Gardner, J. W. (1995). Leadership in large-scale organized systems. In: Wren, J. T. (Ed.), *Leader's Companion: Insights on Leadership Through the Ages* (pp 297–302). New York: The Free Press.

Heifetz, R. A. (1994). *Leadership Without Easy Answers*. Cambridge, MA: The Belknap Press of Harvard University Press.

Kotter, J. P. (1995). What leaders really do. In: Wren, J. T. (Ed.), *Leader's Companion: Insights on Leadership Through the Ages* (pp. 114–132). New York: The Free Press.

Levine, H. A. (2000). *Organizing for Project Management: Part I. Basic Organizational Structures*. PlanView, Inc. [Online]. Available at http://www.myplanview.com/expert51.asp.

Longenecker, P. D. (1998). Managing nurse managers. *Nursing Management, 29*(3), 35–38.

Moss, R., & Rowles C. J. (1997). Staff nurse job satisfaction and management style. *Nursing Management, 28*(1), 32, 34.

Porter-O'Grady, T. (1987) Shared governance and new organizational models. *Nursing Economics, 56*, 281–286.

Porter-O'Grady, T. (1990). Nursing governance in a transitional era. In: Chaska, N. L., *The Nursing Professional: Turning Points* (pp. 432–439). St. Louis: CV Mosby.

Waterman, R. H. (1990). *Adhocracy: The Power to Change*. New York: W. W. Norton & Co.

3 Managing Resources Responsibly

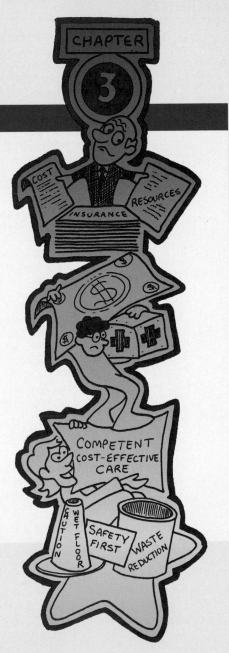

CHAPTER 3

Learning Outcomes ▪ ▪ ▪ ▪ ▪

After completing this chapter, you should be able to:

1. Discuss the various sources of health care funding and how their cost-containment measures have affected health care delivery.
2. Identify the major factors responsible for rising health care costs.
3. Explain the relationship between cost awareness and cost containment.
4. Develop specific strategies nurses can employ that will help limit health care costs, including those related to human and material resources.
5. Discuss the relationship of legal and ethical issues to cost containment.
6. Outline steps in a budget process and identify how a staff nurse could influence this process.
7. Analyze an item to determine whether its cost would be assigned to an operating or a capital budget.
8. Identify major issues related to time management and discuss why each is a concern.
9. Formulate a personal plan for time management based on personal time assessment and identification of strategies that would improve personal use of time.
10. Apply time management techniques to help a group of care providers work more effectively and efficiently.

Key Terms ■ ■ ■ ■ ■

assignment
brain sheet
budget
budget hearings
budget processes
budget variance
capital budget
capitation
control procedures
cost awareness
cost containment
cost-effectiveness
cost-shifting
delegation

diagnostic related groups
   (DRGs)
effectively
efficiently
fee-for-service
fiscal year
health maintenance
   organizations (HMOs)
managed care
Medicaid
Medicare
multidisciplinary team
multitasking
operating budget

patient classification
   systems
preferred providers
prioritize
procrastination
prospective
   reimbursement
socializing
third-party payer
time management
value analysis
variance
zero-base budgeting

According to FIRSTGOV for Seniors (2003), health care costs in the United States are projected to reach $3.1 trillion in 2012, which will reflect an average growth in costs of 7.3%. Health care costs in 2012 will be 17.7% of the gross domestic product (GDP) as compared with 14.1% of the GDP in 2001. This is true despite the United States being the only major industrialized country that does not provide health care coverage for all its citizens. In 2000, the cost for health care in the United States was $4631 per person; this is 83% higher per capita than Canada and 134% higher than the average for industrialized nations (Davis & Cooper, 2003).

As the cost of health care continues to escalate, society expects that all health care professionals will be active participants in managing health care resources. Although resources are most often thought of in dollars, resources in health care must be seen in terms of buildings, equipment, supplies, personnel, and time as well. Each of these areas must be considered as you try to understand how to manage resources effectively.

All members of the health care team must confront the escalating cost of health care. Nurse managers, such as directors or vice presidents of nursing, supervisors, and unit managers, have a significant role in collaborating with others in an organization on resource allocation and are often involved directly in making budget policy decisions. They also have a major role in developing and managing the specific budget for nursing. Staff nurses cannot control all the elements that impact on health care costs; however, they do have control over certain resources in the clinical setting, and to keep costs down they must use these resources responsibly. They are directly involved with and control utilization of resources for each patient. Nurses should be aware of what things cost, how they are paid for, how they are budgeted, how waste creeps in, how feelings affect results, and how money influences services. Nurses must maximize the resources available and recognize when they are inadequate and when patient safety is jeopardized.

■ FACTORS AFFECTING COSTS OF HEALTH CARE

Many different aspects of the system have been cited as creating the increasing costs: overuse of medical resources by patients, administrative costs, and fear of litigation leading to unneeded diagnostic tests (Liebowitz, 2003). Other aspects cited are the increasing health needs of an aging population, the increased cost of prescription drugs, the push for higher wages for hospital workers, and new and expensive technologies (Davis & Cooper, 2003).

Increased Demand for Health Care Services

An increasing older population that has more chronic and acute illnesses and therefore needs more health care resources is often cited as a major factor in increasing costs. The fastest growing segment of the population is over 85. However, this may not be as much of a factor as many believe. Currently, many older adults are reaching 65 years and more with better health than those of similar ages in previous years. According to Strunk and Ginsberg (2002) aging plays a limited role in health care cost trends. However, the overall demand of the population may be very important. Liebowitz (2003) argues that when consumers do not pay the cost of health care services and do not know what they are, they overuse resources. This includes demanding care by specialists when not warranted, asking for the latest and most expensive drugs, requesting costly diagnostic tests that may not be indicated, and not objecting to costly treatment that has limited potential for success. One woman stated, "Going to the doctor is cheaper than having my hair cut!" This woman was only aware of her own copay and had never considered the full cost of the doctor's visit.

In some instances, consumer demand results from greater knowledge about health services and options. For example, the demand from consumers in the 1970s led to the inclusion of the End Stage Renal Disease Program in the Medicare program, thus increasing costs. Consumer demand has had both positive and negative effects. The positive effect is that people are becoming more self-directed with regard to their health. The negative effect is that individuals are demanding the newest, most expensive, and most high-tech solutions without an understanding of realistic alternatives or of the effect that this has on overall health costs.

Technological Advances

Advances in technology resulted in the survival of patients who might otherwise have died, but these patients experienced higher levels of acuity than before. The increased acuity level of patients during their shortened stay created a greater demand for caregivers. At the same time, the shift to outpatient procedures and convalescence in the home increased the need for nurses outside of the hospital. The new technologies that increased costs in one area decreased costs in the management of many surgeries. The advent of laparoscopic procedures made it possible to do many more surgeries as outpatient procedures. Microscopic technology made surgical incisions smaller and minimized recovery time. The simple X-ray has been augmented by the computerized axial tomography (CAT) scan, magnetic resonance imaging (MRI), and the positron emission tomography (PET) scan. Whereas a chest X-ray costs approximately $50, an MRI costs nearly $2000 (Regence Blue Shield, 2003). From cardiac bypass surgery, which averages $57,000 (Regence Blue Shield, 2003), to organ transplantation, new technologies have made it possible to prolong life, but at high cost. Intensive care and trauma care have become more specialized and more costly. Additional hospital beds are being built to accommodate the increase in demand. The feeling that unlimited medical care should be available to all is supported. Costs for care continue to escalate as high-technology advances became the standard. Although there are periodic attempts to provide controls and decrease the government's bill for health care, costs of both Medicare and Medicaid have continued to escalate.

Increased Pharmacological and Medical Equipment and Supply Costs

New drugs are constantly being developed; spending on prescriptions is growing faster than all other health care services (Davis & Cooper, 2003). Although many new drugs offer clear therapeutic advantages, some offer only marginal differences, but their cost is many times higher than the drugs they have replaced. Equipment and supplies have also increased in cost. The simple drip intravenous (IV) has been replaced by complex computerized IV pumps. Again, they offer important advantages but have escalated costs.

Increases in Health Care Personnel Salaries

Because health care is a labor-intensive endeavor, health personnel incomes affect overall health care costs. Nursing moved from a low-wage occupation as recently as the 1970s to firmly within the midrange during the nursing shortage of the 1980s. According to the National Sample Survey of Registered Nurses, "staff nurses in March 2000 earned an average annual salary of $42,133.40 ranking nurses 115th among the 292 major occupational groups in the Bureau of Labor Statistics National Compensation Survey" (Martin, 2003, p. 77). A response to the nursing shortage in the twenty-first century has been an increase in nurses' salaries, and efforts to recruit and retain nurses are adding to personnel costs. Nurses are needed to care for high-acuity patients receiving complex interventions. As acuity levels rise, there is demand for more nurses. Other health care professionals are also in short supply, and this drives up wages. Many more specialty technicians are required to manage and maintain the high-technology services and they add to personnel costs. Physicians' annual incomes increased at a rate far above the average for the population throughout the last half of the twentieth century. Specialty physicians have significantly higher incomes than do general practitioners; thus, the increasing reliance on specialties further increases costs.

Increased Hospital Costs

Increased hospital costs result from several factors. Hospitals are paying more for the underlying technology, drugs, and personnel costs described previously. In addition, hospitals have been pushing for higher payments from health plans, which reverses the trend that managed care created in the 1990s. Hospitals have been maintaining that they cannot remain financially solvent without a change in reimbursement. In addition, there has been an increased use of hospital services since 2000. Strunk, Ginsburg, and Gabel (2002) suggest that this has resulted from a decrease in managed care and fewer requirements for precertification and other strategies to limit treatment in hospitals.

Increased Litigation

An upsurge in litigation against physicians and hospitals raised costs through the increase in liability insurance premiums. Physicians responded by a practice of "defensive medicine," in which additional diagnostic tests were ordered for legal protection rather than for a real belief that they were needed for diagnosis. Patients had tests they might not have needed to rule out esoteric diagnoses. This has added to the overall cost of health care.

■ REVENUE SOURCES FOR HEALTH CARE

In the majority of developed nations, health care is provided through a national (or provincial) health system that covers everyone. In the United States, a complex system of governmental programs and private health plans provides financial support for individual health care. In the distant past, all health care was paid for by individuals. Even today, some persons can afford to "pay as they go" and prefer not to pay the premiums for an insurance policy. However, the costs of a major illness are so high that very few individuals have adequate resources to meet these expenses should they occur.

This led to the development of charitable organizations that provided health care for the poor. Many of these organizations, such as Shriners, religious orders, and voluntary organizations that focused on a particular health problem still exist, although their resources do not begin to meet the needs of those without the means to pay for health care.

The Advent of Health Care Insurance

Although health care insurance was first introduced in the 1930s, the great majority of individuals continued to pay privately for their health care until the 1950s. At that time, consumers began to purchase health insurance in large numbers. A fixed sum was paid to the insurance company each month. The company anticipated that the money paid out for the health care provided to subscribers would be less than the income from the premiums. When a person used health care resources, a bill was sent by the provider to the insurance company for payment of the insurer's share of the cost. A second bill was sent to the subscriber for a portion of the bill that was the individual's responsibility to pay. As health care coverage was added to employee compensation, the individual's share of the bill often was decreased and the insurance paid most or sometimes all of the cost. This type of reimbursement in which the service is performed and then a bill is sent for the fee is termed **fee-for-service.** Fee-for-service plans were historically focused on care for illness and hospitalization rather than preventive services. The consumer was able to choose any provider and determine in collaboration with the physician when services were needed.

Any source of payment by someone other than the provider or the patient is referred to currently as a **third-party payer.** When the hospital bill is sent directly to the insurance company or managed care plan, the consumer is often unaware of the true cost of health care services. When workplace benefits include payment of health care insurance, the individual may not be aware of even the cost of the insurance premiums.

Today, most Americans who have health insurance (third-party coverage) are included in group policies through their places of employment. Although group policies vary with regard to the benefits provided and the services that will be reimbursed, they usually offer fairly comprehensive health coverage. All third-party coverage has limitations: insurance companies often exclude those with preexisting illnesses. The policies may have high deductible expenses that must be paid by the patient, or they may limit access to providers.

Individual health insurance is an alternative available to those who are retired or self-employed, or who are employed in businesses that do not offer health insurance as a benefit. However, individual policies are much more expensive than group policies.

Governmental Programs

The greatest single source of health care dollars is invested by the federal government. These governmental programs have specific eligibility requirements. The **Medicare** program was introduced under the Social Security Act of 1965 to provide health care insurance to people 65 years of age and older and to the disabled. For the first time, health care was seen as a right of all older Americans. **Medicaid,** a federal program administered through the states, provides care for those who meet specific low-income and eligibility requirements. Grant funding for research and development of new products and methods of providing care are also provided by the federal government. Various other federal programs provide care to those in the military, merchant seamen, and Native American populations. Most states have developed programs that provide for care of those with tuberculosis and mental illness (often in large, custodially oriented institutions). These governmental programs are funded with tax dollars.

Access to Health Care

A person's access to health care is dependent on a wide variety of factors: (i) whether the person has some means of supporting the cost of health care, (ii) whether the type of health care needed is geographically accessible, and (iii) whether the potential care is viewed as culturally sensitive.

ECONOMIC ACCESS

An increasing concern is the large number of individuals, including many full-time workers and their families, who are not covered by any insurance or governmental program and who cannot afford health care. Often, these people receive no preventive care and little treatment for chronic or common problems. They delay seeking care until serious problems arise or an emergency exists. They then go to costly hospital emergency rooms, where laws require that everyone who comes to the hospital be treated. The hospital must absorb the costs of this care by charging more to those who are able to pay. This is termed **cost-shifting.**

Because of the many problems with the current system, a variety of approaches to health care reform have been proposed. In most of these proposals, a major aim is to meet the needs of the uninsured population. Although there is currently no nationwide plan for health reform, some states have instituted health care coverage on a statewide basis, which seeks to alleviate this problem.

Some philanthropic organizations still provide free, charitable care to special groups, such as children with burns. In the present health care settings, these groups are often in a position to support care after the limits of any insurance have been reached.

GEOGRAPHIC ACCESS

Health care resources are not evenly distributed across the country. Low-income and rural areas have fewer primary care providers. These settings are often unattractive to those establishing offices and clinics because economic viability depends on having clients who have the financial resources for care. The result is that even clients with financial resources may find themselves unable to access care where they live, because it is not considered a desirable location. Rural locations place many demands on primary care providers, and there are no support resources for their practice. Therefore, fewer individuals are interested in rural or small community practice.

 ## CULTURAL ACCESS

Individuals are more likely to seek care, continue with care, and follow prescribed therapeutic regimens when the individual care providers and the systems in which they work demonstrate cultural sensitivity. The person whose language needs are discounted and who feels disrespected by individual health care workers will often not seek care until a life-threatening emergency demands it. From this viewpoint, the client is facing a problem of lack of access to culturally appropriate services. Chapter 11 discusses the concerns related to cultural competence of health care workers.

■ COST CONTAINMENT

Cost containment includes all efforts directed toward preventing the steep rise in costs of health care. One aim of cost containment is to reduce waste of limited resources and time. Another is to find more cost-effective means of accomplishing the desired health care outcomes. Thus, the goal is to provide safe, effective care at the lowest cost per patient need.

Using Reimbursement to Control Costs

Periodically, all participants in health care were admonished to control costs. Because these voluntary efforts to control cost were not successful, the Tax Equity and Fiscal Responsibility Act was passed in October 1982. It changed the financial structure of health care institutions significantly by altering Medicare and Medicaid payment policies. Limitations were placed on payments in a variety of areas, including outpatient services. In 1983, **diagnostic related groups (DRGs)** created a prospective reimbursement mechanism for Medicare and Medicaid. **Prospective reimbursement** is a predetermined payment schedule for a given surgery or episode of illness based on a type of statistical average. DRGs identified the average number of days of hospitalization and costs for a specific group of diagnoses. A specific payment amount was made for any diagnosis included in the DRG. This payment covered the expected costs for laboratory fees, various therapies, and surgery, as well as nursing care. If a patient stayed more than the predetermined number of days or had extra costly care, the hospital was expected to absorb the cost. Only a few exceptions were made. The costs incurred by those staying more than the average number of days were expected to be offset by those with shorter-than-average stays. The providers now had an incentive to limit the costs of care, because in most instances they would not receive increased payment for increased costs. If costs were less than average, the hospital kept the profit. Hospital administrators began changing practices to decrease costs and encourage early discharge.

Private insurance companies and managed care plans also began instituting prospective reimbursement. Prospective reimbursement has revolutionized the health care delivery system, resulting in fewer patient days of stay per diagnostic category. These changes in hospital stays and reimbursement have been accompanied by an increased need for home health care and outpatient diagnostic tests and surgery. Thus, we are seeing a shift in the environment in which care is delivered, accompanied by an expectation of greater involvement of the family in the provision of care.

Many insurers and providers have taken a more active role in managing the costs associated with medical and hospital costs, paying discounted rates for the care provided by **preferred providers.** Preferred providers are physicians, hospitals, and other health care providers who have contracted for a specific, usually lower, payment for their services and thus have an incentive to decrease the costs. In addition, health plans designate many procedures as outpatient procedures, and if they are performed as inpatient procedures, the health plan denies reimbursement or limits reimbursement to that which would be provided for outpatient services. Some health plans require prior approval for the use of costly tests, procedures, and surgeries. In some instances, a second medical opinion is required before a surgery can be performed. However, these measures have created controversy regarding their effect on quality and timely care.

Managed care refers to any health plan system in which care is actively managed by the third-party payer who sets the ground rules for care and determines where, how, and by whom care will be provided. In a managed care plan, there are increased benefits for preventive services, ambulatory care, and even prescription drugs. In return for this expansion of care, the consumer must accept management of his or her care needs by the plan. There are limits on the providers that may be accessed. Specific hospitals are designated for services. Prescriptions must be filled by designated pharmacies and there is usually a specific list of drugs, called a formulary, that must be used unless special permission is sought. These individuals or groups become preferred providers for members of the health plan. To gain a contract, providers must be competitive in terms of cost, quality, and the comprehensiveness of services available. A small number of managed care plans have been in existence since the 1930s.

Third-party coverage for health care costs began to change rapidly after Congress introduced the Managed Competition Act of 1992. This act encouraged the development of an increasing number of **health maintenance organizations (HMOs)** and other managed health plans. Managed care plans quickly replaced many traditional insurance policies. Currently, concerns are being expressed that the many attempts to control costs through managed care may be diminishing the quality of care because decisions are based on cost rather than medical need.

In the 1990s, an increasing segment of the managaed care market moved to what are called **capitation** payments. In capitated health plans, the plan contracts with a provider organization that can provide all levels of care. The provider organization is paid a flat amount for every individual enrolled regardless of whether services are used. If the provider organization can keep people well, keep them out of the hospital, and avoid high-cost care, the organization will make more money. The provider assumes the risk that an individual consumer might need very high-cost care. This type of plan creates an incentive for the provider organization to work at health promotion and disease prevention strategies. For example, a program for supporting individuals with diabetes in effective disease management has the potential to create better health while avoiding costly complications of diabetes. Although capitated plans have the disadvantage for the consumer of dictating where and how care occurs, they also have the potential to increase the health status of those enrolled. HMOs were the first capitated plans.

In the 1990s, to meet the demands of controlling costs, health care provider institutions began to restructure their organizations (see Chapter 2). By decreasing professional staff, adding unlicensed assistive personnel (UAPs), and altering management structures, the organizations hoped to maintain quality and decrease costs. Limitations were placed on the autonomy of physicians to order high-cost care. Some of these strategies were successful, and some were not. In other instances, reducing the number of registered nurses was found to lead to increased rates of complications and thus increased rather than decreased costs.

In 1997 through the Balanced Budget Act, the federal government mandated the use of a prospective payment system (PPS) for nursing home costs (Infante, 1998). The implementation of PPS began in 1998 with the designation of seven categories of resource utilization groups (RUGs) (Harris, 1998). The assessment data gathered by nurses became the critical base for determining the reimbursement group into which a resident was placed. Increasing constraints were placed on home care agencies to demonstrate that skilled care was needed before reimbursement would be authorized. Reimbursement for home care began to be based on the assessment of the nurse. The total number of home health visits allowed under Medicare was curtailed. Thus, nursing was more significantly involved in the financial status of all health care agencies.

As we move into the twenty-first century, health care reform requires that the provision of health care become more cost-effective and efficient. Accountability will be a hallmark of the first decade. A balance among cost of care, quality of care, and patient satisfaction must be achieved. The complexity of these goals escalates when we consider ethical questions related to distribution of scarce resources among an ever-increasing number of individuals.

Cost Awareness in Nursing

Cost awareness is the first step for nurses in effectively participating in cost-containment strategies. You can begin by understanding the costs of nursing staffing and the costs of supplies and equipment used for nursing care. Then you can successfully participate in and even initiate cost-containment strategies in nursing.

COST OF NURSING STAFF

The overall nursing department budget often accounts for 50% to 60% of the total hospital operating budget and is made up primarily of salaries and supply costs. The percentage of each of these items in the budget varies with the type and quantity of supplies and the number of people needed on a given unit. Prevailing wages in an area heavily impact the amount of money budgeted for salaries by an institution. Traditionally, the cost of nursing care has been included on the patient's bill as an integral part of room and board, as have housekeeping, maintenance, and other services. Determining the actual costs of nursing care, independent of other costs, provides valuable information for decision making. For example, research demonstrating that more hours of registered nursing care decreases the incidence of complications supports the need for a nursing staff with more registered nurses.

Exacting tools have not been developed to identify specific nursing care costs for each patient. Most frequently, an institution determines direct nursing costs and total nursing costs. Direct nursing costs reflect the intensity of nursing care that can be measured in time required to provide the care. They include assessing, planning, implementing, and evaluating nursing care. Total nursing costs include the cost of supplies, as well as support personnel and services, (including staff development, de-

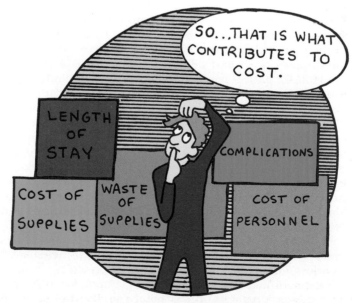

Cost awareness is the first step for nurses in participating in cost-containment strategies.

partment supervisors, and liaison nurses), and specialty nurses, such as enterostomal therapists.

Some organizations are now working on developing systems for charging for nursing care. Most of these projects use patient acuity classification systems as a basis for determining the level and hours of nursing care required. The administration then computes the cost of care by multiplying the number of nursing hours anticipated by the average hourly nursing salary. **Patient classification systems** also can be used to determine appropriate staffing levels. The average number of nursing hours required per month can be used to project the number of full-time-equivalent employees (FTEs) needed.

Although controversy exists on whether nursing services should be billed separately, it is clear that identifying the cost of nursing services is essential to increase accountability for efficient and cost-effective care. In addition, when resources are scarce competition for them increases. To be more competitive in this environment, all aspects of the organization must demonstrate the ability to generate income. In economic terms, the nursing department must demonstrate that it is a profit center rather than a cost center.

Another aspect of understanding nursing costs relates to the full picture of personnel costs in nursing. The cost of each FTE includes both salary costs and benefits, which often equal 20% to 30% of the salary cost. An FTE is a position that can be equated to 40 hours of work per week times 52 weeks, for a total of 2080 hours per year. An FTE can be divided into parts. For example, half an FTE (0.5 FTE) is equivalent to an employee working 20 hours per week for the year. The important part of this equation is that one FTE is equivalent to 40 hours of employment per week whether worked by one full-time person or several part-time workers.

The total hours for an FTE include both productive and nonproductive time. Productive time is the time spent working on the unit. Nonproductive time is that for which the employee is paid but during which the employee is not working, such as vacation time, holidays, and sick leave. Nonproductive time varies, depending on the benefits of the employing institution. If there are 272 hours of nonproductive time, for example, the hours must be covered by another worker and must be considered in the budgeting process. The nonproductive time subtracted from 2080 (the usual hours of work per year) yields the productive work hours. Only the productive time is available for patient care, and, therefore, when hours of care available per patient are computed, only productive hours can be used (Display 3-1). An additional factor for hospitals and nursing homes is that they must provide nursing care 24 hours per day and seven days a week. Therefore, the overall number of FTEs needed greatly exceeds the number of nurses available at any one time. This phenomenon across a hospital results in three or four employees for each patient bed.

Total nursing salary costs are affected by the patient care delivery model selected by the hospital. You may already be aware of strategies to manage the patient care workload. The patient acuity system assists in determining the patient care hours needed on a unit. Patient care delivery models provide a systematic approach for identifying the appropriate caregiver during those hours. Team nursing, primary care, and patient-focused care are examples. Restructured models now tend to bring services closer to the patient, in some cases bringing satellite pharmacies and laboratories to the patient care area (see Chapter 2).

One of the ongoing problems in planning for nursing is the fluctuation in acuity and census of patients on a hospital unit. If a unit is staffed for maximum acuity and full census, then the cost per patient is greatly increased if the census is low or acuity

DISPLAY 3-1	**Calculation of Nonproductive Time**

52 weeks × 40 hours = 2,080 hours for one full-time equivalent employee (FTE)

NONPRODUCTIVE TIME
2 Weeks vacation: 40 hours × 2 = 80 hours
12 Sick days: 8 hours × 12 = 96 hours
10 Holidays: 8 hours × 10 = 80 hours
2 Staff development days: 8 × 2 = 16 hours
Total "nonproductive" time = 272 hours

PRODUCTIVE TIME
2,080 hours (1 FTE) − 272 hours = 1,808 hours for direct patient care

is less. However, if the unit is staffed for an estimated average number of patients, at times of high census there will not be enough care providers. The economic impact of various staffing models also contributes to concerns about workplace satisfaction for nurses.

If the acuity level increases overall, requiring additional hours of care, a float pool of nursing staff or temporary nurse pools can be used to meet the projected need. The effectiveness of this type of system, although generally initiated by administration, depends on the direct input of the nurse who provides patient care and who determines the patient's acuity level at least once a day. Input must be accurate, because the system is only as good as the information it receives. New acuity systems are being investigated that better reflect activity associated with shorter lengths of stay and that require more frequent monitoring.

Some labor costs are considered fixed; others may vary, depending on the number and acuity of patients. Each hour counts and must be used wisely for cost containment. You can easily see that time is money and that those who arrive late, take extended lunch periods and coffee breaks, and are in the lounge when they should be working are misusing resources.

NONSALARY COSTS OF CARE

Another area of concern is buying and distributing supplies. Economies of scale, otherwise known as volume buying, are important in reducing costs, as is appropriate conservation of supplies. Staff may be unaware of the cost of everyday supplies, such as reagent strips used to measure capillary glucose in a diabetic patient or specialized dressing materials. When individuals are unaware of costs of supplies, they are sometimes less careful regarding waste.

Repairs are another concern in a health care setting, wherein much of the equipment, such as electronic thermometers and infusion pumps, must meet exacting standards of accuracy and reliability. A dropped electronic thermometer, a carelessly handled electric eye, or an electrical cord caught in a bed mechanism might each be costly to repair.

Hospitals that maintain a trauma center have very high costs associated with the 24-hour availability of highly trained personnel and complex technology. An added expense is the provision of high-cost services to victims of trauma after the initial emergency response. Many trauma victims exhaust personal health care financial resources and continue to need costly care. Efforts to contain these costs have been successful but have required the participation of everyone involved in care (Taheri et al., 1998).

COST-CONTAINMENT STRATEGIES FOR NURSES

Although many of the system-wide cost problems cannot be affected by the individual nurse, there are things that contribute to the expense of care to individuals on which nurses can have an important effect. Cost containment, in terms of time and materials, begins at the bedside. The employing institution, or even the nursing unit, might adopt cost-containing polices and procedures, but in the end the individual nurse must implement them. Commitment to reducing expenses is supported by the philosophy that if each person does his or her part, the cumulative effect will be great. It is therefore important for you to do your part, no matter how insignificant it seems.

DECREASING TURNOVER OF STAFF

The cost for orienting new staff is high. Maintaining staff by increasing retention of employees decreases the need for orientation sessions. Although the employing agency must place new graduates carefully to maximize potential and encourage job satisfaction, you have an impact by choosing a job carefully. When you are satisfied with your job, you are more likely to become committed to the organization. As you remain in the position and feel comfortable, you begin to develop short-term and long-term professional goals (see Chapter 12).

When you become a more experienced nurse, the manner in which you help to orient new nurses, include them in decision making, and help them become integrated into the staff makes a significant difference in turnover. If you are on a unit with high turnover, it is often useful to begin asking yourself what is occurring that causes individuals to leave. When these are issues beyond your control, you may take your concerns to your unit manager to initiate action.

You can help decrease the turnover of assistive personnel also. Satisfaction in a job often relates to the interpersonal relationships present in the setting. How an individual is treated by a supervisor, the perception of fairness, and a willingness to see each employee as an individual contribute to decreasing staff turnover (see Chapter 5).

MANAGING SUPPLIES

The judicious use of supplies and use of the correct product for the need are essential to cost-effective patient care. Ask yourself, "Is it necessary to open a dressing kit when I need a four-by-four?" or "Are sterile gloves called for or will clean do?" However, nurses must guard against false economy with supplies. The failure to use sterile supplies when called for may save some supply money but open the door to an infection. Managing a major wound requires both the knowledge of dressing materials and the knowledge of costs. "What is a cost-effective approach to healing this wound?" is the important question, and not simply "What is the least expensive care method?"

Purchase of supplies is also important. Nursing and purchasing departments must communicate well to determine the best product for the intended use. The lowest bidder may provide a product that breaks easily, is difficult to open, is undependable, or needs to be repaired frequently. If those who work with the equipment do not inform them of problems, people in the purchasing department will remain unaware of these concerns. In fact, the lowest bid may in the long run be more expensive in terms of wasted time and frustration. Providing clear product specifications for those who purchase the products is the first step in a cooperative effort toward **cost-effectiveness.**

As a nurse, you need to be familiar with the method of charging supplies, whether by bar code directly into a computer, a charge slip, or stickers on a Kardex (but not on your uniform pocket), and you must follow through with the process. You also must document accurately procedures and equipment used, indicating a clear relationship to patient need. Even when items are not charged to the individual, hospitals must be able to track the cost of caring for specific patients in order to calculate the costs of the contracts that are a part of managed care environments. If the institution does not know what it costs to care for a particular health problem, then it cannot determine whether providing the desired care at the cost offered will create a profit or a deficit.

EXAMINING PROCEDURES AND PROCESSES

Many experts feel that direct caregivers can make the greatest impact on quality of care and cost containment. Independent of the larger organization, the nurse manager of a unit, with staff input, can develop efficient systems for an individual unit. Successful innovations that begin on an experimental unit can then be used on other units.

The nurse's ability to adjust to new policies, such as those related to streamlining charting practices, providing reports in ways that save time yet are more meaningful (such as walking rounds), and adapting to new technology, plays an important part in cost containment. Awareness is the first step in decreasing work hours and increasing efficiency. The development of management and communication skills, which allows the nurse to successfully motivate others to use their time and effort efficiently and become more aware of costs, has become a necessity. (see Chapter 5).

PARTICIPATING IN PREVENTION SERVICES

More and more managed care organizations and the health care providers that are contracting with those organizations are developing health promotion and disease prevention programs as both a marketing strategy and to control costs (Schauffler & Chapman, 1998). The overall impact of this on health care costs across the nation has not yet been evaluated in a comprehensive manner. However, many individuals are hopeful that this may strongly contribute to cost containment. Nurses have been at the forefront of developing effective health promotion activities and also have begun examining all interactions with patients from a viewpoint of health promotion.

EFFECTIVE ASSESSMENT AND PATIENT CARE MANAGEMENT

Increased length of stay and complications are great contributors to increased costs (Meding et al., 1998). Each day that a person stays in the hospital or nursing home increases costs. As cited earlier, when reimbursement is fixed by a DRG or contracted reimbursement, extra days contribute to overall costs without providing increased income.

Complications increase costs by requiring longer stays and also by requiring more costly treatment. An infection with a resistant organism may require treatment with a new antibiotic that costs $100 per dose. Preventing that infection saves the cost of the treatment as well as the costs associated with the extended stay that the treatment might require. A pressure ulcer requires added nursing care hours as well as costly dressing materials and a longer stay. The cost of caring for and healing a Stage III or IV pressure ulcer is estimated to be between $14,020 and $22,925, with hospitals spending an average of $400,000 to $700,000 annually on their care (Beckrich & Aronovich, 1999). Because of the high cost of treating these two complications and the strong potential for prevention, the incidences of nosocomial infections and of pressure ulcer development are both used as indicators of quality of care by the Joint Commission on Accreditation of Healthcare Organizations. Preventing complications is a part of effective patient care management. Nosocomial infections are very costly for an institution. The health care worker who is careless about handwashing, does not follow standard precautions, and is careless about carrying items from one patient room to another is a serious cost liability to the employer. When one patient has a known infection, it becomes an even more critical issue. Nurses need to differentiate appropriately between cost-control measures that are useful and those that create the potential for more problems. Nowhere is this more apparent than in infection control. If one patient has vancomycin-resistant enterococcus (VRE) and the protocol calls for using gowns when providing care, reusing the same gown and potentially contaminating your uniform saves a small amount on gowns but may cost a very major amount in transmitting the infection to another patient.

The role of the nurse in anticipatory management, which is reflected in the ability to assess a patient astutely and recognize problems before they become major, is critical to cost efficiency. The nurse is accountable for accurate assessment and planning of care. Although this is fundamentally an obligation to the patient, failure to carry out this role is costly to the institution.

Assuring patient safety also is cost-effective. By developing approaches to such issues as decreasing patient falls, decreasing patient injury, and decreasing medication errors, hospital liability is also decreased. Patient injury may result more directly in increased length of stay and additional costs for the care involved.

Critical Thinking Exercise

Develop a measurable objective related to cost containment against which nurses could be evaluated in an annual performance review. Use this as a basis for a small group discussion on the relationship of cost containment and accountability.

Legal and Ethical Aspects of Cost Containment

Ethical questions arise with regard to the quality of care that limited funding can support. Do we as a society believe that there is a right to health care? Some parts of our society support this, but others do not subscribe to idea of adding more rights. If we believe that health care is a right, what should be included? Most people are comfortable with including immunizations for children, treatment of acute trauma, and response to life-threatening events such as cardiac arrest. However, where to draw the line between everything an individual might want and want a society can economically provide is not simple. When analyzing this precarious balance, the quality, efficiency, effectiveness, and cost of care must all be factored into the decision.

Legal and ethical standards for nursing care require adherence to standards of care defined by the profession. Standards of care and patient safety must not be compromised in the name of cost containment. A nurse who is aware of influences on the costs of health care can readily demonstrate to the organization that the use of old or contaminated supplies that cause the patient additional complications is not practical. The nurse carefully balances the quality of care with conservative management of available resources. It is the legal responsibility of the nurse to maintain the standard of care and not jeopardize patient safety.

Many issues are less clear-cut. Sending an 85-year-old compromised individual home to be cared for by an equally compromised 84-year-old spouse raises questions of safety. At what point does the nurse intervene and say, "This may be the standard practice, but it is not the correct practice in this situation"? Does the nurse have the power to intervene? For the larger society, the questions about denial of services, limitation of services, and refusal to allow referral to specialty resources are creating major ethical dilemmas. Funds for health care are limited. Unrestrained spending is not possible. What then can be provided? Where are lines drawn? Who gains? Who loses? These ethical questions will continue to challenge all of health care.

Critical Thinking Exercise

Identify a cost-containment strategy that you believe has ethical implications. Analyze the strategy by using basic ethical principles as a standard.

■ USING BUDGETS TO MANAGE FINANCES

The viability, or survival and growth, of an organization can only be maintained by having more income than expenses. Most health care organizations are nonprofit, which means that all excess income over expenses is used within the organization to improve services or expand the physical plant through capital investment. Some health care organizations are owned by stockholders who expect to earn a profit on their investment after the needs of the institution are met and care is provided. Whatever the status of the organization, effective budgeting is essential to meeting these demands.

Basically, a **budget** is a formal plan for managing financial resources. The budget document indicates the expected income and expected expenses of an organization, department, or individual. It provides a method of tracking costs and therefore a way to examine where savings could be made. Just as you balance your income and expenses each month, the health care organization must balance its budget.

Many beginning nurses find the subject of budgeting for a health care facility boring and difficult to understand. As a result, they may fail to take advantage of opportunities to affect matters that are very important to the care they are able to provide. This brief overview of organizational budgets is aimed at helping increase your understanding of the processes you find in your place of employment and facilitate your ability to be actively involved.

Capital versus Operating Budgets

The total organizational budget is composed of the operating budget and the capital budget. Organizations differentiate their operating and capital budgets because funds for them must be accounted for separately and may be raised independently.

The **operating budget** is concerned with items that cannot be reused and that are needed for the daily operation of the institution. Salaries are a large part of the operating budget. The operating budget also covers supplies such as medications, dressing supplies, gloves, syringes, linen, and even pens and pencils. Unexpected items often included under supplies include copying and equipment rental. The basic costs of the institution, such as heat, lights, and cleaning, are also considered operating costs.

The cost of direct care supplies, including medications, presents a constant challenge to a health care institution. The ongoing costs of gloves increased dramatically when standard precautions were introduced. New mandates to prevent needle-stick injuries are resulting in escalating costs for equipment. As previously discussed, new pharmaceutical agents are much more costly than older drugs. Decisions regarding which drugs to include in the hospital formulary are made by a pharmacy and therapeutics committee composed of physicians and pharmacists working together.

Capital budget expenditures include major equipment expected to last for a significant period of time and changes in the physical plant, including modification, renovation, or construction. The budget manual for an organization stipulates an arbitrary amount that constitutes a capital expenditure. For instance, if the amount were $1000, any equipment item that cost more than that would be included in the capital budget. Remodeling costs above $1000 might also be capital expenditures. If, for example, doorways needed to be widened to allow wheelchair access, renovation costs might be reflected in the capital budget. As facilities address the problem of back injuries among nursing care staff, the demand for mechanical lifting devices is growing. These will represent a significant capital expenditure for any institution.

Budgets and Organizational Evaluation

The budget allows the organization to plan and manage programs and control spending. Meeting the objectives of the organization within budgetary limits often serves as a criterion to evaluate the overall performance of health care administrators, managers, and specific programs. Managers who fail to keep spending within the budget guidelines or fail to manage the budget to assure that goals for care are met are likely to be removed from their position.

Budget analysis also enables organizations to determine whether certain services should be dropped because they are not cost-effective or others expanded because they are a significant revenue source. In some instances, an institution will decide to continue offering a service that consistently loses money because of the importance of that service to the community. In such a situation, there must be other services that bring in more revenue than they cost to offset the service that operates at a deficit.

Budget Planning

Budget planning for a large institution is a lengthy process involving many steps and taking place over months. Budget-planning procedures vary among organizations. However, some parts of the process are common to all organizations. Operating and capital budgets may be on the same or on different schedules.

The finance or budget office prepares materials, sets time lines, and assures that the process meets the policies of the institution. These **budget processes** include gathering information regarding current expenses, expected or planned changes, expected salary increases for personnel, and forecasts for inflation. Budget planning itself usually starts about 6 months before a new budget must be adopted.

The finance office uses the information gathered to establish an overall preliminary budget for the institution. This office then sends out budget-planning materials to various departments, which include a preliminary budget for each department. In many institutions, a preliminary budget shows the same budget for a department that it had the previous year. The department will be asked to reallocate resources to fit current needs and must justify all new resources requested. When there are economic difficulties, the preliminary budget may indicate that each department must strive to cut expenses by a specific percentage. A few institutions practice what is termed **zero-base budgeting.** In this instance, every department starts from zero and must justify all budget requests and not just new or increased requests.

Each department develops its individual budget requests and submits them by a specified date. The accreditation standards developed by the Joint Commission on the Accreditation of Health Care Organizations (2003) require evidence of collaboration among the various disciplines and departments in developing and implementing budgets. Nursing participation in some facilities is focused on nurses in management positions, but many facilities invite wide participation by everyone in the organization. If you have a budget request, providing a rationale and backup information regarding your recommendation will be helpful, because with your help the manager can then be well prepared to defend the budget request. Once you are familiar with important dates in the budget review for the organization with which you are involved, you can provide timely input. There are few things more frustrating than being told that additional personnel or supplies cannot be obtained because they are not in the budget and it is too late to add anything. This frustration can be decreased by thinking "budget" all year and planning ahead.

After all budget requests are submittted to the finance office, an administrative group or committee reviews all budget requests and their justification and develops a proposed system-wide budget. Budget requests that are based on objectives or goals of the organization are more likely to be funded. The budget for supplies is usually calculated by using the previous year as a baseline, determining a projected expansion or decrease in associated services, and adding a predetermined expected rate of inflation. The budget for supplies can be significantly affected by increasing attention to conservation, decreasing the supplies needed, or decreasing the cost per unit. Health care institutions and agencies often combine efforts to increase volume purchasing and decrease the cost of each item. As the overall budget is developed, funds may be transferred from one department to another, requests may be consolidated, and cuts made in some areas.

Value analysis is a systematic approach to the evaluation of products, including supplies, equipment, pharmaceuticals, and new technology, that are used in providing patient care. It requires careful consideration of the implications associated with all expenditures. Questions such as these are asked: "Are there other departments that use this product?" "Can we develop criteria for the purchase interdepartmentally?" "Is this the best price we can get?" "If we change products, what are the additional costs associated with change?" "What is the comparable repair rate on the equipment being considered?" The effect on patient care quality is an important consideration. The cost–benefit relationship is another important factor. Although purchasing an IV infusion system that does not require a needle for access is expensive, costs related to accidental needle sticks are saved. Nurses are becoming increasingly involved in the value analysis process and in the teams formed to make the decisions.

Even when budget needs are thoroughly documented and justified, there may not be enough money to cover all the requests. The responsible person or committee must prioritize the requests and determine what will be included in the overall system-wide budget to be forwarded to the board of trustees or other governing bodies.

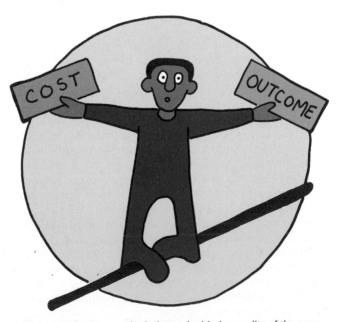

The cost of care must be balanced with the quality of the care.

When the comprehensive budget is brought to the board of trustees, there is again a discussion of the various expenses and a determination of institution-wide priorities. The board of trustees may request additional changes or review. The budget is generally brought forward several months prior to the expected date of implementation, so that adequate time is provided for changes. If revisions are made, the board will review the document again. The final document is approved by the board of trustees, which then authorizes expenditure of funds for the next **fiscal year.** The board of trustees is ultimately responsible for the overall financial health of the institution.

EXAMPLE *Budget Process of Community Hospital*

Let us use a hypothetical hospital named "Community Hospital" to help you see the budget planning process in action. The budget year for Community Hospital extends from July 1 to June 30. This is their fiscal year. At Community Hospital, the board of trustees has an annual fall retreat to review its mission and goals for the coming year. At its January meeting, it formally approves the revised mission and goals for the next fiscal year, which will begin July 1.

Community Hospital's actual budget process begins in January. The finance office prepares the budget packets for distribution to department managers. These budget packets contain all the instructions and forms that must be completed in order to request a specific budget for the coming fiscal year. The budget packets are distributed on February 1 and must be returned to the finance office by the end of March.

In February, each department at Community Hospital begins work on its new budget. Most departments form a departmental committee to gather information and develop the budget. The nursing department of the Community Hospital forms a committee composed of unit nurse managers to prepare the budget. Each nursing unit identifies what is happening in regard to its patient census, changes taking place in care practices and standards, and desired improvements. Each unit manager asks the staff for its input and suggestions in regard to the budget plan for the coming year. Meetings are held on each unit to help in establishing priorities and assure that these priorities are reflected in the budget request. This is the best time for staff nurses to provide input. Wes Miller and Jean Wilson, registered nurses on the neurology unit, have cooperated in studying back injuries and identifying effective lifting devices. They prepared a written request for specific lifting devices for their unit. They included extensive justification for their nurse manager to take to the budget meetings.

When finally submitted, the nursing department's capital budget request includes lifting devices for all nursing units and not just for the neurology unit. After their extensive value analysis, nurse managers agree that staff retention and safety will be enhanced throughout the institution by the use of lifting devices. The justification prepared by the two staff nurses is extremely valuable in their deliberations. Wes and Jean are excited to learn that their input resulted in the hospital adopting a new strategic objective in regard to employee back safety and that lifting devices are going to be purchased for all units.

Critical Thinking Exercise

For a health care organization with which you are most familiar, identify the fiscal year dates, critical dates in the budget cycle, and the definition of supplies and equipment from the budget manual. Using this information, plan an appropriate strategy to have an IV monitor that costs $1500 included in the budget. Consider the following:

  1. What is the justification for the purchase?
  2. Would this be considered an operating or capital expense?
  3. What is an appropriate time line for planning this purchase?

Monitoring the Budget

To assure that the budget is followed, every organization has procedures, commonly referred to as **control procedures,** that are used to monitor expenditures. Increasingly, health care agencies must track costs not only by department or unit but also by patient or resident. This allows the administration to examine details and modify procedures and protocols in a systematic way with costs in mind (Lubarsky, 1998). Control procedures include the work of the unit manager, who supervises ordering and work assignments. The accounting department provides a monthly document that contains detailed information on expenditures to enable the management staff to monitor expenditures for which they are responsible. The manager determines whether there is any **variance** between the budgeted expenditures and the actual expenditures or between expected and actual revenue. A **budget variance** is simply the difference between the planned and the actual expenditures or income.

A variance is considered positive if it increases the organization's available funds. For example, a higher revenue than expected is a positive variance in revenue. Lower expenditure than was budgeted for expenses is also viewed as a positive variance, because more funds are available for use. Unfilled nursing positions result in spending less salary for nurses. Therefore, actual expenses will be less than budgeted expenses. This is referred to as a positive variance, because expenses are lower than planned. A negative variance decreases the available funds. When there are many illnesses among staff, and regular workers must be supplemented with per diem staff (those who work only on the days when they are called), the actual expenditure is higher than that which was budgeted, because the regular staff are paid for sick days and the per diem staff must also be paid. Therefore, there is a negative variance in expenditure. If fewer patients are admitted than expected, the revenue is reduced, and there is a negative variance in income.

The board of trustees (or its designated committee) monitors the overall budget at least monthly and identifies variances between the projected and actual revenue and expenses. The board makes its final overview of expenditures compared with the budget at the completion of the fiscal year. The progress of the organization in using the established tools and meeting its objectives in a cost-effective manner is evaluated, and the assumptions about the future are reviewed. The process then begins again—the budget process is constant and ongoing.

Critical Thinking Exercise

At a facility in which you have clinical experience, research how costs for specific commonly occurring disorders or surgeries are tracked. Identify one example (such as myocardial infarction or fractured hip) and gather information on the costs associated with care for the problem. Report on your findings to your clinical group.

■ MANAGING TIME

Time is a valuable resource. The way you organize your own time as well as the way you delegate to those assisting with nursing care affects the cost of care. Regardless of the clinical setting in which you are working, one common denominator is that you are expected to organize and provide care to your patients effectively and efficiently. **Effectively** means that the care the nurse gives makes the situation better. **Efficiently** means that the nurse gives care in an organized pattern that maximizes the use of time, resources, and effort. You may also be engaged in delegating tasks to others and to helping others in the **multidisciplinary team** (including therapists, lab personnel, diagnostic imaging technicians, social workers, and nutritionists) work in efficient ways. Families and personal caregivers may also need your assistance to be able to effectively organize care needs in coordination with other life demands.

Cost-effectiveness is a primary driving force behind the need to accomplish more in less time. Most nurses find that the current organizational structure provides fewer licensed staff and more responsibilities for the registered nurse. Without effective skills in managing time and organizing care, it becomes impossible for the nurse to accomplish all that is demanded.

The art of **delegation** of appropriate nursing tasks must be mastered (see Chapter 6). Appropriate supervision of those to whom you delegate responsibilities is essential. Developing a team approach and commitment to quality care will help in getting all members of the team to recognize the importance of using time efficiently. Keep in mind that employees who do not give a full day's work for a full day's pay cost the institution (and eventually the patient) additional money. The focus of our effort is to decrease costs associated with waste, rework, unnecessary complexity, and unreliability.

Nurses can make valuable recommendations on routines that may be outmoded or no longer needed. Repetitious paperwork might be reduced, especially with the introduction of computers. You, as a staff nurse, can make recommendations to streamline the system at the grassroots level. You are the best person to evaluate existing systems and anticipate needed changes.

STRATEGIES FOR EFFECTIVE TIME MANAGEMENT

At first, going through the steps necessary for establishing better **time management** may seem difficult and actually wasteful of time that could be spent in other ways. However, once you have learned actions to help your personal organization and management of time, you will find that good organization becomes second nature. You may already be a very good time manager, but everyone can become better. By learning one new action, you may save a significant amount of time for other activities. Some people report that when they feel time-stressed by the number of activities they must fit into a given period of time, they recall time management principles and modify their actions. Knowing and adopting a time management program can help all of us reduce stress imposed by time constraints, so that we can accomplish more in less time. We recommend that you first do a personal assessment of how you use time and then identify areas in which you might improve.

TIME ASSESSMENT

An interesting and essential first step in beginning to manage time more effectively is to identify how you use time. Only through examining how you spend your time can you begin to set priorities, eliminate time barriers, and incorporate aids to better time management. Most people are surprised by the following time assessment exercise because they have never looked closely at their time expenditure during one or more days. You may know whether you are a morning or evening person, that is, at which time your energy is highest, because you get more done during these hours. Few people are able to maintain a high-energy level consistently throughout the day. The time assessment chart in Table 3-1 should validate for you when your energy level is highest. It may suggest that you are not using your high-energy hours wisely and can identify when it is best to work on projects.

Time assessment can also help you discover time wasters of which you are not aware. People often find that they have obvious time wasters that can be eliminated. It is also important to recognize your particular time savers. These may be simple behaviors that collectively save time.

Begin your time assessment by setting up a chart similar to that in Table 3-1. List on the right side of each column, by the quarter hour, exactly how you spend your time throughout one or more days. Be very specific. The list will not be as useful if the language is too general. Record everything you do, including minor interruptions and time spent socializing. Try to keep the form up-to-date as you move through each day, because accuracy in recording decreases as you become distracted with the next activity. You may want to vary the form. For example, if you work evenings or nights, you need to change the time designations. This information is only for your use, and it is not necessary to share it with others unless you wish to do so.

The next step is to analyze your log. Mackenzie (1990) encourages you to look at questions such as these: When did you start the activity that was number one on your list? Could you have started it earlier? Were you distracted while working on it? Could you have avoided that distraction? What was your longest period of uninterrupted time? During which period of time were you most productive? Did you accomplish all the activities you wanted to complete during the day?

Looking at your time assessment, identify your time savers and time wasters. This exercise often proves revealing. For example, if you are on a nursing unit in which a good friend is also a staff person, you may not realize how much time you spend socializing. On the other hand, you may have many strengths in time management that you can build on. You may note that in certain instances you negotiated with another staff member to share tasks, thus saving time for both of you. You might conclude that you have been unrealistic in the number of tasks you

TABLE 3-1	TIME ASSESSMENT		
	DAY 1	**DAY 2**	**DAY 3**
	6:00	6:00	6:00
	6:15	6:15	6:15
	6:30	6:30	6:30
	6:45	6:45	6:45
	7:00	7:00	7:00
	7:15	7:15	7:15
	7:30	7:30	7:30
	7:45	7:45	7:45
	8:00	8:00	8:00
	8:15	8:15	8:15
	8:30	8:30	8:30
	8:45	8:45	8:45
	9:00	9:00	9:00
	9:15	9:15	9:15
	9:30	9:30	9:30
	9:45	9:45	9:45
	10:00	10:00	10:00
	10:15	10:15	10:15
	10:30	10:30	10:30
	10:45	10:45	10:45
	11:00	11:00	11:00
	11:15	11:15	11:15
	11:30	11:30	11:30
	11:45	11:45	11:45
	12:00	12:00	12:00
	12:15	12:15	12:15
	12:30	12:30	12:30
	12:45	12:45	12:45
	1:00	1:00	1:00
	1:15	1:15	1:15
	1:30	1:30	1:30
	1:45	1:45	1:45
	2:00	2:00	2:00
	2:15	2:15	2:15
	2:30	2:30	2:30
	2:45	2:45	2:45
	3:00	3:00	3:00
	3:15	3:15	3:15
	3:30	3:30	3:30
	3:45	3:45	3:45
	4:00	4:00	4:00
	4:15	4:15	4:15
	4:30	4:30	4:30
	4:45	4:45	4:45
	5:00	5:00	5:00

Continue on into late afternoon or evening

attempted in a given period of time and that you are now ready to write a more re-alistic plan.

Another value of your time log is helping you to be realistic about the length of time a task really takes. For example, if you are responsible for providing hygiene care to a patient, how long does that really take? Sometimes as a student, you become used to having a limited number of clients for whom to care and think of the hour you spent in the patient's room as essential. In reality, the actual tasks were completed in 15 minutes. If you keep thinking that providing hygiene requires 1 hour, you will not start because you will not ever have 1 hour available, and thus you will never be able to finish your assignment effectively.

WRITING THINGS DOWN

Although most of us think we have a very good memory, it is more efficient and time saving to develop the habit of writing things down. You need a method of writing down the tasks you need to accomplish. A written record is also essential for your assessment data, which must be documented and must also be used as you make decisions.

One answer for a written plan of action is to use a worksheet for planning and use the same worksheet to make your notes. Many practicing nurses call this a **brain sheet.** The term *brain sheet* is used because most nurses find it impossible to "hold in their brains" (maintain in their memory) all the details they need to remember for the day. Whatever its title, the worksheet records these details.

To create your own worksheet, you may find it easiest simply to write down tasks in a "to-do" list, adding to it as you think of additional tasks. You may begin with information communicated in the intershift report and then expand the list with information from the plan of care, care pathways, protocols, and physician's orders. Some items on the list will have to be done at specified times. For example, you will note the times when medications and treatments must be administered. Other activities, such as health teaching, can be done at any time that is convenient for you and the patient. After looking at the AM care needs, you could quickly decide that the best time for teaching would be immediately after the patients finish their lunch. Some agencies provide a general form that nurses can use to write out a worksheet (Display 3-2). Some forms are developed by computer and have patient names and identifying information preprinted to facilitate use.

PRIORITIZING ACTIVITIES

After you have written your list, you can refine and **prioritize** the items. Prioritizing places things in order of their importance. If you don't prioritize, you may run out of time before an important task is done or you may not attend to a task that needs prompt attention. As you become more experienced, you will find it easier to sort priorities as you identify tasks. However, priorities will change throughout the day as new events occur. Remain open to adding and deleting items and reordering your priorities.

To determine priorities, a useful question to ask is, "Is this task critical to the well-being of the patient?" See Display 3-3 for a list of priority-setting criteria that may be useful to you. You might designate items as essential on your list by circling them, highlighting them, or writing them in red ink. Some things must be done at specific times, which you can note on your worksheet. When time is at a premium,

DISPLAY 3-2	Sample of an Agency Worksheet

ROOM/PATIENT	DX	ACTIV.	DIET	I/O	IV	MEDS	TX	TESTS	OTHER
414A M Spencer, G. 82	CHF	Chair BRP	2 Gm Na	√	D5.S → 1100	9-111 1-7 7pi lidcom	O₂ @ bl.	ECG	
B M Jeffers, K. 79	®CVA	Chair	Isocal 30 ml/hr.	√		9-11 1-11	√ Skin		Discharge to Rehab.
415 G Winston, M. 72	Intract. Angina	Cardiac Level 3	Cardiac	√		NTG 9-1 1-1			Severe last night

setting priorities becomes even more critical. Setting priorities helps you to guard against the tendency to do those things that are immediately apparent and neglecting those that are actually more important to patient well-being.

Next, identify the second-priority tasks. These are tasks that are important but not urgent. You might put a question mark above these items. Tasks designated as lowest priority are neither as important nor as urgent as first- and second-priority items. The lowest-priority items are often the "hope to accomplish" items, so leave them unmarked. If you need to add more items during the day, you will have to review and revise your priorities.

Another aspect of setting priorities is to be sure that your priorities fit with the priorities of your supervisor (Mind Tools, 2003). Your manager may want to assure that the care planning documents are done in a timely manner. If you put this at the bottom of your priority list, you will find yourself in conflict. Sometimes nurses are so oriented toward helping others that their own responsibilities take second place. Although helping the nursing assistants with their tasks may create a good feeling in the team, if it results in the neglect of duties that require a registered nurse, you have not used your time well.

LEARNING TO DO A TASK MORE QUICKLY

One contributing factor in an expert nurse's completion of tasks is simply working faster. For example, when you first started hanging IV medications, each might have taken you 20 minutes to prepare and administer. As you become more proficient, you can move more rapidly. Sometimes you may need to analyze tasks to determine

---

DISPLAY 3-3   Criteria for Setting Priorities

1. *Items critical to maintaining life:* Think in terms of your CPR basics
   Essential assessment
   Airway management
   Breathing support
   Circulation needs
   Neurological stability
2. *Critical symptom management:* What is most important to the patient?
   Pain management
   Relief of nausea
   Relief of diarrhea
   Relief of severe anxiety
3. *Items needed to progress in health restoration:* What orders has the physician written? What nursing plans have been developed?
   Medication and intravenous fluid administration
   Completing treatments
   Preventing complications
   Meeting nutritional needs
4. *Items needed to move toward self-care*
   Teaching
   Contacting referral needs
   Meeting psychosocial needs
5. *Creating comfort and feelings of well-being*
   Bathing
   Changing linens

---

whether there is a more efficient way to accomplish the same task. You will be working smarter and not just faster. One of the hallmarks of the scientific management movement of the 1930s and 1940s was the use of time and motion studies to increase production in factories. The aim was to eliminate wasted effort. Although health care is different from a factory, there is a lesson to be learned in the idea that we may continue to do something in an inefficient method because we have never examined it closely.

ORGANIZING TASKS

When you were enrolled in your first nursing courses and planning your first patient care, your instructor probably encouraged you to anticipate the equipment and supplies you would need for your patient's care, to collect them, and to take all of them with you as you started the care. Having to leave the room to get a roll of tape, an extra needle, or a particular instrument can steal much important time. Being organized in this fashion requires thinking ahead, or visualizing what you will be doing. For example, if you are going to change a dressing, what will you need? Is there a dressing tray? Is everything on the dressing tray that should be there? What additional supplies might be needed? What instruments are needed? Where are the gloves? This type of mental review can save many extra trips to retrieve forgotten items.

In addition to organizing individual tasks, another component of organization is to group tasks together to save steps. If you are starting down the hall to a patient's room, ask yourself, "What is needed in that room?" You may make one trip taking supplies for multiple needs at the same time. Before you leave a room, pause and assess the room to assure that details are taken care of, and, if not, complete them at that time. Ask the patient if he or she needs anything before you leave the room. This may save additional trips to the patient's room. If the patient needs a PRN medication, check the medication administration record to see whether any routine medications can be administered at the same time, saving another trip. (Remember that there is a time frame in which medications can be given.)

Multitasking is being engaged in more than one task at a time. This may include planning for several tasks at one time, preparing for several tasks at the same time, or actually having several tasks in progress at the same time. Traditionally, individuals were encouraged to finish one task before beginning another. In the health care environment, that may not be possible or even desirable. When you cook a meal, you must attend to each item you plan to serve in a manner that assures that all are completed to serve together even though they take different preparation times. In a similar manner, in health care you must be making progress on multiple goals simultaneously if the overall goal of discharge on a specified day can occur. You must also be making progress for multiple patients at the same time.

Multitasking may be as simple as learning to do tasks with enough assurance that you can converse with the patient at the same time. You may be gathering information or doing simple teaching at the same time that you are doing a routine task. Multitasking may also involve more complex planning with more than one patient. See the following case study for an example of complex multitasking.

EXAMPLE   *Multitasking on a Nursing Unit*

John Wilson is assigned to care for Edmund Jones, who has been newly diagnosed as having diabetes. Mr. Jones will be discharged soon. John Wilson has several patients to care for and therefore decides that he must integrate teaching of Mr. Jones with his other work. When he arrives to check the patient's blood glucose, he gives Mr. Jones a pamphlet to read about the blood glucose monitoring device he will be taking home. John asks Mr. Wilson to follow the steps while he is doing the procedure this time. After the procedure is completed, John asks Mr. Jones to review the pamphlet independently during the morning. Because John had planned ahead, he brought the next IV fluid bag to the room, and while the Mr. Jones begins reading this pamphlet, John proceeds to hang the next IV fluid bag. Leaving Mr. Jones to continue reading, John returns to the desk to document the glucose measurement and the IV administration. While at the desk, he begins the discharge process for a second patient by notifying the pharmacy of drugs ordered for the patient to take home. He then moves to the next room to complete the essential assessment on a third patient. When this assessment is completed, he returns to Mr. Jones's room. John discusses the pamphlet content with the patient, answers questions, and plans with the patient for him to try this skill with help at 11:30 a.m. John then picks up the pharmacy order that is now ready at the desk so that he can move to discharge teaching for one of his other patients.

Keeping multiple tasks organized and on track requires that you attend to central principles. Remember that accuracy or safety can never be compromised for speed. You must be careful to correctly estimate how much time a given task will take so that your time plan is realistic. If you tell a patient you will return, you must do so in a timely manner to maintain trust. When you are with a patient, be sure to focus your attention on the person for that time. The feeling that the nurse is always poised for flight rather than attending to the current patient's concerns often leaves patients feeling neglected and uncared for even when tasks are done competently. For this reason, you should also try to sit down when teaching or interviewing a patient. This action communicates a personal focus and facilitates the nurse–patient relationship.

If you have too many tasks going, you may feel scattered and may forget some aspect. Therefore, start out with grouping or balancing two different tasks and move to additional tasks only when these work well together. As you become more skilled with thinking of multiple tasks at the same time, you will save steps through fewer trips up and down the corridor. You will feel satisfaction at making progress toward the multiple objectives of your day. Further, you will feel less overwhelmed by the volume of work to be accomplished and more in control of your day.

DELEGATING

In most care settings, the registered nurse will be working with a variety of nursing personnel with different backgrounds. Licensed practical (vocational) nurses, UAPs, and nursing students may be working with you. In some settings, the housekeeping people are considered part of the unit staff and not a separate department. In these settings, the nurse must develop skill-appropriate delegation. Failure to delegate leaves many new graduates feeling overwhelmed and makes it impossible for them to complete their care. Chapter 6 focuses on the process of delegation.

ORGANIZING WITH THE TEAM

When you are responsible for a nursing care team, you can use these same strategies to help the team work more effectively. An **assignment** includes all the tasks and aspects of care for which an individual is responsible. Making assignments for members of the team is usually the responsibility of the registered nurse. Although an efficient system for making assignments may be in place, it is also possible that no one has carefully examined the system. The geographical layout of the unit, the care needs of the patients, and the skills of the individuals on the team should be a part of your decision making in regard to assignments.

You can help your team members with their organizational skills within their assignments. You might be able to suggest ways they could organize tasks in a time-saving manner. Sometimes you may want to help people to work together on some tasks. By observing the manner in which time is used and how people work together, you may find ways to help them feel more productive and less stressed.

Often, the nurse is responsible for coordinating the efforts of a multidisciplinary team. For example, schedules for diagnostic tests, physical therapy, and special treatments must occur appropriately in relation to the overall plan of care. When this is your responsibility, you will want to be certain you understand what is necessary for the patient's progress. Does one diagnostic test need to be scheduled before another? Will the diagnostic test interfere with the patient's physical therapy?

Communicating with the appropriate team members may require telephone calls, individual meetings, or sometimes multidisciplinary team meetings. For example, in the long-term care setting, the multidisciplinary team meeting includes the major care providers in the institution and the family members in planning for effective and personalized care.

When working within a home care agency, you may find that the leader of the multidisciplinary team is a physical therapist if rehabilitation is the primary reason for health care. When the patient's nutritional status is the major concern, the multidisciplinary team may be led by a nutritionist. In such instances, you will need to understand your own responsibilities in communicating with the team leader or case manager. The highest-quality care will be provided when you understand the goals and priorities for individual clients.

CREATING EFFECTIVE MEETINGS

As a registered nurse you will find yourself participating and even leading a variety of meetings from shift report to institutional committees. Mackenzie (1990) identifies four reasons for having meetings:

1. To coordinate action or exchange information
2. To motivate a team
3. To discuss problems on a regular basis (as in a staff meeting)
4. To make a decision

These four kinds of meetings all occur in a nursing unit at one time or another.

Meetings are expensive and must be planned carefully. If there are eight people in an intershift report and the report takes 45 minutes instead of 30 minutes, there has been a loss of 2 hours of care. Remember that a 1-hour meeting with eight people amounts to 8 working hours, or 1 working day. This same 1-hour meeting of eight registered nurses who earn an average salary of $22.00 per hour costs at least $176.00. If these nurses are not replaced on the unit during the meeting, this cost will be reflected in decreased care or overload of others.

Meetings bring the best results when certain guidelines are followed. First, they should be called only when necessary. Meetings are essential if you want a group of individuals to solve a problem together; if all have information that must be communicated to the others; or if there must be an opportunity for questions, answers, and explanations. If the purpose is simply providing information, it might be accomplished just as well with a memo, e-mail, or posted notice for the persons who need the information.

Second, follow an agenda. We tend to think of agendas as somewhat formal pieces of paper that provide a list of items to be discussed and sometimes state the time allowed for the discussion and whether action is needed. However, agendas can be much less formal than that. Any consistent approach or routine way of addressing an action might be considered an agenda. Think back to the shift reports we mentioned earlier. Why do some reports take 30 minutes whereas others take 45 minutes? Why have some facilities chosen to use dictated reports? Taped or standardized report forms are usually designed to focus the report on important items and encourage an organized presentation of information. As you become increasingly responsible for giving reports, think ahead to what information you want to share. Develop a format for sharing the information that is complete yet concise. Use it consistently and stick to your format. Don't let others distract you with comments that do not relate to what you are sharing.

The third suggestion for useful and meaningful meetings is to start on time. Much valuable time is wasted waiting for stragglers. If you hold up meetings for these latecomers, you reward them in a sense, suggesting that their presence is so critical that you can't start without them. At the same time, those who arrived on time for the meeting may be harboring dissatisfaction because the meeting did not begin when it was scheduled. Once you have established a pattern of beginning on time, fewer individuals will be inclined to appear late. This applies to intershift report and team meetings as well as to committee meetings.

The last part of starting on time is ending on time. If we are reasonable in developing our agenda, most of what we have to accomplish is done within the time frame that is allowed. Have you ever noticed how much is accomplished in the last 10 minutes of a meeting? Why do you think that occurred?

Barriers to Effective Time Management

Some people resist the concept of time management. These individuals often suffer from the notion that they work better under pressure. The stress that this creates may seem to be an impetus for action, but if any unanticipated problem or obstacle occurs, tasks may not be completed when needed. The constant feeling of stress begins to undermine feelings of well-being.

Other people believe that time management is basically just using good sense, and as long as things are going well, give little thought to how they could be even more productive or find more leisure time to enjoy relaxing. They may believe that a "to-do" list is all that is necessary to manage time effectively. These people do not value learning new time management skills.

The discipline required by time management discourages some who believe that "spontaneity is the key to creativity and success," whereas others say that time management takes the "fun out of life" (Mackenzie, 1990, pp. 10, 11).

SOCIALIZING

Probably nothing steals more work time than the **socializing** that occurs while on the job. Whether in the form of an extended conversation that is initiated at the water fountain or a discussion of plans for the coming evening that occurs in the medicine station, socializing causes valuable time to be lost each day. No one intends to waste time socializing—it just occurs. It occurs as an immediate antidote to stress, as a need for a change of pace, as a need to be informed, as curiosity, and as a component of a naturally gregarious personality. Personal telephone calls received while at work might also be considered socializing, unless they are of an emergency nature.

You can take actions to spend less time socializing and more time in productive work. When you find yourself involved in a conversation that is taking more time than you have, you can say, "I must check on my patient now, but let's meet for coffee after work, when we'll have more time to talk." This may also help to remind your colleagues that they also have patients who need attention. Monitor your own social needs and activities. If you really want to discuss a personal issue with a colleague, see whether you can arrange to take a coffee break or lunch at the same time.

PROCRASTINATION

Procrastination is defined as a chronic delay in implementing actions that are necessary to accomplish important tasks. Although there may be times when delaying a task does not have adverse consequences, in most instances consistently putting things off and not getting responsibilities completed is very detrimental to accomplishing goals.

Researchers have found that people procrastinate for a number of reasons. The development of procrastination has been explained in many different ways, such as childhood experiences, self-esteem, and fear of failure. Different reasons may underlie procrastination in different people, and it is possible that the same person may procrastinate in some circumstances and not in others. Here we will focus on changing the behavior rather than trying to explain the reasons for the behavior.

An important step in handling procrastination is to make a personal commitment to change your behavior so that you complete tasks on time. This commitment will be easier to make if you realize that you are the one who can take control of the situation—it is something you have the power to change. Set realistic deadlines for yourself and adhere to them. And once you have met your goals, give yourself a reward. The reward can be a special time with your family, a luxurious bath, a hike in the woods, a shopping expedition, or whatever appeals to you. The important thing is having a tangible reminder (and acknowledgment) that you met your goal.

Many techniques can help procrastinators if they recognize that their behavior is a problem. With this in mind, you can address your problem. One strategy is to make tasks more manageable by breaking them into pieces and doing one part at a time. A project does not seem so overwhelming when you use this technique. For example, as a student, if you have a paper that is due, you may decide to review the literature as one step, discuss the relevance of the literature review to your topic as another, and make a summary statement or draw conclusions as the final step in preparing your assignment.

As a nurse, you may need to identify ways in which large projects can be broken up into smaller segments. For example, if all residents on the long-term care unit for which you work must have new care-plan forms prepared to accommodate a new record system, you might set a goal of preparing two forms each day until all have been completed. When you divide work into segments that can be accomplished in a shorter period, the entire project seems more doable.

OTHER TIME WASTERS

Some activities that waste time are found in any situation or organization. All may rob you of feelings of control over your time and the self-esteem that comes from accomplishment. Mackenzie (1990, p. 55) has identified 20 of the biggest time wasters and makes suggestions on how to minimize them (Display 3-4). Some are most applicable to and are products of the work environment. Others reflect, to a greater extent, personal factors or characteristics over which we have control. Many of the time wasters he has noted are directly applicable to nursing and the provision of patient care. As you review these time wasters, consider which are applicable to you and your setting. Each person finds different time wasters a personal concern. You may want to read more about some of these.

DISPLAY 3-4	**20 Common Time Wasters**

1. Management by crisis
2. Telephone interruptions
3. Inadequate planning
4. Attempting too much
5. Drop-in visitors
6. Ineffective delegation
7. Personal disorganization
8. Lack of self-discipline
9. Inability to say "no"
10. Procrastination
11. Meetings
12. Paper work
13. Leaving tasks unfinished
14. Inadequate staff
15. Socializing
16. Confused responsibility or authority
17. Poor communication
18. Inadequate controls and progress reports
19. Incomplete information
20. Travel

From Mackenzie, A. (1990). *The Time Trap* (p. 55). New York: American Management Association. Reproduced with permission.

Critical Thinking Exercise

Review the time wasters discussed. Which of these time wasters do you identify as affecting the nursing environment? Which ones do you see as directly related to the way you manage your personal life? Which ones overlap, reflecting traits that characterize the way you manage your personal life as well as your professional life? What might you do to change your own time management and eliminate time wasters?

■ KEY CONCEPTS

- Costs in health care have grown because of aging of the population, increased use of technology, new and expensive treatment modalities, and rising salaries and profits.
- Health care is funded through government programs, insurance and managed-care options, self-pay, and charitable care.

- Health care financing has changed from the 1930s, when most care was privately financed; to the 1950s, when insurance plans grew; to the 1960s, with the development of Medicare; to the 1980s, when prospective payment changed lengths of stay; and to the 1990s, when managed health care became widespread.

- Cost awareness requires that you understand the many factors that contribute to the cost of health care, including length of stay, complications, waste of supplies, and cost of personnel. Identifying the specific costs of nursing care for an individual client is gaining increasing attention as a way to support the maintenance of nursing staff.

- Nurses have a responsibility to use resources, including money, buildings, equipment, supplies, personnel, and time responsibly.

- Nurses can effectively contribute to reducing waste and finding more cost-effective means of accomplishing desired health care outcomes. Conserving supplies, delegating tasks, giving a full day's work for a day's pay, maintaining patient safety, preventing complications, and planning with others are all ways nurses can manage resources. Becoming involved in the budget process assists nurses in becoming more effective in the system.

- The nurse is legally and ethically responsible for providing competent care. If the care provided is below established standards, it is not cost-effective.

- Understanding the budget provides a foundation for participating effectively in planning for and managing nursing care.

- The budget process involves people at all levels, from the board of trustees to those who deliver care. It requires assessment of the environment, establishment of goals and objectives, and development of specific budget requests.

- Budget monitoring is done by the individual manager as well as by the accounting department and the finance committee in order to effectively maintain control of spending and plan for the future.

- Time management is an essential skill in enabling the nurse to accomplish all the differing tasks that are required. While on-the-job experience supports time management, this is a skill that can be learned.

- Barriers to effective time management include the myth of working better under pressure, not valuing the skill of time management, and resisting the loss of spontaneity.

- General principles of time management include understanding yourself and asserting control over your own time. Further, you must learn to plan your activities, handle paperwork efficiently, and create effective meetings.

- Effective time management begins with a thorough self-assessment. Identifying personal time wasters is also an important part of this process. You also need to look at whether you demonstrate personal disorganization, whether socializing is a problem, and whether you procrastinate. You will become more productive if you look at how you are using your time, when you carry out certain activities, how you plan your time, and what occurrences commonly waste time.

- Techniques to help you with time management include using worksheets, developing skill in prioritizing tasks, writing things down, and learning to do tasks more quickly.

- Multitasking is a mechanism for working on multiple goals or outcomes for different patients simultaneously.

- Time management skills are also useful when working with a multidisciplinary team and organizing many aspects of the client's care.

REFERENCES

Beckrich, K., & Aronovich, S. A. (1999). Hospital-acquired pressure ulcers: a comparison of costs in medical vs. surgical patients. *Nursing Economics 17*(5), 263–272.

Davis, K., & Cooper, B. S. (2003). *American Health Care: Why So Costly?* Invited testimony, Senate Appropriations Commitee, Subcommittee on Labor, Health, and Human Services, Education, and Related Agencies, Hearing on Health Care Access and Affordability: Cost Containment Strategies [Online]. Available at www.cmwf.org.

Harris, C. J. (1998). RUGs: a new bridge to payment. *Provider, 24*(7), Special Section 2, 11.

FIRSTGOV for Seniors. (2003). *Health Care Costs Expected to Rise to $3.1 Trillion Over Next 10 Years* [Online]. Available at www.seniors.gov/articles/0203/health-costs.htm.

Infante, M. C. (1998). PPS weighs in with legal concerns. *Provider, 24*(7), Special Section 6-7.

Joint Commission on Accreditation of Healthcare Organizations. (2003). *Hospital Accreditation Standards and Survey Process.* Oakbrook Terrace, IL: Author.

Liebowitz, S. (2003). *Policy Analysis: Why Health Care Costs Too Much* [Online]. CATO Organization. Available at www.cato.org/pubs/pas/pa211.html.

Lubarsky, J. M. (1998). Putting costs under a magnifying glass. *Provider, 24*(7), Special Section 3-4.

Mackenzie, A. (1990). *The Time Trap.* New York: American Management Association.

Martin, S. (2003). Show bedside nurses the money? *American Journal of Nursing, 103*(4), 77, 79, 81.

Meding, J. B., Keating, E. M., Faris, P. M. et al. (1998). Maximizing cost effectiveness while minimizing complications in total hip replacement. *American Journal of Orthopedics, 47*(4), 295–298.

Mind Tools. (2003). *Time Management Skills: Making the Most of Your Time* [Online]. Available at www.mindtools.com/page5.html.

Regence Blue Shield. (2003). *How Much Things Cost* [Online]. Available at http://bcbshealthissues.com/healthplans/costs.

Schauffler, H. H., & Chapman, S. A. (1998). Health promotion and managed care: surveys of California's health plans and population. *American Journal of Preventive Medicine, 14*(3), 161–167.

Strunk, B. C., & Ginsburg, P. B. (September 2002). *Aging Plays Limited Role in Health Cost Trends,* Data Bulletin No. 23. Washington, DC: Health Services Council.

Strunk, B. C., Ginsburg, P. B., & Gabel, J. R. (2002). *Tracking Health Care Costs: Growth Accelerates Again in 2001.* Health Affairs, Nov/Dec, 2002. [Online]. Available at www.healthaffairs.org/WebExclusive/Strunk_Web_Excl_092502.htm.

Taheri, P. A., Wahl, W. L., Butz, D. A. et al. (1998). Trauma service cost: the real story. *Annals of Surgery, 227*(5), 720–725.

Supporting Quality Care

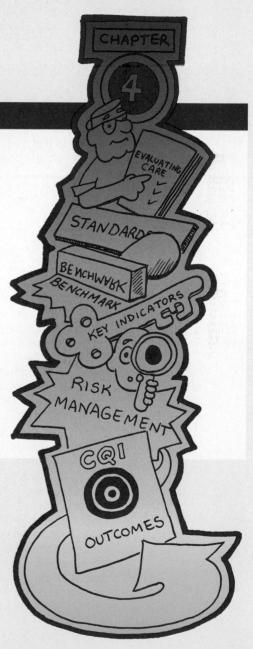

Learning Outcomes

After completing this chapter, you should be able to:

1. Explain the various sources of standards for evaluating care.
2. Differentiate among structural, process, and outcome standards and explain the focus of each.
3. Discuss the use of key indicators to measure performance.
4. Discuss the strengths and limitations of goals and objectives for evaluating care.
5. Explain how data can be gathered for the purpose of evaluation and the differences in the data derived by different methods.
6. Describe key aspects of a quality improvement program and the problems inherent in such systems.
7. Analyze the ways in which risk management strategies relate to quality assurance, quality improvement, and other evaluation approaches.
8. Participate effectively in the evaluation and improvement of patient care.

Key Terms ■ ■ ■ ■ ■

audit

benchmark

concurrent audits

continuous quality
  improvement (CQI)

cost standards

cost–benefit ratio

cost-effectiveness
  standards

discoverable

evaluation standards

goals

key indicators

objectives

outcome standards

performance improvement

performance standards

proactive

process standards

proximal cause

quality assessment and
  improvement (QAI)

quality assurance (QA)

quality assurance reports

quality circles

quality improvement (QI)

quality indicators

rapid process
  improvement

retrospective audits

risk management

root cause analysis

structural standard

total quality management
  (TQM)

Maintaining and improving the quality of care requires the active involvement of everyone in the health care system. In 1999, the Institute of Medicine (IOM) released a report on measuring the quality of health care (IOM, 1999). This report focused on the need to evaluate health care in its totality, identifying whether there has been underuse of needed, effective, and appropriate care; overuse, i.e., excessive or unnecessary care; or misuse, including flaws and errors in care. The report identified that everyone in health care must be engaged in evaluation activities for it to be effective and of high quality. Accreditation standards for health care agencies from organizations such as the Joint Commission on Accreditation of Health Care Organizations (JCAHO) now require that an ongoing evaluation plan be in place that addresses all aspects of the organization.

Although each agency has an individualized plan for evaluating and improving the overall care provided, several approaches are commonly used. As you become familiar with these various approaches to evaluation, you will be better able to function effectively within the unique plan of an individual agency in which you are employed. All nurses have responsibility within these plans for monitoring the quality of nursing care delivered and responding to results of evaluation by improving practice to improve outcomes for clients.

Common attributes of any evaluation system include the standards to be used for evaluation, methods of collecting data, the analysis of the data, and the use of the information generated in the analysis. This chapter helps you understand these standards, where they originate, how they are used, and some of the systems in place designed to facilitate the evaluation process.

■ STANDARDS FOR EVALUATING HEALTH CARE

Any evaluation process needs to be conducted in relation to standards. You are familiar with being evaluated in your nursing program in relation to the standards required for a specific grade. The faculty established these standards based on its knowledge of nursing. There is a standard that designates A-level work. To achieve that A grade, you need to know what is required. To participate effectively in health care evaluation, you need to understand the types of standards that are used for health care evaluation and the sources for the standards, just as you have needed to understand the standards for achieving an A grade. Standards define activities and outcomes as well as the structural resources needed for care. As authoritative statements set forth by a group with power, standards establish the expected level of care or performance.

Types of Standards

Three types of standards are traditionally used for evaluation in health care: structural standards, process standards, and outcome standards.

Structural standards establish guidelines for organizational patterns and support structures for providing health care. Structural standards include the physical plant, equipment, number of personnel, their educational backgrounds, and assigned

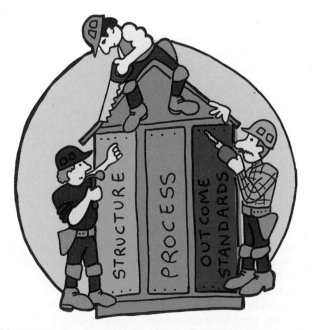

Most evaluation plans include a similar framework for standards.

responsibilities. Standards for physical facilities include heating and ventilation and infection-control capabilities. Policies that guide action are also considered structural standards. Structural standards for an intensive care unit might specify the number of square feet per patient, the equipment to be available at the bedside, and the availability of specially trained nurses at all times at a ratio of one nurse to two patients. Another structural standard might specify the standards for emergency equipment and supplies available on the general medical surgical unit.

Process standards describe methods of providing services. Process standards are also referred to as **performance standards.** A process standard might specify that each resident admitted to a long-term care facility have a minimum data set (MDS) form completed within 4 hours of admission. Another process standard might state that the initial nursing care plan be established within 24 hours of admission. Protocols and procedures are examples of process standards. Process standards are receiving increasing attention as a way to systematize care and eliminate the inappropriate deviation from what have been identified as best practices.

Processes to be used for evaluation constitute one type of process standard. Some writers have identified evaluation as being so important that they have placed processes for evaluation in a separate category entitled **evaluation standards.** The purpose of separating them is to assure that all aspects of the organization are included in a well-done evaluation plan. Increasingly, evaluation standards require that patient/consumer input be included.

Outcome standards are used to evaluate the results of actions and processes. These might be patient outcomes, including aggregate outcomes, such as the incidence of nosocomial infection for the hospital as a whole, or individual outcomes, such as the time by which the postoperative hip replacement patient is expected to be ambulating with assistance. One difficulty with using outcomes as a measure of effectiveness is that patient outcomes are the result of a wide variety of inputs, such as patient compliance, underlying disease processes, and individual responses, as well as the health care provided. Outcomes are used also for evaluating internal processes. In fact, because all processes have some type of results, almost every process can be evaluated both by whether the process was conducted appropriately (a process standard) and whether the desired outcome of the process was achieved (an outcome standard). The IOM has identified that process and outcome must go hand in hand. Effective processes increase the likelihood of appropriate outcomes. However, if outcomes are not met, it may mean that processes need to be changed (IOM, 1999).

 ## Sources of Standards for Care

There are multiple sources of standards for health care. Most of the organizations and agencies that formulate standards focus on the processes in place. Some also may provide structural standards. Outcome standards are a relatively new part of standards developed by organizations and governmental agencies. Often, agencies reviewing health care organizations require that a health care organization set its own outcome standards for evaluation.

Two of the sources of standards for nursing that could be considered process standards are the Nurse Practice Act and the American Nurses Association (ANA) standards. The Nurse Practice Act of each state or province identifies legal standards for the practice of nursing. These standards are specific and detailed in some states.

When questions as to the legal standard arise, the board of nursing usually studies the situation and determines how the law applies to that circumstance. You will want to understand clearly the legal standard for care where you practice.

The ANA has adopted the Standards of Clinical Nursing Practice (ANA, 1998), which outlines both standards for client care based on a nursing process approach and standards for professional performance focusing on the nurse's responsibilities as a member of the discipline of nursing. These standards were first formulated in 1991, apply across the nation, and are broad and general in nature. They are now in their second edition. Each standard is accompanied by a set of specific criteria that can be used for evaluating whether that standard has been met. In addition to its general standards, the ANA also publishes standards for specific areas of clinical practice, such as psychiatric mental health nursing and for nursing administrators, that represent more than 20 areas of specialty practice. Many specialty nursing organizations, such as the National Intravenous Therapy Association, also publish specific standards of practice for their own specialty.

Regulatory agencies, such as state health departments and the federal government working through Medicare and Medicaid rules of participation, also set standards for health care institutions. These standards have always included structural standards, for example, the types of care providers required and the physical plant. The health department (or its equivalent) must approve any inpatient health care agency in regard to the safety and appropriateness of the physical plant before the agency can provide care. Processes, such as the frequency of assessment and other services offered to clients, were developed more recently. These organizations are currently requiring that specific outcomes of care be met. Health care organizations are approved according to specific criteria based on the kind of care they will be providing, such as acute care or long-term care. The approval bodies examine records and also send individual inspectors to agencies. Medicare and Medicaid standards for reimbursable care have changed the way care is delivered in home care and in long-term care agencies.

Accrediting groups such as the JCAHO, have standards for all aspects of institutional care, structure, process, and outcomes. These standards must be met for an agency to be eligible for JCAHO accreditation. JCAHO reviews documents and also sends a team of on-site evaluators to examine the institution in relation to the standards. You may have experienced the tension that occurs in a hospital when an evaluation visit is expected. These visits may also be unannounced. JCAHO plans that all visits will be unannounced in the future to assure that the same quality of care exists on a day–to-day basis as occurs during a visit.

An increasing number of clinical practice guidelines (CPGs) are being established through the Agency for Healthcare Research and Quality (AHRQ), formerly the Agency for Health Care Policy and Research (AHCPR). This agency of the federal government convenes expert panels to review the research, consult with authorities in the field, and synthesize the information into a recommended set of guidelines for health care clinical practice. Some of these guidelines are very extensive, such as the ones published in regard to the management of pain. These guidelines are focused on processes of care that have been shown to create better outcomes of care. Each health care facility also sets its own standards of practice. These standards must conform to the general standards identified previously, but they speak to the specific needs of the clients served and the specific setting in which the nurses practice. Committees or task forces of nurses working together most commonly establish agency nursing standards.

The AHRQ has established a set of databases called the Healthcare Cost and Utilization Project (HCUP) for collecting and aggregating data across many institutions in order to inform decision making in those institutions (AHRQ, 2003). These databases allow researchers to track and analyze data in order to identify trends and patterns of care for all population groups. The size of these databases makes it possible to track information for uncommon conditions as well as for commonly occurring health problems. Institutions may then set standards based on this information.

Benchmarking

Many institutions are moving to an approach to setting standards called benchmarking. A **benchmark** is a specific quantitative standard, usually the highest standard, with which you compare your own institution. Benchmarks may be used with any type of evaluation system to establish the standard for an outcome, a structure, or a process. The aim is to meet or exceed the benchmark.

An institution may establish its own benchmarks based on its past performance. For example, an institution may review its records for care of individuals with a total hip replacement. Based on this review, the institution establishes benchmarks for outcomes, such as the cost of care for an individual with total hip replacement, number of days of hospitalization, and level of function at discharge. To use the last category, a standardized functional assessment tool must be used for each patient at discharge. Then, individual cases as well as aggregate data may be compared with these benchmarks to determine whether the care is meeting the desired standards.

Another way of establishing benchmarks is to aggregate data from multiple institutions. A large health system with multiple hospitals, clinics, and long-term care facilities may aggregate data within its own system. Benchmarks derived from the aggregate data are used to measure individual institutions or agencies within its system. These benchmarks may be the best performance of any institution within the system or some statistical measure related to it, such as within a standard deviation of that measure.

Insurance companies and the Health Care Finance Administration (HCFA) of the federal government have set standards by aggregating data regionally and nationally. They aggregate data from many institutions and identify the average length of stay, the number of nosocomial infections per 100 patient care days, the average cost of treating a myocardial infarction, and other important indicators of quality of care. Institutions can then compare themselves against these benchmarks. The diagnostic related groups (DRGs) for Medicare payment were originally set by benchmarking the average length of stay and average cost of care for the conditions included in the group.

Sometimes a large institution establishes its standard, and other institutions use that as a benchmark against which to measure themselves. This might occur when a particular institution becomes a center for a specialty service, such as oncology care. If this institution established benchmarks for its internal use, it might be asked to share the benchmarks to help smaller institutions direct their efforts toward the same standards. Some agencies may advertise themselves as agencies that serve as the benchmark for others.

Outcomes related to cost are so important in modern health care organizations that they are identified as a separate category of **cost standards,** also termed

cost-effectiveness standards. Cost-effectiveness standards are increasingly important as constraints on health care financing become more acute. Cost-effectiveness refers to the ratio of the cost in resources to a given health care outcome. It is also referred to as a **cost–benefit ratio.** It is not enough to say that a given strategy produced a positive outcome for the client. Costs may be simple to calculate; however, effectiveness or benefits are not. One of the difficulties is how to include "soft" areas in the discussion of benefits. Benefits may include satisfaction, quality of life, alleviation of anxiety, and comfort. People sometimes disagree on whether a change in process that reduces cost also reduces quality. Another concern is how much is reasonable to spend to achieve a particular outcome. Setting benchmarks for cost-effectiveness is very complex and causes considerable controversy.

■ COLLECTING DATA FOR EVALUATION

Collecting data for evaluation is costly to an institution. Therefore, decisions on what data to collect and how to collect them are critical. Data are collected in a variety of ways, which include quality assurance reports, audits, and planned observations and questionnaires directed to health care consumers. Data gathered for system evaluation are not considered **discoverable** for the purposes of litigation. This means that the institution cannot be required to present those data to someone who is suing the institution. The concern is that if hospitals and other care providers were required to provide the records of their own evaluation processes to those who bring suit against the institution, the institution would hesitate to identify problems or concerns that need improvement. This would be detrimental to the entire process of improving health care.

Key Indicators

Because it is impossible to track every aspect of care, an effort is made to identify specific data that will provide information about the whole situation. These specific data that have been shown to relate to overall quality are termed **key indicators.** Key indicators may reveal a problem in care or simply the need for more extensive data collection. An example of a key indicator in the care of a person with diabetes is obtaining a quarterly hemoglobin A1c level. If this test is done, it enables a great deal of other effective disease management to be addressed. Absence of this test indicates that the patient is not being monitored in what has been demonstrated to be an effective manner.

Data on key indicators are collected and tracked on an ongoing basis. For example, the surgical wound infection rate in a hospital is considered by most approval authorities to be a key indicator of surgical services. To monitor this key indicator, every wound infection would be identified, the organism involved would be noted, and statistical information compiled. This process facilitates early identification of any pattern that might indicate a need for further investigation. Accrediting organizations mandate the use of some key indicators (such as infection rates). The health care institution itself chooses others.

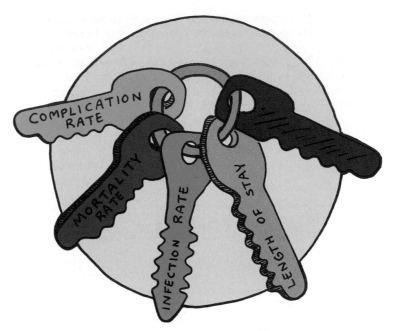

Key indicators are used for evaluating health care services.

Quality Assurance Reports

Quality assurance (QA) reports provide a way to track the occurrence of untoward incidents. Whenever an untoward incident occurs, a report (commonly referred to as a QA report) is completed and circulated to the appropriate individuals within the institution. This report provides a complete factual record of the incident to those responsible for monitoring safe practice. The individual who identifies the problem is usually responsible for preparing the report. Some nurses are reluctant to prepare reports because they mistakenly believe that doing so is an admission of personal error. In fact, the person completing the report is simply identifying the problem and the relevant facts and not accepting accountability for the problem. The report is not part of any patient record; it is entirely an internal agency document. When you are responsible for completing a QA report, you should strive to be very objective and factual; you should not include conjecture, blame, or assumptions. The entire process of QA is discussed later in this chapter.

Audit

An **audit** is another method used to monitor standards. An audit is a systematic data collection process that commonly focuses on documentation. Audits can be used to examine structure, for example, reviewing documentation of the recharging of all fire extinquishers; process, for example, reviewing the records to determine that the appropriate pain assessment was completed on all postoperative patients; or outcomes, such as looking for evidence that the patients treated with cardioversion were discharged with a normal sinus rhythm. Audits in regard to patient care are conducted by examining patient records. **Concurrent audits** involve examining records of clients who are still receiving care and are sometimes referred to as real-time audits. **Retrospective audits** involve examining records after clients are discharged.

When records are audited, it is assumed that actions not documented did not occur. When patient care demands are high, care providers may neglect documentation. Poor documentation may have adverse consequences, because data collection through audit would make it appear that care was not provided. You need to understand the importance of your documentation. Although the results of audit are not discoverable, the patient record would be if the patient were to sue. The same conclusion drawn in the audit, that care was not provided, would be drawn in the legal proceeding. Documentation provides evidence of the nursing process in action and legal evidence of the quality of care provided.

In a very large institution, an audit may examine a random sample of records. However, for client problems that are not common, the records of every patient with a specific problem might be examined. Medical records personnel might perform the audit by examining records, recording the data, and developing statistics of the results. Computerized records make it possible to include all records in an audit. This is one of the strong driving factors in the move to computerize documentation systems.

EXAMPLE *Using an Audit for Improvement*

An audit review committee composed of a nurse, a physical therapist, and a pharmacist was charged with the task of reviewing the care of the patients having a total hip replacement who did not conform to the expected length of stay. As part of the data, they were given the records of several patients with long lengths of stay. As they reviewed the chart and discussed the care of Mr. Jones, they sought information regarding factors that had contributed to the increased length of stay. They noted that he was ready for discharge at the appointed time, but that the discharge planner had been unable to place him in a Medicare unit for rehabilitation until 48 hours later. As they reviewed additional patient records, they noted that the same pattern had occurred several times. They also identified two patients who had had multiple coexisting illnesses that had resulted in complicated recovery. The committee's conclusion was that resolving the transfer problem would contribute significantly to assuring that the length of stay met the desired target. This was communicated to the discharge planning office so that they could develop an action plan for change.

Where computerized record-keeping systems are in place, concurrent audits are becoming more frequent and systematic. The computer may automatically audit documentation of all medications on an hourly basis and provide a report of discrepancies noted. The purpose of these automatic auditing systems is to enable the staff to correct potential errors before they actually occur. A missed medication is immediately brought to the attention of the staff so that it can be given. This same automatic ability is one of its drawbacks. Computers do not make inferences or judgments; they only report data. If the medication is being held awaiting consultation between a nurse and a physician, some systems continue to report an error message, although withholding the medication is an appropriate nursing action. The basic programming of the computer system must be extraordinarily complex to take into consideration all the individualized actions that can occur. This is why most computer audit systems require that a person review all data to make judgments regarding the meaning of the data.

Computerized audits are facilitated by the use of standardized language. Medical records departments are able to categorize all medical diagnoses through the use of the international classification of diseases, thus facilitating retrieval of medical data. Nursing is only recently moving to the use of standardized nomenclature for nursing actions and phenomena. The nursing minimum data set (NMDS) for assessment, NANDA nursing diagnosis classification system for problems identified, nursing interventions classification (NIC) for nursing actions, and the nursing outcomes classification (NOC) for the results of nursing care together provide a comprehensive nursing terminology. These classification systems are discussed in Chapter 14.

Critical Thinking Exercise

A retrospective audit was conducted on documentation of PRN medication administration. The audit revealed that in 30% of the cases of administration of the PRN medication, there was no documentation of the assessment that led to medication administration. In addition, the effectiveness of the PRN medication was charted in only 50% of the cases. You have been asked to be on a committee that will examine this problem and make suggestions for improvement. What interdisciplinary team members would be valuable on this committee? What is the standard toward which your committee should aim? What data do you need in addition to these statistics? Where might you look to determine the underlying causes of the problem? What might be a corrective action to be taken relative to each possible cause?

Direct Observation and Interview

Direct observations and interviews are sometimes used to gather information related to standards. Specific standards are designated for study. A guide for the interview must be designed that will facilitate collecting the same information from every patient. The nurses who complete the interviews must be trained and interrater reliability established so that the use of multiple nurses does not affect the reliability of the data. The use of direct observation and interviews is very valuable in concurrent review of standards but is costly in terms of personnel time.

EXAMPLE   *Improving Pain Management*

Community Hospital decided to study whether the patient-controlled analgesia (PCA) pumps recently introduced were having the desired outcomes related to pain management. A nurse researcher was asked to design a process to study this question by using interviews with patients. The nurse identified an interview that had been used in several other hospitals that had initiated the use of this same brand of PCA pump. She asked for three nurses who would interview a random sample of patients. The nurses were trained in the use of the interview tool and checked for interrater reliability. Seventy-five patients were interviewed and the results of the interviews were analyzed by the research nurse. The results showed that the patients who understood how they were safeguarded and used the pump correctly had excellent pain relief. The results also identified that some patients did not understand the pumps, used them rarely, and were not happy with their pain control. Based on the patient's responses, a decision was made to institute a standardized teaching protocol for patients being started on the PCA pump. A further plan was made to repeat the interview strategy after the new protocol was in place.

Surveys

Surveys or questionnaires gather information regarding the perceptions and feelings of individuals in the system. Surveys of employees may provide insights into both strengths and weaknesses of the organization. Health care institutions are also asking consumers to evaluate services. Patients can rate their personal satisfaction with care and the adequacy of supports provided to meet their needs, and they can point out any problems they encountered. Some agencies use simple checklists or rating scales that are given to the patient at the time of discharge. Again, the development of valid and reliable surveys requires time of the personnel who understand this process. If the survey contains numerical rating scales or other such quantitative data, cumulative statistics from the completed surveys can be obtained in order to determine satisfaction with care. Areas that demonstrate a consistent pattern of dissatisfaction are then investigated. Narrative data from client questionnaires are often more difficult to analyze because of the variety of standards that these individuals may be using for evaluation. A critical evaluation based on early discharge might be made by a patient who used as a standard of comparison a hospital stay in the 1960s, when hospital stays were much longer. On the other hand, a similar criticism might be based on a patient's evaluation of personal readiness for self-care. This second adverse evaluation might be much more important to follow up. Such things as patient satisfaction and quality of life are difficult to put into a cost–benefit equation. This is especially true because response rates on patient satisfaction questionnaires tend to be very poor and may not represent the entire range of patients (Spooner, 2003).

■ ANALYSIS OF DATA

Analyzing the data collected includes the use of simple descriptive reports, percentage and numerical reports, and sophisticated statistics. Trends in data over time can reveal significant changes that might not be noted with a one-time data collection. One of the hallmarks of the current large health care organizations is the increasing sophistication of the data analysis techniques used. Charts, graphs, and statistical calculations are used to translate the data gathered into useful information. To complete cost–benefit analyses, an agency must have the capability of tracking and analyzing a wide variety of data. Long-term care facilities are using data relative to nursing hours required, supplies used, and cost of medications and therapies to correlate with reimbursement systems. As more and more health care institutions are entering into contracts with managed care organizations to provide a specified type of care for a flat fee, this kind of tracking is essential to the economic viability of the organization.

Analysis of the data includes identifying discrepancies between the desired outcomes and the actual outcomes and areas that are opportunities for improvement. When there are discrepancies, they must be remedied in order to meet the outcomes as identified. Opportunities for improvement are areas of satisfactory function for which a potential exists for moving toward excellence.

■ ACTION PLANS

Action plans are detailed approaches to making changes. Successful action plans are similar to successful nursing care plans. They are specific, identify the person responsible for each action, and set a time frame for implementation. Without action plans for change and improvement, evaluation lacks effectiveness.

■ USING GOALS AND OBJECTIVES IN THE EVALUATION PROCESS

Evaluation may also be based on specific, targeted goals and objectives. This may be part of an overall plan for management by objectives. Let us review the definitions and various components of goals and objectives.

First, goals may be developed. **Goals** are the broad statements of overall intent of an organization, department, unit, or individual. They are usually stated in general terms. Based on the community's health needs, the institution forms goals. Within that framework, various departments and units form their own overall goals.

Objectives are the specific accomplishments that help achieve a goal. They usually have a related time deadline. Some organizations choose to develop specific objectives without overall goals. The effective nurse manager may use institutional goals and objectives as a basis to develop specific unit goals and objectives that conform to those expectations. Thus, the manager is helped to set priorities and establish plans of action. Unit goals and objectives are usually developed with the cooperation of the entire staff. This helps the staff to determine priorities for time and attention and to share a realistic picture of the workload. When evaluation is based on goals and objectives to which everyone contributed, the evaluation may be viewed as helpful and fair.

One of the strengths of using goals and objectives as an approach to evaluation is that all individuals clearly know their direction. When everyone knows what the goals and objectives are, their individual behavior is more likely to change to facilitate meeting the goals and objectives. Evaluation is very clear—you can identify what was accomplished and what was not. Whether as individuals or as an entire agency, people respond well to clearly defined expectations.

Using goals and objectives for evaluation does have limitations. First, setting goals and objectives cannot be done in isolation. They need to be made in relation to standards of care. If this is not done, the goals and objectives may be accomplished without anyone investigating whether a high level of care was achieved in an economically viable manner.

In addition, it is impossible to address all the areas of function of a major health care agency in a few specific objectives. Sometimes the areas for which goals and objectives have been formulated do very well, but other areas are neglected or overlooked in the process. On the other hand, if a great many specific objectives are identified, it is difficult for individuals to keep them in mind and they may just ignore them. Often, goals and objectives are used for areas in which change is being planned and not used for general evaluative purposes.

Another problem is that conflict over goals may occur within an institution. Although the nurse manager does not often have direct responsibility for resolving an institution-wide conflict, nurses should understand the nature of such conflicts as well as some of the techniques for conflict resolution (see Chapter 9).

Critical Thinking Exercise

Your unit has been asked to develop goals and objectives for the coming year. Who should participate in making this decision? What information do you need to begin planning? What process might be used to accomplish this? How will you evaluate the goals and objectives that are developed?

■ QUALITY ASSURANCE AND IMPROVEMENT

Quality assurance and improvement are the focus of most evaluation activities mandated by accrediting agencies. Again, terminology may vary and quality improvement may be identified as **performance improvement.**

Quality Assurance

Quality assurance refers to activities that are used to monitor, evaluate, and control services provided to consumers. The goal of QA is to identify areas in which standards have not been met and correct them. QA programs were the first major movement to examine health care delivery in a systematic and comprehensive manner. These programs have provided a clear pathway to examining important components of the system and have helped identify areas in need of change. When organizations carry out these activities, criteria or standards are set, information related to the standards is collected, and then, if there is a discrepancy between the standards and the information, corrective action is taken. Setting standards and collecting data have been previously discussed.

Identifying areas in which there are errors is a part of quality assurance. In 2000, the IOM released a major report that discussed the incidence of error in the health care system as found by several different research studies. The data identified what many believed to be a staggering incidence of errors. Not only did errors occur, but deaths occurred because of some of these errors. Historically, action plans for remedying errors in health care focused on changing the behaviors of the health care providers. The IOM report made multiple suggestions for creating a safer health care environment. These included leadership issues, error-reporting systems, setting performance standards, and creating a safe system (IOM, 2000). These are issues that can be addressed through a comprehensive QA program.

SENTINEL EVENTS

Sentinel events are defined by the JCAHO (2002) as "unexpected occurrences involving death or serious physical or psychological injury, or risk thereof. Serious injury specifically includes loss of limb or function. The phrase "or the risk thereof" includes any process variation for which a recurrence would carry a significant chance of a serious adverse outcome. Loss of function includes sensory, motor, physiologic, or intellectual impairment. Sentinel events signal the need for immediate investigation and response. Thus, sentinel events include both errors and what are commonly referred to as near misses. Some examples of sentinel events are

- Death resulting from a medication error or other treatment-related error
- Suicide of a patient in a setting in which he or she received around-the-clock care.
- Surgery on the wrong patient or body part regardless of the magnitude of the operation
- Hemolytic transfusion reaction involving the administration of blood or blood products having major blood group incompatibilities
- A near miss, which might include the erroneous administration of a drug that paralyzes musculature to a nonintubated patient who was successfully intubated and treated.

Root Cause Analysis

An important aspect of QA is taking action to correct situations in which standards have not been met. The JCAHO requires that institutions establish root cause analysis when a sentinel event occurs. A **root cause analysis** is a comprehensive, often complex, process that seeks to identify all the contributory factors to an error and identify their share of causation. This is in contrast to the common approach of identifying the **proximal cause** of an error. The proximal cause is the individual action that was in error. For example, a nurse makes a medication error. The proximal cause is the nurse's failure to check one or more of the five rights of medication administration. A root cause seeks to find out what led to the error by this nurse and could lead to errors by other nurses. This analysis would examine the medication labeling, the storing systems, the patient identification system, the prescribing procedures, and so forth. Because root cause analysis is time consuming and therefore costly, it is usually done only in response to major errors such as sentinel events or the identification of multiple similar errors.

The Veterans Administration National Center for Patient Safety (VA NCPS) (2003) has created a nationwide program targeting patient safety. One aspect of this program is conducting root cause analysis whenever an error or a near miss occurs. According to the VA NCPS,

The goal of a Root Cause Analysis is to find out
what happened
why did it happen
what do you do to prevent it from happening again.

Root cause analysis is also a tool for identifying prevention strategies. It is a process that is part of the effort to build a culture of safety and move beyond the culture of blame. In root cause analysis, basic and contributing causes are discovered in a process similar to diagnosis of disease, with the goal always in mind of preventing recurrence (VA NCPS, 2003).

Techniques such as root cause analysis strive to address the need for both structural and process changes. For example, if two medications with similar names and similar containers but very different actions and dosages have been mistakenly administered, either structural or process changes might be needed to correct the error. A root cause analysis would strive to determine which strategy for correction should be adopted. A structural change would be to change the storage of these two medications so that they are no longer stored in the same area. Changing the structural pattern of the storage itself might eliminate future errors. A process approach to this problem would be to set up specific checklists or perhaps bar codes for the use of these medications.

ACTING TO PREVENT ERROR

One problem with QA has been the tendency to focus on clinical outcomes only and not on other aspects of the organization's functions. The emphasis on corrective action has often been on changing the behaviors of the health care providers. The need for changes in the systems rather than changes in individual care providers was often neglected. The most recent efforts of the IOM and JCAHO have been aimed at addressing system problems.

In 2002, the JCAHO began making recommendations in regard to patient safety goals. In January 2003, they announced six patient safety goals along with strategies toward reaching these goals. These strategies were based on expert analysis to identify common system problems in need of improvement. Display 4-1 gives the 2004 safety goals.

Another criticism of the QA programs in health care has been that the programs often focused on minimal standards. These standards were set by accrediting agencies and state health departments. Minimum standards may have a place in eliminating bad care, but they will not assist in providing excellent care. This drawback of QA has led to the emergence of the quality improvement movement.

The Quality Improvement Movement

The **quality improvement (QI)** movement or performance improvement movement incorporates all the activities of QA and moves beyond them to include a wide variety of programs aimed at improving the quality of health care. The QI movement actually began with the work of Deming, an American who went to Japan after World War II as an adviser to businesses. Businesses focused on zero defects, meeting customer needs, and constant improvement. In addition, responsibility, accountability, and authority for maintaining quality were placed in the hands of those

DISPLAY 4-1	**Joint Commission Patient Safety Goals for 2004**

1. Improve the accuracy of patient identification.
   a. Use at least two patient identifiers (neither to be the patient's room number) whenever taking blood samples or administering medications or blood products.
   b. Prior to the start of any surgical or invasive procedure, conduct a final verification process, such as a "time out," to confirm the correct patient, procedure, and site, using active—not passive—communication techniques.
2. Improve the effectiveness of communication among caregivers.
   a. Implement a process for taking verbal or telephone orders that require a verification "read-back" of the complete order by the person receiving the order.
   b. Standardize the abbreviations, acronyms, and symbols used throughout the organization, including a list of abbreviations, acronyms, and symbols *not* to use.
3. Improve the safety of using high-alert medications.
   a. Remove concentrated electrolytes (including, but not limited to, potassium chloride, potassium phosphate, and sodium chloride >0.9%) from patient care units.
   b. Standardize and limit the number of drug concentrations available in the organization.
4. Eliminate wrong-site, wrong-patient, wrong-procedure surgery.
   a. Create and use a preoperative verification process, such as a checklist, to confirm that appropriate documents (e.g., medical records, imaging studies) are available.
   b. Implement a process to mark the surgical site and involve the patient in the marking process.
5. Improve the safety of using infusion pumps.
   a. Ensure free-flow protection on all general-use and PCA (patient controlled analgesia) intravenous infusion pumps used in the organization.
6. Improve the effectiveness of clinical alarm systems.
   a. Implement regular preventive maintenance and testing of alarm systems.
   b. Assure that alarms are activated with appropriate settings and are sufficiently audible with respect to distances and competing noise within the unit.
7. Reduce the risk of health-care-acquired infections.
   a. Comply with current CDC hand hygiene guidelines.
   b. Manage as sentinel events all identified cases of unanticipated death or major permanent loss of function associated with a health-care-acquired infection.

From Joint Commission for the Accreditation of Healthcare Organizations (2004). Available at http://www.jcaho.org/accredited+organizations/patient+safety/04+npsg/04_npsg.htm.

closest to the product. Deming emphasized workers as humans, not cogs in a wheel (Oberle, 1990). Three of the most widely quoted experts in this field are Deming (1986), Crosby (1979), and Juran (1988). Donabedian is credited with being the first to apply QI techniques to health care organizations (Elliott et al., 2000). The essential attributes of the QI movement are now being widely applied to the health care environment.

The latest accreditation standards from the JCAHO include one that focuses on QI as well as the activities of QA. The JCAHO (2003) has designated these activities as **quality assessment and improvement** (QAI). QAI is defined as the ongoing activities designed to objectively and systematically evaluate the quality of patient/resident care and services, pursue opportunities to improve patient/resident care and services, and resolve identified problems. Standards are applied to evaluate the quality of an organization's performance in conducting QAI activities.

Critical Thinking Exercise

The administration has announced that the regular JCAHO accreditation visit will take place in 6 months. Committees are being formed to examine all the various standards set by JCAHO and to evaluate whether the institution is meeting those standards. In areas in which a discrepancy is noted, the committee is to plan for remedial action to ensure that the institution meets the standard by the time of the visit. What are problems and advantages for an institution with this approach to meeting accreditation standards? As a staff nurse, how might you contribute to the success of this process? If you were the charge nurse on days, how might your contribution be different from the staff nurse's contribution? How might this process affect patient care standards?

CONTINUOUS QUALITY IMPROVEMENT

Continuous quality improvement (CQI) is a process in which ongoing analysis and improvement lay the foundation for change. In this process, **quality indicators** are continuously examined. Quality indicators include those data that would indicate that high standards of care are being maintained.

However, planned data collection and working on key indicators are not the only aspects of the organization that are subject to examination. Central to the idea of CQI is the need to "tinker" constantly to improve any process. No human endeavor is ever perfect. If everyone is committed to the effort, incremental changes can be made that will improve quality. Some institutions, by their very natures, have supported individuals and groups in efforts toward CQI. With the JCAHO criterion regarding QI now in place, organizations that are accredited by the JCAHO will need to take action in this realm. See Display 4-2 for steps in the CQI process.

In CQI (or PI), an individual or group may identify a process that could be improved. When this is brought to the attention of a manager, a team or task force is assigned to quickly examine the issue, gather data, suggest a plan for improvement, and initiate the plan. After the new process has been implemented, data are again gathered to determine whether improvement has occurred. In organizations that emphasize **rapid process improvement,** this may all take place in 1–2 weeks. The idea is to move quickly to change what needs to be changed. Because the team represents

DISPLAY 4-2   **Steps in the CQI Process**

1. Carry out planned data collection
2. Identify an area to improve
3. Form a task force of stakeholders
4. Plan a change in systems or processes
5. Implement the change
6. Collect data again to evaluate the change

the stakeholders, they are empowered to move ahead with change. The focus is on constantly improving performance and all workers empowered to collaborate in change.

EXAMPLE *A Quality Improvement Process*

At Community Hospital, the nurses identified that initiating total parenteral nutrition (TPN) often required many hours. Some of the community physicians did not always remember the details of ordering TPN and might have neglected to include information that was essential to filling the prescription. If the nurses did not detect the discrepancy in the order and contact the physician right away, the order was sent to the pharmacy. After the usual delay in filling a pharmacy order, the pharmacist would discover the discrepancy, call the unit, and the nurse would need to call the physician. Then there was sometimes a delay before the physician was located. The order was always followed through: the patient did receive the correct TPN, and no error occurred. Changing this system was seen as an opportunity to move from satisfactory performance to excellent performance.

When this was brought to the manager's attention, she quickly contacted the pharmacy and the chief of the medical staff. Each appointed a person to be part of a team to develop a new process that would expedite the patient's receiving TPN. The team met; determined that the desired outcome was that TPN would be initiated within 2 hours of the order being written. Together they designed an order form to be used for all TPN orders that included preprinted options for each item that needed to be included in the order. There was a way for each item to be individualized if the physician did not choose one of the preprinted options. By the end of one week, a sample form had been printed by the records department and circulated to all staff physicians for comment. Sample forms were placed on each nursing unit and nurses asked to comment on the form. A similar process was used in the pharmacy.

At the end of the second week, the team met again, reviewed all suggestions, and identified the final format of the order sheet for TPN. This was sent for printing, and by the end of the third week after the team was formed, the new TPN order sheet was available on each unit. Time of filling of orders and administering IVs were a routine part of the patient care record. At the end of 3 months, an audit was done to determine the time from the writing of the orders to the hanging of theTPN. All reviewing the report were pleased to learn that the maximum time from writing to implementation of the order was now 2 hours and 15 minutes, but the average time was now 1 hour and 40 minutes.

TOTAL QUALITY MANAGEMENT

Total quality management (TQM) is an overall management program to implement CQI. TQM includes the use of structural, process, and outcome standards for QA as previously described plus additional specific programs designed to improve quality. The emphasis is on interdisciplinary collaboration and on examining and changing administrative as well as clinical practices. Green (1992) suggests a model for TQM in the health care environment that involves dividing each of the areas of standards into three domains: the patient or clinical domain, the staff or professional domain, and the administrative or system domain. Her model assists individuals in examining the system and understanding the quality management process.

 # Key Aspects of Quality Improvement Programs

There are numerous specific QI programs in which health care agencies and institutions are participating. Each program has a somewhat different emphasis and some different techniques. However, all the programs involved in QI include similar values and concerns. A key starting point for QI programs is a commitment by management at all levels to work with employees to empower them in their work. (See Chapter 1 for a discussion of empowering staff.) Instilling pride and creating an atmosphere in which individuals can be creative and innovative are key goals of QI. The opinions and suggestions of employees must be valued, and employees must feel comfortable in making suggestions. To be effective, QI requires skills of working in groups and teams: listening, collaborating, and reaching consensus. It also requires an endorsement of the concept that failure is acceptable. Not all new ideas will work, but often the viability of new ideas won't be known until they are tried. If failure is not tolerated, then many positive ideas are lost also.

When problems occur, a QI approach does not seek people to blame but rather examines the system to identify what in the system may be interfering with achieving goals. QI should encourage people to develop new approaches to problem situations. Employees must be encouraged to identify problem areas so that corrective action can be taken. However, the goal is not just to correct errors, as in QA programs, but also to identify ways to improve care. CQI organizations attempt to become learning organizations in which everyone is learning, changing, and improving.

Obtaining sufficient data to accurately identify any problem or to plan for change requires that systems be established to gather the information needed. Ongoing systems that identify quality indicators and methods of collecting information are central aspects of most quality management programs. Analysis of information must be carefully done so that the real root of any problem is identified. For the information to affect planning, data obtained by the monitoring program must be communicated to the employees who are most closely involved. As health care organizations have moved to greater computerization of information, additional avenues for effective monitoring of data have become available.

The use of teams for problem solving is a hallmark of quality efforts. Teamwork provides a variety of viewpoints on each problem area. Teams may be small within a department or may be multidisciplinary in nature. Managers are not always in charge of the teams, which often are self-directed and self-limiting. Some programs use **quality circles** (see Chapter 6), which are teams of workers who meet regularly and whose purpose is to identify ways of improving quality within their own work setting. To free individuals to use their creativity and not to be constrained by the potential for evaluation of their efforts, these quality circles do not include management personnel.

Everyone must focus on meeting the needs of the customer. For many health care workers, the customer is the patient or client. Understanding the clients who are in your facility is critical to creating quality care for each individual. To do this, data are needed on the various demographic aspects of your client population. What are the age, sex, cultural or ethnic background, and usual sources of payment for services? These data support efforts to adapt care strategies to meet individual needs. For example, if you have a large group of clients whose primary language at home is not English, then quality care would include the provision of translation services to assure that these individuals participate fully in their care.

There are also internal customers. Surgeons and nurses are customers of the housekeeping department that cleans the operating rooms. Unless the housekeeping department meets the needs of the surgical personnel, the patients cannot receive the care they require. The X-ray technician is meeting the needs of the patient-customer for quality care in the department, and is also meeting the needs of the radiologist-customer for technically excellent X-rays. When clearly identified, an internal customer can be asked to help identify quality.

Eliminating waste is another key aspect of quality programs. A balance of cost and effectiveness is critical in a health care system that has limited resources. Waste contributes to costs without enhancing effectiveness. Those closest to the situation can most easily identify waste. Time, materials, and space may be wasted if those who use them most frequently do not feel responsible for monitoring waste. QI seeks to make those closest to the use of resources responsible for eliminating waste. For example, in one institution, a clerk in the records department identified forms that duplicated information and saved the facility thousands of dollars in the immediate cost of forms plus untold hours of staff time in completing them.

Both TQM and CQI place a major emphasis on empowering individuals within an organization to work toward quality. Individuals are encouraged to contribute, innovate, and participate. The quality movement is helping focus efforts on major changes needed as health care reform becomes a reality. The desired result is improved care for clients within realistic economic constraints. When applied effectively, the QI movement may engage the best that all health care providers have to offer and set the stage for positive inclusion of the client-consumer in the processes of care.

Barriers to Quality Improvement

The costs of QI efforts are significant. An organization developing a CQI program might spend $20,000 to $200,000 initially for program development and training (McLaughlin & Simpson, 1999). There is the cost of staff time, computer programming, and documentation. The goal is that the efforts of CQI will improve the functioning of the organization to such an extent that these costs are more than made up; however, this may not occur.

No program, whatever its focus, can by itself create quality. Quality health care originates with individuals at all levels of the organization and requires commitment at all levels. If every level of administration is not fully committed to quality, then the organization will not be able to change. If quality programs are just another fad or set of phrases and slogans, they will quickly be dropped because they are not relevant to the demands of health care. Any change this inclusive takes time to design and to implement. Those who are looking for a quick fix through QI programs are not likely to find what they are looking for.

Critical Thinking Exercise

Margaret Neal, the administrator of Harbor Home Health Agency, has always operated within a traditional authoritarian management framework. Yesterday, she announced that a consultant in TQM has been asked to assist in restructuring the entire way the agency operates. What are some of the concerns that you and other staff members might have about this project? What factors currently at work might make TQM difficult? What changes will be needed in the organizational operation to make TQM work effectively?

■ RISK MANAGEMENT

Another aspect of a health care organization's evaluation and planning activities involves minimizing the risk to the institution or agency from an error or problem that could result in legal action or liability. This is referred to as **risk management.** Part of the use of QA data is to lower the risk to the institution of being involved in lawsuits from consumers and the public when standards are not met. To oversee this activity, health care institutions employ a risk manager, who studies the QA findings with this perspective in mind. Although most errors or problems do not result in litigation, the potential exists and can be very costly to the institution. If problems have been noted and not corrected, both the chance of a judgment against the health care institution and the size of a legal judgment may be increased. The public is concerned about safety in health care and reacts adversely to any indication that safety has been compromised.

Another focus of risk management is to think ahead about defense when a legal action is contemplated or actually occurs. The risk manager might review the documentation system, focusing not only on what is needed for quality of care, but on what would be needed to demonstrate that appropriate care did occur so that litigation would not be initiated or for defense in litigation. This reflects the concern about charting that actions not charted will be considered not done. Although this emphasis sometimes seems annoying to health care professionals, it is essential in today's society.

Risk managers also attempt to be **proactive** in identifying and eliminating areas of risk for the institution. Through knowledge of what is happening to other institutions, review of court cases, and education, the risk manager tries to help the institution avoid problems that others have encountered. For example, classes that focus the attention of the staff on situations of risk, such as the overly critical patient and family, and how to effectively manage this problem might be used as a strategy for lowering risk.

As a new graduate, you can participate in risk management most effectively by assuring that all your patients receive quality care that meets the standards established by the profession. This also includes establishing and maintaining rapport and complete and thorough documentation of that care. If these criteria are met, patients and their families usually feel well cared for, and litigation may not be instituted even if an error were to occur. In addition, understanding the concerns of risk management may be helpful to you as you attempt to institute a change in practice. Often, costly changes that benefit patient care are more readily instituted if they are seen as also minimizing risk to the institution. Further, an understanding of risk management is essential to protecting yourself as a professional. This is mentioned throughout the text, but a more comprehensive discussion of legal issues in individual nursing practice can be found in texts or online education resources on legal issues.

■ EVALUATING NURSING CARE THAT YOU MANAGE

An understanding of all the concepts related to evaluation will be of personal use to you in evaluating the nursing care in which you participate. You can identify specific standards of care that you will strive to meet and determine ways of improving care. Using standards to evaluate care can be an ongoing part of your professional life. You might share standards developed by nursing organizations with others at your place of work and encourage discussion of how well care in your setting meets those standards. When requesting continuing education, needed equipment, or changes in policies or procedures, you can use standards of care to help you determine what is needed in your setting.

Goals and objectives may be established informally with a team even when the setting does not have a formal process in place. For example, you may say to those on your team, "Let's see if we can complete our taped reports by 2:45 p.m. every day to make sure we have plenty of time for last-minute care needs." Meeting this specific objective will require you and your team to plan strategies for organizing care and completing report. You could also involve staff in planning goals and objectives by saying, "What goal in regard to patient care do we want to set for this year?" The staff could then discuss its own perceptions of the situation and work cooperatively to set appropriate goals.

A philosophy of continuous improvement can serve as a guide to your entire professional life, regardless of whether your organization has a formal QI plan. You may look for ways to improve your own practice and better serve clients for whom you have responsibility. You may actively participate at your place of employment in committees or task forces assigned to improve policies and procedures. Your own reading and study can serve as the foundation for actively seeking improvements in practice. As an individual focused on improvement, you may stimulate others to adopt this same philosophy and thus may help produce an environment that supports excellence in nursing practice.

■ KEY CONCEPTS

- ■ Standards for evaluation may include structural, process, and outcome standards. Processes include evaluation standards as well as other processes in the organization. Outcomes include costs as well as patient outcomes and outcomes of the various internal processes.
- ■ Standards are developed by a variety of sources, such as accreditation organizations, professional standards of practice, governmental regulations, and individual facility planning.
- ■ Benchmarking refers to setting specific measurable standards against which an agency or institution will compare itself. Benchmarks are established through data collection across agencies or by the accomplishments of excellent health care agencies.
- ■ Data for evaluation are collected through incident or QA reports, retrospective audit, concurrent audit, direct observation or interview, and questionnaires.
- ■ Analysis of data requires that an agency be able to develop statistical reports as well as simple numerical and descriptive reports. Cost–benefit analysis is important to the financial viability of any health care organization.
- ■ QA activities mandated by many official agencies use structural, process, and outcome standards to evaluate health care practice. QA focuses on using key indicators to identify problems and then instituting corrective actions for those that fall short of standards.
- ■ The QI movement seeks to improve care continuously. TQM provides a framework for CQI through the use of such strategies as identifying quality indicators, establishing group efforts in the form of quality circles, meeting the needs of both internal and external customers, and eliminating waste.
- ■ Goals are broad statements of overall intent that lend direction to actions at every level in an organization. Objectives are specific accomplishments that indicate that a goal is being met.
- ■ Goals and objectives can be used as a guide in planning appropriate actions and in evaluating the effectiveness of the actions.
- ■ Advantages of using goals and objectives for evaluation are that individuals clearly know their direction and that behaviors are more likely to be purposeful.
- ■ Limitations of using goals and objectives include conflict over goals and the inability to address all essential areas effectively.
- ■ Risk management focuses on correcting problems that have been identified, supporting the mechanisms by which an institution can defend itself in any legal action, identifying potential legal risks, and changing practice to minimize those risks.
- ■ As an individual nurse, you can use these strategies to evaluate the care in which you participate and to seek improvement in health care delivery.

REFERENCES

Agency for Healthcare Research and Quality (AHRQ). (2003). *Databases and Related Resources from HCUP* [Online]. Available at www.ahcpr.gov/data/hcup/datahcup.htm.

American Nurses Association. (1998). *Standards of Clinical Nursing Practice*. Kansas City, MO: Author.

Connor, P. E. (1997). Total quality management: A selective commentary on its human dimensions, with special reference to its downside. *Public Administration Review, 57*(6), 501–510.

Crosby, P. B. (1979). *Quality is Free: The Art of Making Quality Certain.* New York: McGraw-Hill.

Deming, W. E. (1986). *Out of Crisis.* Cambridge, MA: Center for Advanced Engineering Study, Massachusetts Institute of Technology.

Elliott, C., Shaw, P., Isaacson, P. et al. (2000). *Performance Improvement in Healthcare.* Chicago: American Health Information Management Association.

Green, E. (1992). Teaching a new approach to quality improvement. *Journal of Continuing Education in Nursing, 23*(1), 20–23.

Institute of Medicine (IOM). (1999). Measuring quality in health care. In Donaldson, M. S. (Ed.), *National Roundtable on Health Care Quality.* Washington, D.C.: National Academy Press.

IOM. (2000). *To Err is Human: Building a Safer Health System.* In Kohn, L. T., Corrigan, J. M., and Donaldson, M. S. (Eds.), *Committee on Quality of Health Care in America.* Washington, DC: National Academy Press.

Joint Commission on Accreditation of Healthcare Organizations (JCAHO). (2002). *Sentinel Event Policies and Procedures* [Online]. Available at http://www.jcaho.org/accredited+organizations/hospitals/sentinel+events/se_pp.htm#1; revised July 2002.

JCAHO. (2003). *Comprehensive Accreditation Manual for Hospitals: The Official Handbook.* Chicago: Author.

JCAHO. (2004). *Joint Commission Patient Safety Goals for 2004* [Online]. Available at http://www.jcaho.org/accredited+organizations/patient+safety/04+npsg/04_npsg.htm.

Juran, J. M. (1988). *Juran on Planning for Quality.* New York: Free Press.

McLaughlin, C. P., & Kaluzny, A. D. (1999). *Continuous Quality Improvement in Health Care.* Gaithersburg, MD: Aspen Publications.

McLaughlin, C. P., & Simpson, K. N. (2000). Does TQM/CQI work in health care? In Lighter, D. E., and Fair, D. C. (Eds.), *Principles and Methods of Quality Management in Health Care* (pp. 34–56). Gaithersburg, MD: Aspen Publications.

Spooner, S. H. (2003). Survey response rates and overall patient satisfaction scores. *Journal of Nursing Care Quality 18*(3), 162.

White, A. W., & Wager, K. A. (1998). The outcomes movement and the role of health information managers. *Topics in Health Information Management 18*(4), 1–12.

Veterans Administration National Center for Patient Safety (VA NCPS). *Root Cause Analysis* [Online]. Available at http://www.patientsafety.gov/tools.html. Accessed July 27, 2003.

unit 2

MOVING INTO A PROFESSIONAL ROLE

Before being able to function effectively as a manager of nursing care, it is critical that a novice to a career in nursing possesses an understanding of the roles the professional nurse occupies in the health care delivery system. Unit 2 focuses on the more important of these roles. The unit begins with a discussion of the nurse's role as a communicator, teacher, motivator, and team builder. Vital to all aspects of the management role is the ability to use communication skills adeptly. Selecting communication techniques appropriate to the situation and developing the ability to be an active listener are important to functioning in a leadership role. Of equal importance is the ability to communicate effectively in confrontational situations. Nurses also use communication skills to motivate members of the nursing team. Being able to motivate others to do their best job and to remain challenged by everyday responsibilities may make the difference between an effective manager and an ineffective one. An overview of theories of motivation is provided to serve as a foundation for presenting this important role. Team building and teaching are also important skills that require the ability to communicate effectively. Chapter 5 concludes with a discussion of skills needed in these areas. Knowing what to delegate, when to delegate, how to delegate, and to whom to delegate nursing tasks become critical as nursing teams increasingly are composed of registered nurses and unlicensed assistive personnel. Of equal importance is mastering the art of decision making, because nurses use decision-making skills in all aspects of patient care, but particularly when assigning duties and prioritizing care. Chapter 6 focuses on these skills. Chapter 7 explores the nurse's role as supervisor and evaluator. Evaluation of peers and employees is an ongoing process. When you function in the role of manager, carrying out evaluation of employees and providing feedback on their performance may be a significant part of your job. This chapter includes a discussion of the instruments most commonly used in evaluation of health care personnel and discusses the performance appraisal interview. The chapter concludes with a discussion of progressive discipline and the steps to be followed in the process.

Nurses also have active roles as client advocates and in the process of change, in which they may be cast as change agent. In today's complex health care environment, the ability to serve as an advocate for clients and to teach them the essential aspects of advocating for themselves has never been more important. Being able to manage change confidently and effectively is becoming even more critical in our ever-evolving health care environment. Selecting strategies for change that fit the situation will make a difference in the cooperation that is engendered from others affected by the change process. Understanding human reactions to change and the change process is also a critical element to bringing about change. With increasing frequency, nurses find themselves in the role of negotiator and mediator, whether it relates to personnel issues, concerns about limited resources, scheduling conflicts, or interpersonal conflicts. This unit concludes with a discussion of conflict management and the nurse's role as negotiator and mediator.

5

The Nurse as Communicator, Teacher, Motivator, and Team Builder

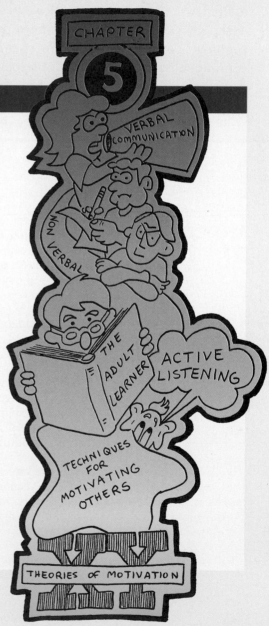

CHAPTER 5

Learning Outcomes

After completing this chapter, you should be able to:

1. Describe the essential components of effective communication, including various approaches to interpersonal interaction.
2. Identify aspects of communication that are critical to functioning effectively as a manager, including using communication skills to motivate and teach.
3. Compare four popularly held theories of motivation, and explain how each can be applied when working with others in a health care setting.
4. Identify and describe behaviors that will strengthen the team.
5. Discuss the team-building process and why it is important in the health care environment.
6. Outline the nurse's role in creating a climate for learning and providing practical support for continued learning in the workplace.
7. Discuss factors to be considered when working with adult learners.
8. Explain how principles related to teaching and learning can be applied to adult learners in the workplace.
9. Identify factors to consider when planning a learning experience, including assessing needs, writing objectives, and planning teaching strategies.
10. Describe problems that may occur in staff teaching, analyze why these may occur, and develop possible solutions.

Key Terms ■ ■ ■ ■

achievement
achievement motivation
active listening
affective learning
affiliation
assertiveness
cognitive learning
communication
confrontation
dissatisfiers or hygiene
    factors

extrinsic
feedback
hierarchy
intrinsic
learning style
motivation
motives/motivators
physiological needs
psychomotor learning
reinforcement
safety needs

satisfiers or motivators
self-actualization
teaching/teaching role
team building
Theory X
Theory Y
trust

The ability to communicate skillfully is probably the most important of all the areas in which one needs expertise in order to manage effectively. We use **communication** when we teach, direct and delegate, motivate, evaluate, and build teams, as well as in many other day-to-day activities involved in the management role. This puts the ability of a manager to communicate skillfully at the core of working effectively in a management role.

Communication, which is the process people use to exchange information, occurs constantly between all people (Videbeck, 2001). Included in the information exchange are ideas, attitudes, and feelings. Effective communication is vital to many activities that we have come to take for granted. You have only to observe the chaos that occurs when one of the avenues of communication used in day-to-day operations fails to realize how significant communication is. Have you ever tried to register for a course when the computer was "down?" Have you ever looked for an address when the street signs were missing or hidden from view? Have you tried to call home during a bad storm or natural disaster, such as an earthquake, when the telephone lines were clogged? Have you ever had laryngitis and tried to communicate without speech? Have you tried to care for a patient when physicians doing morning rounds had the chart in use? Communication, which is an interpersonal process, requires good interpersonal skills, including sensitivity to and respect for others. It also involves far more than simply giving or receiving information. It involves reading, writing, speaking, and listening. We rely on effective communication in all these modes to support quality care.

All nursing programs provide instruction in basic communication skills, as a result of which you already have a good grasp of elements that constitute communication and factors that influence the effectiveness of it. Display 5-1 summarizes some of the concepts with which you are already familiar and serves as a review of the topic. We build on your basic understanding of communication in the content that follows.

DISPLAY 5-1 | **Major Communication Concepts**

- Communication may be intrapersonal, interpersonal, group, or societal.
- Communication involves a sender, a receiver, a message and a mode by which the message is sent. *verbal, nonverbal written,*
- Communication takes several forms or modes, primarily verbal, nonverbal, and written.
- Verbal and nonverbal forms of communication can either complement one another or be contradictory in nature.
- Therapeutic communication is that which has purpose and direction and is employed to achieve established objectives that focus on the needs of other people.
- Effective communication involves active listening.
- The words with which we communicate can mean different things to different individuals.
- A number of factors influence communication, including a person's perceptions and values, culture, and life situation. *Filters*
- Communication involves feedback that allows the sender to know which messages were received and correctly understood.
- Blocks to communication occur when responses are made that are not helpful and in one way or another demean or disparage another.
- Communication is culturally sensitive and culture bound and results from experiences one had in early childhood that left impressions of how the world is structured.

Adapted from Ellis, J. R., & Hartley, C. L. (2004). *Nursing in Today's World: Trends, Issues and Management* (8th ed.). Philadelphia: Lippincott Williams & Wilkins.

■ COMMUNICATION IN AN ORGANIZATIONAL SETTING

Most of the information you have learned about communication was probably directed toward patient interactions. When we apply the principles of communication to the organizational setting, we add new dimensions to the process.

Factors Affecting Organizational Communication

In Chapter 2 we discussed formal and informal organization, chains of command, and channels of communication. The communication patterns of the organization need to be in harmony with these other aspects of the institution if the organization is to function effectively. What aspects of the organization have an effect on communication patterns?

First, the formal structure of the organization affects communication patterns. If the organization employs a tall structure and is bureaucratic in nature, workers at the bottom of the organizational hierarchy may receive little communication from those in the top positions. It is impossible for managers in large organizations to communicate with each employee personally. Much of the communication therefore comes through others or in written format.

The informal structure of the organization also affects communication. In large organizations, subgroups may alter or translate messages to suit their purposes, values, and allegiances. The resulting communication network of the informal organization is often referred to as the grapevine. This communication network flows unsystematically among individuals and often may carry misinformation. This is due in part to the speed with which it travels throughout the organization and the fact that messages are primarily distributed verbally. As such, they are subject to the distortions of individual values and perceptions. Those sending the messages have little accountability for the statement that is communicated.

In an organization, the flow of verbal communication is in several formal directions in addition to the grapevine. It flows downward as the manager communicates with subordinates and it flows upward as subordinates report to the manager. It flows horizontally when managers from different units communicate with one another. It flows diagonally when a manager from one department communicates with staff in other departments, as might be seen in a situation in which a pharmacy manager communicates with staff nurses on a unit. The many directions in which messages flow in organizations add to the complexity of the process.

Many of the communications that occur within organizations, regardless of the direction they flow, are not face-to-face. Written messages, either in the form of memos or e-mails, are commonplace. Verbal messages also may not be face-to-face. The majority of them take place via telephone, in which nonverbal cues are missing. If telephone messages are intercepted by answering machines, additional factors are added.

Desirable Qualities in Organizational Communications

There are several desirable qualities of communications that occur in an organizational setting that apply regardless of the mode used to send the message. All communications must be accurate, straightforward, and unambiguous. The persons receiving the message must be able to easily and correctly understand it. Messages should not overwhelm the receiver either in terms of the number received or the language of the message. Today, with e-mail so readily available in most business situations, it is easy for managers to become inundated with messages. Thinking carefully about what needs to be included in a message can assist in keeping the communication clear and focused and free of extraneous information that may not be relevant to the situation.

 VERBAL COMMUNICATIONS

Verbal communications take several forms. They often occur in a face-to-face environment. In organizations, they also frequently occur via the telephone. We use verbal communications when delegating and giving directions, in interviews, in team building, and a host of other organizational activities. Verbal communications should be direct, concise, easily understood, and culturally and developmentally appropriate. When communicating verbally, it is important to remember that words can mean different things to different individuals and at different stages of development. For

---

DISPLAY 5-2   **Statements That Ask for Perceptions of the Recipient of Communication**

- "Now can you please explain how you are going to do that?"
- "Would you please repeat what I just told you?"
- "Would you tell me in your own words how you will determine whether or not Patient Y is able to manage in the shower?"
- "Let's stop for a moment and have you summarize the instructions you have been given."
- "Please tell me in your own words what you understand I said."

---

example, nurses who have been in nursing many years may refer to a Levine tube whereas nurses with only recent experience may never have heard this designation for a nasogastric tube. Coworkers for whom English is a not the native language may have difficulty with expressions that seem common usage to those who have been raised understanding and speaking English. Someone might say "If we don't get this IV started right away, we may be 'up a creek without a paddle.'" This idiom refers to being without an effective alternative and comes from the idea of being up a stream without a way to navigate the waterway.

When you are speaking, think of the person to whom you are sending your message. Is your language clear and direct? Is the vocabulary appropriate to the circumstance? (For example, you may have to delete idiomatic expressions and uncommon vocabulary when talking with someone for whom English is a second language.) Does your nonverbal message match the words you are using?

Perception of another person's communication is almost always incomplete. Words represent generalized symbols that must leave out unique details in order to be efficient. Because this is a characteristic of language, you will need to seek feedback regarding the messages you send. Verifying with others that they perceived your communication as you intended it is a critical element in communicating effectively.

You can take several actions to verify that the message you sent has been correctly perceived. To begin with, it is judicious to avoid asking "yes" or "no" questions to confirm correct reception of the message, because you may not receive enough information. Rather than asking, "Do you understand what I mean?" you might say, "Can you tell me what I have just asked you to do?" Display 5-2 gives examples of phrases that you could use to help obtain this information. In this way, you can help assure that accurate communication occurred.

NONVERBAL COMMUNICATION

Nonverbal communication is usually considered the message that we send through our physical appearance and movements, or everything an individual does that we can observe. It encompasses a wide variety of elements, including facial expression, appearance (e.g., clothes worn), body language (e.g., postures and gestures), eye contact, and the use of touch. The message transmitted nonverbally may be read much more keenly than the verbal message, and if the verbal and nonverbal messages are dissimilar, the nonverbal message is often the one that is received. Therefore, nonverbal and verbal messages should be congruent.

Nonverbal forms of communication carry different values in different cultures. Think, for example, of the handshake. It can be firm or it can be a gentle clasp. Some cultures view a firm handshake as connoting confidence, honesty, and forthright behavior. Other cultures interpret a firm handshake as a symbol of aggressive behavior. Similarly, most Americans think of the ability to maintain eye contact as an important characteristic signifying sincerity and inviting interaction. However, in some cultures eye contact may be avoided because it is viewed as rude or defiant, and casting the eyes downward may be considered a symbol of respect.

When touch is employed in communicating, even greater variables can exist. Some see the use of touch, such as a pat on the back, as reaching out or establishing communication with another. Entire approaches have been developed by using touch therapeutically. But some cultures see the touching of another person, especially without that person's permission, as a serious taboo. Elaborate mechanisms to provide for personal territory free from touch have been developed. With the current recognition that touch can be perceived very differently by different people, in the workplace people should refrain from touching others without first determining that the use of touch is acceptable.

Managers working in a variety of environments work at developing nonverbal skills that will assist them in carrying out their responsibilities. For example, talking to someone with both of you seated conveys the nonverbal message that you are willing to focus your attention to that situation exclusively. Many administrators nonverbally communicate that an interview is over by rising from behind their desks. The very fact that an administrator conducts the interview from behind the desk also sends a message. When a manager asks an employee to meet in the office, the place of meeting conveys a message that the conversation is something that needs to take place in private.

Accompanying your verbal statement with a nonverbal message may reinforce that message. For example, if you say, "I must get back to working on this admission assessment" and turn away at the same time, you have made your message doubly clear. However, at times, individuals send ambiguous or confusing messages by their nonverbal behavior. In the last example, if you said, "I must get back to working on this admission assessment" but continued sitting at the desk by an individual who wanted to talk, that person might assume from your nonverbal behavior that you did not really intend to leave and that further conversation was in order. As you perfect your communication skills, you will want to reflect on the messages you send nonverbally.

WRITTEN COMMUNICATIONS

Written communications are probably used the most frequently in organizations. Some examples of the forms they can take include memos, e-mail messages, job descriptions, performance appraisals, business letters and letters of recommendation, policies, procedures, and protocols.

When preparing to send a written communication, it is wise to think about the message you want to send and how you will structure it. Written messages should be mostly composed of subjects and verbs and few adjectives or adverbs. If action verbs are used, they tend to have a stronger impact. In selecting the words that you are going to use, use common terms and language that is generally understood by all, avoiding emotionally charged words or expressions. If you are using abbreviations (such as NPO, DNR, or ED), be certain that they are ones that have been approved by the agency or organization. To increase patient safety, the Joint Commission on Accreditation of Healthcare Organizations (JCAHO) expects that all agencies it accredits use a list of standardized abbreviations (JCAHO, 2003). Arrange your messages logically and keep the message as short, concise, and to the point as possible. It is desirable, especially when writing memos, to make your main point at the beginning of the message. Finally, it is important that you use correct terminology, spell accurately, and use proper grammar in your communications. If the message is hand written, for example, in the form of charting, be certain that the writing is also legible and clean.

GROUP COMMUNICATIONS

In the organizational setting, many communications occur with a group of people, either large or small, and become more complex as the number of participants increases. Communicating with a group requires special qualities if it is to be most effective. Group communications are also enhanced when the leader has a good understanding of group dynamics. When working with a group, the effective leader is able to encourage the timid, quiet the talkative, motivate the uninspired, and move everyone toward the goals of the organization—no small undertaking. We discuss working with a group in more detail in the section on team building.

When communicating with a group, it is doubly important that you think through the message you want to transmit and the way in which you want the message transmitted or its delivery style. Once you have reached decisions on these items, you will want to consider the words you will use and the best timing for the communication. You will want to be certain that the words carry no emotional overtones and are culturally sensitive and easily understood.

Other Essential Communication Skills

A number of other behaviors that result in more effective communication should be used by all individuals working in an organization. Perfecting these skills can result in being a more valuable employee and having greater job satisfaction.

ACTIVE LISTENING

As part of your nursing education, you have undoubtedly learned the techniques of **active listening.** These listening techniques are an essential foundation to working effectively with others on the health care team. Many people feel that listening is even more important than speaking.

Active listening means that you value what others have to say and their contribution to the situation at hand. When you listen to another staff member, listen for the feelings, values, and opinions being expressed as well as the facts being communicated. These may have a greater effect on working relationships and accomplishments than do facts surrounding the situation.

Some of the techniques that convey active listening include making eye contact, focusing your attention on the individual, and making time to hear the concerns. In the busy health care arena, it is easy to be distracted or feel so rushed that you listen with your attention divided between the person and other issues. This may result in perceiving only a part of the message and may make the speaker feel devalued. In other instances, some persons begin to form their response to a message before the message is completely delivered. This also interferes with active listening.

When someone interrupts you to talk about a problem or concern, you may need to assess the situation as to its urgency. If you determine that the situation is not urgent, you can arrange to meet later in order to give the person your full attention. By carefully responding to them, you can help staff learn what concerns require your immediate attention and what should wait until you are not involved in another task. The nurse who responds to staff with irritation may find they become reluctant to interrupt even though the situation may be urgent.

While listening, remember the general leads you have learned that encouraged patients to talk and conveyed your interest in what they had to say. These same general leads of nodding, making brief responses of "Um-hmm" or "Go on," will help the reticent staff member to explain more fully.

In some situations, your listening ear may be all that is needed. Staff members want someone to be aware of their feelings. Once you are, they feel valued and are comfortable. Often, staff members are able to solve problems independently after having had a chance to talk out their concerns. You can encourage this by your response to what they have to say.

ASSERTIVE COMMUNICATION

Assertiveness is "the right of the individual to behave in a way that meets his needs as long as he does not intrude on the needs and rights of others" (Sundeen et al., 1998). Assertiveness differs from aggressiveness; aggressive behavior infringes or intrudes on the rights of others. It also differs from passiveness, in which the individual disregards personal needs and rights in order to accommodate others. Assertiveness is an essential skill for nurses, both for working with clients and with other members of the health care team. Without effective assertive behavior, you may be overwhelmed by the demands of others, because of your passivity or conversely may alienate others by your aggression.

Nonverbal messages of assertiveness have characteristic behaviors. The first involves looking the other person in the eye during conversations. We mentioned eye contact previously in the context of genuine listening and in terms of what it means to different cultures. Eye contact also communicates that you see the other person as your equal and allows you to receive and respond to nonverbal messages. In Western cultures, eye contact is important to others perceiving you as a strong, confident, and independent person. For individuals from non-Western cultures, this behavior may be difficult and need to be learned and practiced.

Additional behaviors that you can employ include speaking with sufficient volume to be heard easily. Although raising your voice or talking loudly is perceived as aggressive, if your communication is difficult to hear, you appear lacking in confidence. Speak clearly. If others are not certain of what you said, they may simply discount what you have to say and move on in the conversation. In decision making, others may ignore your input.

Keep your message crisp and to the point. Think ahead to know what you want to say. When you ramble, or take a circuitous route to the main idea, you may lose the other person's attention. Continuing to talk and explain after you have made your point may begin to make you appear less confident.

Nonverbal gestures also must give the image of a confident and independent person. Standing straight and holding your head high reflects pride in yourself. When you make hand gestures, they should be precise and decisive, not "fluttery." Hand gestures communicate a message about self-assurance.

Use "I" statements when discussing feelings or opinions. This does not make the other person feel accused or attacked, but clearly delineates your position. You are asking the other person to consider your viewpoint and/or feelings on the subject.

LEARNING TO SAY "NO"

To establish appropriate professional boundaries with both other health care professionals and with clients, it is essential that you learn to say "no" when that is the appropriate response to a request. Saying "no" is often difficult for many nurses, perhaps because a large part of nursing is focused on meeting the needs of others. Yet it is important that we are able to do so. Chandler (2001) makes the point that saying "no" is taking a stronger stand than is saying "yes"—that it is setting the limits. Because of this, it is powerful, and, when recognized, can motivate us.

When someone requests your time for any purpose, you should think first of whether meeting the request is within your area of responsibility, whether you have the time to meet the request, and whether this is an appropriate use of your skills or energy. Failing to say "no" when it is right to do so may leave you overwhelmed by the additional responsibilities to which you have agreed and probably angry at yourself for allowing this to happen.

Although it is not always easy to do so, saying "no" when you really should say "no" is an assertive response. For example, another nurse asks you to take care of a patient's discharge while she goes to lunch. The patient needs a properly planned discharge, but you do not have the time to carry out this task. In reality, the patient's discharge needs would be better met by the person who understands the problems that have occurred and is involved in care. Assertively saying "no" provides *better* care for the patient by redirecting the task to the person who can best complete this activity.

Another example of the importance of saying "no" is seen if you are asked to do something that is outside your scope of practice or at which you are not competent. Because you are always legally accountable for your actions, you could jeopardize your own license by a failure to say "no."

Practicing techniques for saying no may be useful to you. Simple statements such as, "I'd really like to help you, but I can't;" or "I'm sorry but I can't help you right now;" said sincerely should be adequate. Remain pleasant and cordial while responding to the request. If you feel it is important to do so, you may wish to give a brief explanation of why you are saying "no." However, there is a risk that an explanation may be seen by the person making the request as a point from which to argue against your decision.

EXAMPLE *Opening the Door to Further Discussion*

Maurice Market worked on a busy surgical unit in an urban hospital. He was respected for his ability to provide direction to others. One morning at coffee he was approached by a coworker. The coworker asked Maurice whether he would allow his name to be submitted as a candidate for hospital bargaining representative. Maurice knew such activities would take a lot of additional time. He was planning to enroll at a local university to continue work toward another degree in nursing. This would not allow the time that would be needed to work as a representative. Maurice responded, "No, I'm sorry, that is something I can't do right now. It's not that I don't appreciate the importance of the job. I believe that having good representatives is important and I have always been interested in collective bargaining, but it's not something I can do right now." The coworker interpreted Maurice's continued discussion of the request as an invitation to continue to push Maurice toward allowing his name to be submitted. "You would make a fine representative. You have such good critical thinking skills that are an asset when dealing with issues," the coworker persisted in his efforts to get Maurice to agree.

CONFRONTATIONAL SKILLS

Confrontation is the process of directly addressing a problem situation with the person involved. Confrontation is needed when the problem is one of voluntary behavior that infringes on the rights of others or that interferes with work performance. Some situations that might require confrontation include an individual who is chronically late for work or who persists in taking more than the allotted time for breaks. Confrontation may be required with a coworker who habitually asks you to complete work that he or she was assigned. Sometimes confrontation is appropriate with a client or family. If a client or family has been verbally aggressive or abusive toward a health care worker, the behavior may need to be addressed. Confrontation is more problematic when addressing behaviors of a person who is in authority, such as your unit manager, or someone who has power, such as a physician. However, confronting such individuals may be necessary if you are going to advocate for a client or be able to manage your own feelings and emotional responses about the situation effectively.

People frequently avoid confrontation because they associate it with aggressive behavior. However, confrontation may be handled with assertive rather than aggressive communication. Another reason that confrontation is avoided is the concern about the response of the other person. Some individuals become very upset when confronted with a problem; they may become hostile or defensive. Others show their distress through emotional outbursts or crying. Regardless of the possible responses, some situations demand confrontation in order to move toward resolution. Ignoring or avoiding problem behaviors provides an implied endorsement of their continued expression. You will find the following behaviors helpful when you find it necessary to confront another:

- *Assess the situation.* Before you confront an individual, it is advisable to assess the situation to clearly identify the problem behavior in your own mind and be certain that confrontation is appropriate. You must be able to describe it clearly, be specific about when it occurred, and have identified how it interferes with the effective job performance of others or how it affects patient care. The more specific and clear your own communication, the more likely you are to be capable of creating change.
- *Prepare for the other person's responses.* Preparation for a confrontation also involves considering feelings. Prepare yourself emotionally to cope with the response you may encounter before you begin a confrontation. How will you respond if the individual becomes aggressive? How will you respond if the

person becomes angry? Think through the various possible responses and consider how you will manage each of them.

■ *Consider the timing.* Timing of a confrontation is critical. Sometimes you may delay a confrontation until you are more able to deal with the situation. Ignoring the situation for a time until you can manage an appropriate response might facilitate a more effective response. If you are angry, you usually are not prepared to be objective and dispassionate. If the other person is angry, that individual may not be able to hear what you have to say. However, do not put off a confrontation for too long; problem situations rarely correct themselves.

■ *If possible, conduct the confrontation in private.* A private confrontation is preferable because it is respectful of the other individual's feelings. In addition, privacy allows the other person to listen to you without the distraction and concern about the response of others present in the setting. You might simply say, "This needs to be discussed now, but it would be better if we discussed it in private." If you then indicate a place or even begin walking into an office or conference room, the other person may move with you.

■ *If in public, speak quietly and briefly.* Unfortunately, situations may arise in which behavior must be confronted when it occurs and conducting a private conversation is impossible. Speaking quietly to the person in a brief and direct manner may be necessary. In a critical situation, if you observe incorrect technique, you need to take over the task saying, "I will finish setting up this . . . and we can discuss the process after the patient is stable." Alternatively, you might say, "I have had a lot of experience with this task. I will talk you through the technique and we can discuss it later." In the light of possible legal liability, discussing another person's deficiencies in the presence of patients or family is unwise.

■ *Use assertive communication skills.* Assertive communication is essential during a confrontation. You need to clearly state your concern by using "I" statements. Try to avoid the accusatory "You always" or "You never"; rather, frame your statements in descriptive language such as, "Each day this week, I noted that you took 25 minutes for your morning break" or "Dr. Johnson, when you fail to complete medication orders in writing, it creates the potential for error and harm to the patient and demands staff time that should be available for patient care." Continuing on to describe the correct behavior or policy then sets the framework for your request that this standard be met: "Breaks are scheduled for 15 minutes only." "The hospital policy requires that medication orders include route and timing, as well as dosage."

Critical Thinking Exercise

You were appointed as charge nurse on the evening shift of an orthopedic surgical unit. You have noted that an LPN who has worked in the facility for 20 years tells family and patients that they should talk to the day charge nurse about any concerns because the evening charge nurse (you) is so new that she really doesn't know what is going on. You have decided you need to confront this individual about the behavior. Why is this a concern? What are the possible benefits and costs associated with confronting this individual? Plan a strategy including specific words you will use to talk with the LPN about your concerns.

■ USING COMMUNICATION TO MOTIVATE, COACH, AND BUILD TEAMS

As a team leader or charge nurse, much of your success in directing or delegating to staff will depend on your people-management skills—your ability to motivate those around you to achieve the highest level of job performance.

Motivating others requires skillful use of communication skills. **Motivation** may be defined as encompassing all those individual factors that cause or impel an individual to do something (Ellis & Hartley, 2004). The factors that drive behavior are considered **motives** or **motivators** and may be **intrinsic** if they arise from within or **extrinsic** if they come from outside the person. Intrinsic factors might include such things as desire to be liked, desire for recognition, or need to achieve. Extrinsic motives might include desire to make money, work in a rich environment, or drive an expensive car. It is the extrinsic motivators that involve effective use of communication skills.

Theories of Motivation

The principal objective of any theory of motivation is to explain the choices people make among a variety of possible behaviors. Understanding what factors influence your behavior and the behavior of those around you will provide an ability to enhance your own motivation and the motivation of others.

MASLOW: HIERARCHY OF NEEDS

One of the best-known contemporary theorists on motivation was Abraham Maslow, about whom you may have learned in your first nursing course. Maslow suggests that human needs are ordered in a **hierarchy** from simple to complex. The simplest needs, **physiological needs,** are the greatest behavior motivators until satisfied to the degree needed for sustaining life. Until then, most of a person's activities will be focused at this level. Security or **safety needs** become predominant once physiological needs are met. After these two lower-level needs are fairly well satisfied, **affiliation** or acceptance will emerge as dominant. When affiliation needs are dominant, a person strives for meaningful social relationships. Next, the person experiences the need for esteem, both self-esteem and recognition from others. Satisfaction of these needs produces such feelings as self-confidence, prestige, power, and control. The final need in this hierarchy is the need for **self-actualization**—the need to maximize one's potential (Maslow, 1954). In our society, most people are motivated by higher-level needs.

HERZBERG: MOTIVATION-HYGIENE THEORY

Herzberg et al. (1959) and Herzberg (1966) found that when people felt dissatisfied with their jobs, they focused on the environment in which they were working. Conversely, when people felt satisfied with their jobs, they focused on the work itself. He concluded that humans have two different categories of needs, which are essentially independent of each other and affect behavior in different ways.

Herzberg called the first category of needs **dissatisfiers,** or **hygiene factors,** because they describe our environment and serve the primary function of preventing job dissatisfaction. His use of the word *hygienes* relates to its medical meaning—prevention and concerns for a healthy environment. Hygiene factors are related to conditions under which a job is performed and include variables such as organizational policies, work conditions, interpersonal relationships, salaries, status, and job security.

Herzberg called the second category of needs **satisfiers,** or **motivators,** because they seem to be effective in moving people to superior performance. Satisfiers involve feelings regarding the work itself. They include achievement, professional growth, recognition, responsibility, and advancement—factors that expand job challenge and scope and have a positive effect on job satisfaction, workers' efforts, and output.

Although hygiene needs, when satisfied, tend to eliminate dissatisfaction, they do little to motivate an individual to superior performance. Fulfilling or satisfying the motivators, however, permits individuals to grow in their job performance, and, in turn, increase their abilities. Herzberg suggests that this can be accomplished through job enrichment, by which he means the deliberate upgrading of responsibilities, scope, and challenge in work. The clinical ladder common in many of today's hospitals might be said to reflect this concept. Clinical ladders were introduced to give staff nurses professional recognition and financial rewards for clinical expertise while allowing them to remain at the bedside.

McCLELLAND: AFFILIATION–POWER–ACHIEVEMENT

McClelland and associates (McClelland, 1953, 1961) also studied motivation. They identify three major motivators: affiliation (the desire for friendly, close social relationships), power (the need to be in control), and achievement (the desire to excel, advance, succeed, and grow). They focused much of their writing on the need for achievement and its importance in motivating many individuals.

Achievement-motivated people set moderately difficult but potentially attainable goals for themselves. They like to assume responsibility for problem solving rather than leave the outcome to chance; they believe that their efforts and abilities can positively influence the outcomes of moderately risky situations. Another characteristic of achievement-motivated people is that they seem to be more concerned with personal achievement than with the rewards these achievements may bring. Although rewards are not rejected, they are not as important as the accomplishment itself. Rewards are valuable primarily as a measure of personal performance.

Achievement-motivated people often prefer situations in which they receive concrete feedback on their performance. They tend to value task-related feedback rather than social-attitudinal-related feedback. Social-attitudinal feedback is far more important to people who are focused on the need for affiliation. **Achievement motivation** does not usually operate when people are performing routine or boring tasks in which no competition is involved. When challenge and competition are involved, however, achievement motivation will stimulate good performance. McClelland suggests that achievement-motivated people spend a lot of time thinking about doing things better and that this thinking in achievement terms precipitates positive behaviors.

McGREGOR: THEORY X AND THEORY Y

McGregor (1966) developed the concepts of Theory X and Theory Y. **Theory X** suggests that most people would rather be directed than assume responsibility for creative problem solving. They find work distasteful and are motivated primarily by physical and security needs. They must be managed through close supervision, seek rewards in money and fringe benefits, and are coerced into positive performance with threats of punishment.

Drawing on Maslow's theory of the hierarchy of needs, McGregor concluded that Theory X's assumptions about human nature are generally inaccurate, because most people, having satisfied their physical and safety needs, are motivationally dominated by the needs for affiliation, esteem, and self-actualization. Thus, he hypothesized an alternative way of viewing people at work, which he termed Theory Y.

Theory Y assumes that people are basically reliable and naturally enjoy work if conditions are favorable. It further assumes that people welcome opportunities to make contributions and can be self-directed, creative, and are motivated by exposure to progressively less external control and progressively more self-control.

McGregor believes that broadening individual responsibility is beneficial both to workers and to the organizations for which they work. Giving people the opportunity to grow and mature on the job helps them satisfy more than just physiological and safety needs. It motivates them to seek higher-level needs, to utilize more of their potential, to be more productive on the job, and to achieve more of their own and the organization's needs. This philosophy is often used in organizations focused on increasing worker productivity. The different theories of motivation are summarized in Table 5-1.

The Coaching Role

As the approach to managing others has moved toward greater involvement of subordinates in decision making, the recognition of team effort, and the development of trust and support among all employees, more attention has been focused on the role of the manager as a coach. In many ways, coaching others is not significantly different from being able to motivate them, with the exception that it takes a more humanistic and transpersonal approach. Whitworth et al. (1998) identified coaching as a collaborative process that is focused on actions that will move the client forward though the process of learning. The learning may be associated with job skills, understanding the organization, increasing productivity, meeting new challenges, or other issues specific to an organization. It is the process by which the coach helps persons fulfill their potential. Typically in a coaching situation, an experienced individual works one-on-one with a subordinate to guide their actions and build their skills and knowledge. It may cover an extended period of time and is less intense than mentoring. (See a further discussion of the coaching role in Chapter 7.)

Team Building

Another concept receiving much recognition in management circles is that of **team building.** The goal of team building is to generate a type of synergy in which the outcome of people working together toward common goals has a greater effect that can be realized by the sum efforts of having people work individually. An essential quality of a team is centered on the concept of trust, the confidence that members of the team have that their colleagues' intentions are good. Members of the team must understand and be open with one another. Once trust is established, team building can proceed with having all individuals involved in identifying the goals and establishing the processes that need to be taken to meet that goal. It builds on the concept that those closest to the problem may be able to provide the best solutions to it. The ideas

TABLE 5-1	THEORIES OF MOTIVATION	
Theory	**Description**	**Application**
Maslow Hierarchy of needs	Physiological (food, clothes, shelter) ⇓ Self-preservation (safety, protection) ⇓ Affiliation/acceptance (love, belonging) ⇓ Esteem (self-confidence, recognition) ⇓ Self-actualization (maximum achievement competence)	Managers who facilitate opportunities for employees to meet more than basic needs in the work setting will attract and retain more and better workers.
Herzberg Motivation—hygiene	Dissatisfiers/hygiene factors, which prevent job dissatisfaction focus on work environment and work conditions. **versus** Satisfiers/motivators, which promote superior performance and focus on work achievement.	Managers who provide employees with job enrichment opportunities will increase worker performance.
McClelland Affiliation, power, achievement	Major motivators: affiliation (need to belong), power (need to control), and achievement (need to succeed).	Managers who are aware of employees' unique needs for motivators and provide appropriate opportunities for needs gratification will stimulate superior work performance.
McGregor Theory X Theory Y	*Theory X* Workers are basically dissatisfied and are motivated by fear of the manager's displeasure and by money and fringe benefits. **versus** *Theory Y* Workers are basically satisfied and welcome opportunities to be self-directed and creative.	Managers who broaden employees' responsibility and opportunity for self-direction and input into decision making will enhance workers' job productivity.

of all persons count. All members of the team share in the problems and in the successes, thus building each individual's commitment to the goals of the project. Managers focus on how problems can be corrected rather than on how they occurred or who was responsible for the occurrence. Individual fault-finding is eliminated.

Lencioni (2002) has identified five dysfunctions of a team: (i) an absence of trust, which results in team members feeling vulnerable; (ii) fear of conflict, which limits healthy debate and exchange of ideas; (iii) lack of commitment due to failure to totally buy into the decisions that have been made; (iv) avoidance of accountability, which is related to lack of total commitment, and (v) inattention to results, which occurs when

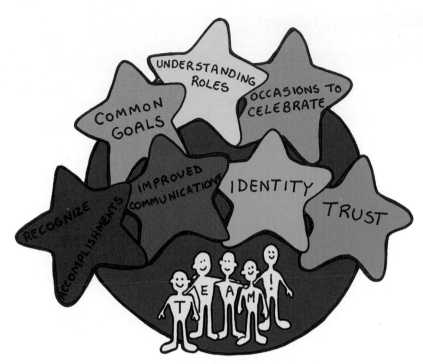

The goal of team building is to generate a type of synergy among team members.

personal egos and values take precedence. He further states the leadership role requires role modeling the willingness to be vulnerable, promoting healthy conflict, pushing for closure around issues and not worrying about making a wrong decision, creating a culture of accountability on the team, and recognizing and rewarding behavior that results in achievement of goals.

■ TECHNIQUES FOR MOTIVATING OTHERS, COACHING, AND TEAM BUILDING

As you begin assuming the responsibility for motivating, coaching, or team building, remember that different individuals will respond to different things at different times in their lives. For the new nursing assistant who is an immigrant, the most important factor may be meeting basic needs through having a much-needed income. Any threat to the number of hours worked or the job itself would be very important. For a registered nurse who has worked at your facility for a year and gained confidence in his or her own skills and abilities, achievement may be the primary motivating factor. You will need to listen carefully to others to understand what inspires them. Following is a discussion of the key factors that you will need to consider in meeting your goal of directing others through motivation, coaching, and team building.

Establish Trust and Respect

First, it is important to have the trust, respect, and thus the confidence of others. People will trust you and find you to be credible when you consistently follow up on problems and when you follow through on all promises. Create a safe environment and demonstrate confidence in what you are doing. Others will learn to trust in your judgment and your ability to provide leadership when you are knowledgeable about patient care, rules, and procedures, and all things that make you a valuable resource to others. You should strive to be respected for your knowledge, integrity, and reliability.

We tend to trust people when they keep us informed about things that are happening that will impact us. We trust them when they share their expertise, admit mistakes, and acknowledge shortcomings. If they cannot answer a question, they do not try to pretend they know or make up a response. They are honest and straightforward about missing deadlines or being unable to do something. If there is a personal problem, they deal with you face-to-face and in private (McKenna & Maister, 2002). One of the best ways to lose trust of colleagues and team members is to pretend that you have a response to a problem or knowledge that you lack. An honest, straightforward approach is always best and one you will want to develop in your professional role.

Be a Good Listener

We have already discussed the importance of active listening. Remember that active listening is the ability to understand, appreciate, and respond accurately to the feelings expressed by the other person. McKenna and Maister (2002, p. 77) identify three critical steps that will help you listen actively: "1) ask questions and encourage dialogue, 2) listen intently, making a written note of the situation, problem or request, and 3) summarize and paraphrase your colleague's situation, problem or request."

Be a Role Model

A **role model** exhibits behavior that is worthy of being copied. The way in which you organize your time (see Chapter 3) and balance your priorities should provide a model for those you want to encourage. As a role model, you can often set the tone and pace for your team. You set the standard for ethical behavior and support the view of what is important. Your own energy level can help energize others. The way you relate to staff, clients, and families models how staff should relate. Many individuals look to the person in a leadership role to determine their approach to the job.

Take an Interest in Others

One of the greatest motivators is caring. All human beings like to feel that someone cares about them. Both Maslow and McClellan focused on the importance of affiliation or acceptance—the need to be loved, to belong, to be accepted. If you are able to meet that need in the others on your team, they will be motivated to achieve the goals of client care that you have set for your team.

To convey caring, the single most important behavior for you to exhibit is a genuine interest in the members of the staff as individuals. Ask how things are going. Take an interest in their careers and help them grow. Include them in decision making regarding concerns with which they deal. When you see that people are ready for a little more responsibility, give it to them. When possible, include your nursing assistants in team discussions about patients. Include as many of your team as possible in staff development programs, even if they are not going to be directly responsible for the information or equipment discussed. This may help enlarge their perspective. Take an interest in the desire of your staff for upward mobility. Encourage them to go back to school and offer to help them by answering questions or rearranging their work schedules when possible.

Support the Competitive Spirit

As mentioned earlier, Lencioni (2002) encouraged leaders to promote healthy conflict. Some would view this as supporting competition. Although some persons may view a competitive environment as hostile or unpleasant, others thrive in such a milieu. The challenge of determining who can do something fastest, who can receive the best rating, or who can demonstrate the greatest capability is very motivating to people with a competitive spirit. These same people who enjoy being first or best, typically enjoy celebrating others' victories. Such competition is productive and the benefit for the organization is obvious.

It is important to distinguish productive competition from destructive fighting or the interpersonal politics that can sometimes be found in organizations. Unfortunately, when too much effort is invested in suppressing competitive ventures and the protection of individual's feelings and sensitivities, tension can result. This tension can often produce a situation worse than the open competition. In these situations sensitive issues must be called out and discussed openly.

Reward Positive Behaviors

Of all the factors that Herzberg identified as motivators, the two that ranked the highest were recognition and achievement. One of the best ways to encourage people is to give recognition for a job well done.

Swansburg and Swansburg (2002) support the idea that one should develop a reward system that reinforces selected values. A simple "thank you" for a task accomplished or a comment on the quality of what was done is rewarding. Your genuine pleasure in another staff member's extra efforts, your thoughtfulness in verbalizing it, your effort to acknowledge the behavior immediately, and encouragement to keep it up are extremely powerful motivators. Moreover, you should not keep good works secret. A public "thank you" is much more effective than a private one. It might even encourage other team members to act in such a way as to receive a similar reward. Never miss a legitimate opportunity to add to a staff member's pride and self-confidence. The word *legitimate* is emphasized because—as with all motivational techniques—appropriateness, honesty, and sincerity are critical. Overzealous or insincere praise is as meaningless as no praise at all.

In working with others, Blanchard and associates emphasize the importance of building trust, accentuating the positive, and redirecting the energy when mistakes occur. They state, "Attention is like sunshine to humans. What we give our attention to, grows." (Blanchard et al., 2002, p. 43).

Consider the following points when you evaluate the significance of rewarding positive behaviors:

- Positive behaviors that are reinforced by praise tend to continue or even increase.
- Negative behaviors that are not acknowledged and from which rewards are withdrawn tend to diminish.
- Positive behaviors that are not rewarded tend to diminish or even disappear over time.

EXAMPLE *The Importance of Recognizing Others' Efforts*

Alice Cheery had been a charge nurse for only 2 months. In assessing her own skills in this role, Alice determined that the staff was not as enthusiastic and motivated as she had hoped it would be. Alice reviewed all the things she might do to change the situation and decided that she would try to find more occasions to recognize the good things the staff did. She offered praise when a patient's room looked particularly nice, when work was completed in a timely manner, when someone went out of their way to help another staff member, and other day-to-day occurrences. Within 6 weeks, the tone on the unit was upbeat and people appeared to be enjoying work.

Share Goal Setting and Decision Making

As mentioned previously, achievement was one of the highest-ranking motivators. Both Herzberg, who discussed achievement in the context of satisfiers, and McClelland, who specified achievement as a motivator identified its importance. All people need to feel important and valued. People perform better when they feel they are accomplishing something important to themselves and to others. They feel a sense of achievement when contributing to a team effort—when they understand how their job fits into the overall scheme of things and how their performance affects the team's performance. If team members do not think they make a difference and instead think of their jobs as inconsequential and menial, they cannot experience job satisfaction or be high achievers. People work better when they can show off their talents, skills, and experiences.

J. M. Juran, one of the "quality gurus," addresses the need for specific goals if quality outcomes are to be achieved (Juran, 1988). Involving others in goal setting and then in making decisions about how to reach those goals help build team spirit and motivation. They help subordinates demonstrate their competence and help the manager identify areas in which teaching will increase satisfaction, both from the clients and from the workers.

To help staff members develop the ability to handle responsibility, mutual goal setting and decision making are useful. The key is to give others an opportunity to articulate their thoughts, their opinions, and even their personal goals and objectives. If staff members have no goals or have not thought them through, here is an opportunity for you to be helpful.

Offer Constructive Criticism

One of the most difficult management behaviors that must be learned by people new to the leadership role is offering constructive criticism. Some fear that if they criticize the performance of their subordinates, they will not be liked, and, consequently, those they supervise will not be responsive to their directions.

Current literature regarding correcting the behavior of subordinates places much emphasis on focusing on the error or problem as soon as possible, being very clear about what was wrong, and eliminating blame. (Review the section on team building.) When identifying an error or problem area, help others see how or why it is a problem. At times it is helpful to shoulder some of the blame for not making the task clear with statements such as, "I should have been clearer about what I expected;" or "I'm sorry I was not more clear in my directions." Then go over the task or procedure in detail to be sure it is clearly understood. Express confidence in the ability of the subordinate to satisfactorily complete the assigned responsibility. Thus, constructive criticism is directed toward the observed behavior and not toward the individual. As previously discussed, criticism should occur in private. A more comprehensive discussion of this process is found in Chapter 7 in the section dealing with evaluation and feedback.

Critical Thinking Exercise

Paul Perry is the day charge nurse on a unit for Medicare patients at Melody Nursing Center. His staff is composed of two licensed practical nurses, each giving medications and doing treatments, and four nursing assistants. He is concerned that the nursing assistants are not motivated to give the best possible care to the elderly patients on this unit. What strategies might he use to increase motivation of this staff? What barriers might he face in this setting? Whom might he enlist as allies in this process?

■ USING COMMUNICATION SKILLS TO TEACH OTHERS

Throughout much of the previous section we have alluded to the **teaching role** of the nurse manager. All good nurses are teachers. Nurses teach not only patients and families but also other nursing staff members. Teaching other nursing personnel is often overlooked as a major responsibility of the registered nurse. Some nurses feel that teaching is the sole responsibility of the staff development or in-service education department. Although this is a major component of staff education in any agency, the staff nurse frequently is required to teach other staff members. For example, experienced nurses on a unit may teach new nurses about unit routines and procedures. A nurse may teach other nurses about dealing with an unusual patient care problem. A nurse who has learned to manage a new piece of equipment may need to teach others those skills. Staff nurses may be expected to teach the assistive personnel with whom they work. As mentors or preceptors, staff nurses provide the support and teaching that helps the novice nurse to move toward expertise and the nursing student to move toward competence. Charge nurses and unit managers have even more extensive responsibilities for assuring that teaching needs are met.

Establishing a Climate for Learning

In Chapter 2, we discussed organizational climate. One part of that climate is the attitude toward learning that is shared by individuals on a particular unit or in a particular clinic. Peter Senge has written extensively about the "learning organization," which supports empowerment of employees through continued learning. Employees are encouraged to learn what is going on at every level within the organization and values and visions are shared (Senge et al., 1994). Historically, because of the nature of their services provided, health care professionals have always had a significant teaching role, whether in hospitals, clinics, communities, or other public environments.

As you move into a professional role, you will find people who value opportunities to learn, convey excitement about enhancing and expanding their practice, and demonstrate enthusiasm about incorporating new information into care patterns. At other times, you may see those who not only act disinterested but also actively resist participating. Encouraging staff to share resources, help one another, and work together as a team sets the stage for a positive climate toward teaching and learning. Are staff members included in planning for staff development in the institution? Often when people become part of the planning, they feel commitment toward attending. This is part of involving others in goal setting and decision making that we mentioned earlier.

The information that follows helps you understand some of the basic principles involved in teaching others and can guide you as you assume the responsibility for teaching others.

Applying the Teaching–Learning Theory

Staff teaching may involve informal or spontaneous incidents as well as formal, structured presentations. Informal situations occur during the day-to-day routine of providing patient care, such as showing the unit charting procedure to a newly hired licensed practical nurse or reviewing the routine for signing for narcotics with a new graduate. Formal teaching situations occur when a prepared instructor offers a specific class, such as a class in cardiopulmonary resuscitation or a class focusing on the effects of a new medication. Regardless of the type of teaching, formal or informal, when you are teaching, the process requires the application of basic the teaching–learning theory. You must understand some basic assumptions about the adult learner, teaching learning principles, and factors affecting the individual's readiness to learn.

ASSUMPTIONS RELATED TO ADULT EDUCATION

Let's begin by reviewing some assumptions related to teaching adults. Knowles (1980) identified several basic assumptions related to adult education. It is helpful to consider these before you set up your teaching situation. The assumptions are as follows:

- Adults can and will learn. In fact, they have a natural potential for learning.
- Learning is an individual experience. Learning will not occur if the individual is not ready or does not want to learn. This assumption mandates that the role of the teacher be that of a helper or facilitator of learning who works with the learner to achieve goals and objectives that the learner sees as important.

- Learning should make sense to the adult learner; that is, learning should relate to what is already known and should meet a need felt, implied, or voiced by the learner.
- Learning occurs best in a situation that tolerates differences, emphasizes growth, and is characterized by trust and respect.

PRINCIPLES OF TEACHING AND LEARNING

Adults learn best those things that they want to know and which they perceive as being meaningful to their work or personal life. Whether a person wants to learn how to play tennis or how to manage the newest infusion pump, the learning experience, regardless of difficulty, may also be enjoyable. However, if the individual has no desire to learn to play tennis or to manage the infusion pump, attempts to learn (as well as teach) will most likely fail.

Active participation in the teaching–learning process facilitates learning. Therefore, any teaching activity must provide ample opportunity for the student to participate in all stages of the process, including the assessment and planning phases as well as the implementation phase. Learners are more committed to the learning process when they have been included in determining the expected learning outcomes and the methods used to measure outcomes. When the learner is actively involved, the mind is more likely to be engaged with the learning. Active learning strategies tend to increase the time that the person is actually engaged in the learning task.

Appropriate sequencing facilitates learning. Learning is easier when it begins with what the learner already knows. For example, if a nursing assistant (NA) needs to learn a special transfer technique, the nurse teaching the nursing assistant would relate this to what the NA already knows about transferring patients. Moving from simple to complex and from concepts related to wellness to those related to illness both facilitate learning.

Feedback as to performance can facilitate learning. When learning a new skill, being coached about what you are doing correctly and what you are doing incorrectly helps you learn. Practicing incorrectly will make it more difficult by requiring that you unlearn before you can relearn. It has been said, "It is not practice alone that makes perfect but perfect practice which makes perfect."

Learning is retained longer when it is put to immediate use and when it is reinforced. Nothing motivates one to learn like success. Being able to use learning immediately not only promotes retention but also gives the learner a feeling of success. **Reinforcement** is something that the learner perceives as positive occurring as a result of performing the desired behavior. Reinforcement might be praise from a manager, a new assignment, or even an opportunity for more responsibility. The personal satisfaction from being able to accomplish the task also reinforces learning.

Mutual respect and rapport make the learning process easier. Good communication techniques are essential for establishing rapport, working through the teaching–learning process, and providing appropriate feedback and reinforcement. Teaching is an interpersonal process, a relationship between two people. Therefore, the emotional climate is important to the learning process. For more information on the conditions of learning, see Display 5-3.

FACTORS AFFECTING INDIVIDUAL LEARNING

Adult learners come to any educational process as individuals. Those who teach must recognize some of the differences that exist among learners that influence their ability to learn.

DISPLAY 5-3   **Conditions of Learning**

The learner
■ Feels a need to learn
■ Perceives the goals of learning to be his/her goals
■ Accepts a share of the responsibility of planning and implementing the learning experience
■ Experiences a feeling of commitment to learning
■ Participates actively in learning
■ Experiences a sense of progress toward goals

The learning environment is characterized by
■ Physical comfort
■ Mutual trust and respect
■ A feeling of mutual helpfulness
■ Freedom of expression
■ Acceptance of differences

The learning process
■ Relates to previous experience of the learner
■ Makes sense to the learner
■ Provides a sense of progress

Based on content from Knowles, M. S. (1980). *The Modern Practice of Adult Education: Revised and Updated.* Chicago, IL: Association Press.

Age. Adult learners may range from the beginning teen with a first job to the older adult at the age of 65 or beyond. Review your knowledge of psychosocial development and consider how the developmental stage of individuals might influence their approach to learning and their responses to you as a teacher. How might you adapt the differences that age creates?

Gender. Both men and women may be found in direct care positions. Gender difference affects both what needs to be taught and your approaches. Although both men and women caregivers may need help in understanding how to establish appropriate boundaries, differences exist in what usually is accepted behavior for men and what is accepted for women. In teaching, men and women will have different experiences and frames of reference that need to be considered.

 Ethnic and Cultural Background. In teaching, one must consider the ethnic and cultural background of the learner. For example, the numbers of assistive personnel who are immigrants or of different cultural and ethnic backgrounds from patients present challenges in the use of language and in understanding customs. Increasing numbers of patients who possess cultural and ethnic backgrounds different from the various care providers are seen in many health care facilities. Education for care providers must take the differences into consideration and help them provide culturally relevant care to all patients. Care providers must also learn to work effectively with other staff members who differ from them.

Educational Level. If you are teaching licensed personnel, you may be able to assume a consistent and standardized educational background. When teaching assistive personnel, you may find a wide range in educational levels. College students or even college graduates may be working in an assistive position as a temporary job. Those whose backgrounds include minimal formal education and few academic skills also may be working in an assistive position. Accommodations need to be made that will give consideration to those differences. For example, certification examinations for nursing assistants in long-term care may be given orally for those who do not read and write English with sufficient ability to take the written examination in English. When teaching these individuals, making reading assignments from text materials would not be an alternative.

Life Experiences. Each student brings to the classroom a wide array of life experiences. The woman who has cared for several family members through terminal illness may have a very different background from which to learn of the care of the dying patient than would the person who has never confronted death in the family. A mother who has changed diapers and cleaned up sick children who were vomiting and had diarrhea responds very differently to being taught how to help patients with such problems than does the person who has never before had to respond to such a situation. The more you understand about the previous experience of an individual, the more you are able to take that into consideration when teaching.

Learning Styles. Different people learn differently. One aspect of **learning style** is the mode of sensory input by which each individual learns most successfully and easily. Some of us learn best from hearing as input and others with visual input; some learn best through actual physical contact and touching. These tactile learners need to have a hands-on approach to learn. Although individuals can learn from all different

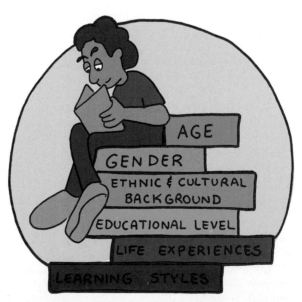

Many factors influence an individual's ability to learn.

modes, they may learn more easily in a particular mode. Using multiple modes of input often facilitates learning when that is possible.

Another aspect of learning style is the method of organizing material that an individual finds most helpful. Some like material presented in a very sequential, linear fashion. Others find such an approach boring and prefer chunks of information that can be put together at the end. The level of abstraction learners prefer may also vary, with some finding abstractions very difficult whereas others find abstract ideas interesting and challenging.

As a teacher, you will not always be able to assess and plan teaching strategies that match the learner's preferred style. However, you can vary your approach and recognize that sometimes the reason your teaching has not been successful relates to a need for different style. You can guard against the tendency to always teach in the way that most facilitated your learning without recognizing that it may not be the most comfortable or easiest for those whom you are trying to teach.

Planning for Staff Education

Planning includes assessing for learning needs, identifying the goals or objectives of teaching, and making a plan to meet those goals. Planning requires consideration of the type of learning that needs to occur as well as developing specific goals and objectives for the learning.

TYPE OF LEARNING

The type of learning that is to occur should be considered during the planning process. There are three types of learning: cognitive, psychomotor, and affective. The type of learning affects all objectives, learning activities, and evaluation strategies.

Cognitive learning involves learning facts and information. Some examples of cognitive learning are being able to name the 12 cranial nerves, listing the signs and symptoms of hemorrhagic shock, and identifying the drug classification of morphine. This information might be gained by reading, through a lecture, through a video, or from a poster. However, most individuals will need to spend personal study time to retain the material.

Psychomotor learning involves learning how to do a physical task, such as giving injections, starting an intravenous (IV) line, or transferring a patient from the bed to a chair. Knowing facts about the procedure does not mean that you can perform it. Just as riding a bicycle requires that your neuromuscular coordination develop the ability to maintain balance, starting an IV requires that your sense of touch, use of fingers, and eyesight all be coordinated. Psychomotor learning does not occur without physical practice.

The third type of learning is **affective learning,** which encompasses attitudes, values, and feelings. This type of learning occurs gradually and perhaps unconsciously. Values and attitudes are difficult to change and even more difficult to measure. However, this type of learning is often necessary if the nursing staff wishes to provide high-quality nursing care. Examples of affective learning are accepting certain ethnic or cultural groups or believing in the rights of patients or clients. It might also include your idea of the ideal nurse. Often, affective learning is "caught" from working with those who espouse these beliefs. Although affective change may be the goal, working on changes in behavior may be the focus of education. For example, you may want nursing assistants to feel respect for elderly nursing home residents. You can teach policies and protocols (cognitive learning) and require specific behaviors, such as addressing the person by the desired name, knocking on doors before entering, and providing privacy for personal care.

The type of learning determines how you will teach as well as how you will evaluate whether learning has occurred. For example, if an LPN were to ask you for help with tracheostomy care, what type of learning should occur in this situation? Obviously, this is an example of psychomotor learning. The LPN needs to learn how to do tracheostomy care and suctioning. If psychomotor learning is to occur, then simply talking about how to do the procedure will probably not accomplish the identified goals. Although reading about the procedure in the hospital manual is helpful, more teaching is needed if the learner is to accomplish the goal of doing tracheostomy care and suctioning. In addition to providing facts about how to perform the procedures, the nurse should provide a step-by-step demonstration of tracheostomy care and suctioning and an opportunity for the LPN to practice the skills.

The type of learning also affects how you evaluate the effectiveness of the teaching–learning activity. In this example, you would expect that the LPN would be able to demonstrate appropriate technique when providing tracheostomy care for the patient.

ASSESSING FOR LEARNING NEEDS

Whenever you are responsible for teaching, you will want to do a prior assessment to determine what needs to be taught; the level of understanding, skills, and abilities the learner already possesses; and factors that will affect the process of learning. Questions you could consider might include: What skills does staff seem to have the most difficulty performing well? How ready is the staff to learn more about these skills? What mandatory programs, such as fire safety, need to be repeated? Are there topics on which staff has requested more knowledge? Are there new standards, guidelines, equipment, or regulations that must be shared with staff?

In an informal teaching situation that occurs when the need arises, such as showing a new employee how to operate a piece of equipment, assessment is still important. You will need to have an understanding of what the learner already knows about that type of equipment and what experience he or she has had with it. Building on past experience is important in staff teaching.

WRITING GOALS AND OBJECTIVES

Another important part of the planning phase is identifying clear, attainable goals. Well-stated goals and objectives are just as essential in teaching as they are in planning patient care. Both give the nurse a clear direction for action and help identify when the goals have been met.

EXAMPLE *Learning About Ineffective Coping*

During morning report, Alice Mayberry, a staff nurse says, "What does the nursing diagnosis 'ineffective coping' really mean? I think we are using it incorrectly or inappropriately." Another staff member says to Jay Conner, the team leader, "Why don't you plan a class for us about nursing diagnosis?" Jay was not certain whether the staff wanted more information about ineffective coping or nursing diagnosis in general. He discussed the request with other members of the staff, learned from his assessment that staff were having difficulty with the application of ineffective coping and planned a formal teaching situation around that topic. As a part of the planning process, he developed the following objectives for the learning experience: Following an in-service presentation about the nursing diagnosis of ineffective coping, the staff will be able to

1. List the defining characteristics of ineffective coping
2. Identify possible etiologic or contributing factors
3. Write a nursing diagnosis for ineffective coping, using the correct problem–etiology–signs and symptoms (P–E–S) format
4. Identify at least three strategies that might be used to help an individual with ineffective coping

As noted in this example, an important characteristic of a clearly stated objective is the identification of who will be learning and under what conditions. In this example, the staff members are those involved in learning, and the conditions are "following an in-service presentation." Another characteristic is that behavior is stated in action verbs that can be observed. For example, Jay would be able to observe if the staff could "list," "identify," and "write." Suppose he had identified the following objective: "Know the etiologic factors related to ineffective coping." Could he observe knowing? Although knowledge (knowing) can be assessed by paper-and-pencil tests, it is difficult to observe visually.

Objectives assist us in identifying what information to present to the group and in providing guidelines for determining the effectiveness of the teaching activity. Before making the presentation, we should share these objectives with the group to be certain that the staff members agree on the identified outcomes.

By using these objectives, the team leader could easily plan a formal presentation about the nursing diagnosis of ineffective coping. An outline for the presentation would include the following:

1. Definition of ineffective coping
2. Etiologic factors that may underlie ineffective coping and would serve as the "related to" portion of the nursing diagnosis statement
3. Defining characteristics indicative of ineffective coping along with other assessment findings that might be present with ineffective coping
4. Strategies commonly used for alleviating ineffective coping
5. Practice or experience in writing a nursing diagnostic statement

Because one of the objectives involves actually writing a nursing diagnosis for a patient experiencing ineffective coping, the nurse must include time for the staff to do so.

Well-stated objectives should also include any standards used for evaluation. Objective 3 provides an example of a standard: "using correct P–E–S format." This standard provides additional information to both the learner and the teacher about the quality of the outcome and provides the basis for evaluating whether learning has occurred.

PLANNING A TEACHING STRATEGY

Selecting teaching strategies (or methods) is an important part of the planning phase. Many strategies are useful in presenting material as well as demonstrating skills. One of the most frequently used teaching strategies is the lecture, in which the teacher tells the audience about the concept to be studied. The lecture approach may be used when specific information must be imparted to the participants. If you select this method, consider handing out an outline or brief synopsis of the lecture. Providing some written information allows participants to concentrate on what's being said without having to worry about taking notes for future use. Lecture format may also be useful when the goal is to share personal thoughts and feelings or to provide motivational information. One drawback of the lecture is that it requires little participation from the audience. For that reason, you may want to consider other approaches that will encourage more participation.

One such approach is the case study. For example, the staff nurse could present information about a patient who has been diagnosed as experiencing ineffective coping. Specific information about the diagnosis could be applied to this patient situation. It really does not matter, for the sake of learning, whether the diagnosis has been made correctly. The staff should be able to meet the objectives of the presentation through examining this case.

Poster presentations are effective ways to present information about a variety of subjects, such as new drugs, unfamiliar medical diagnoses, or new procedures. All nurses on a unit may participate in education through the development of poster presentations. Posters can be placed in conspicuous places, convenient to all staff. The advantage of poster presentations is the effective use of time and the maximum involvement of the individual learner. The disadvantages include the time needed to prepare effective presentations. Figure 5-1 illustrates a poster presentation related to medications.

Keeping reference books in a convenient location on the unit and suggesting their use are other ways to support staff development. Securing subscriptions to journals helpful to staff is still another. Perhaps a committee of nurses from your unit could work together to identify needed books and journals and, if necessary, identify ways to secure funds to obtain these references. Another option is to encourage nurses on the unit to share articles out of journals to which they subscribe. It may be possible to make a copy of an article that can be circulated for people to take home to read.

Games are another interesting teaching strategy. Games encourage participation of the learner, provide a relaxed, less intimidating environment, and are fun. Crossword puzzles, bingo-type games, board games, and card games are just a few of the many types that may be used.

Filmstrips, movies, and videotapes are also effective teaching tools. These media presentations can be used for large group presentations or individual viewing. To be certain that the material matches the objectives of the activity, filmstrips and other media should be previewed before showing. The use of posters has been discussed previously.

Demonstrations are the most useful method for teaching psychomotor skills. The demonstrator should teach the major steps in the process and should emphasize critical processes, especially those related to patient and staff safety. Videotapes and movies may also be used to demonstrate skills. Filmstrips are usually less successful, because they do not show the actual movements that are critical to achieving psychomotor skills.

DRUG: Zantac (ranitidine hydrochloride)

CLASSIFICATION: Antiulcer/antisecretory

USUAL DOSE:

150 mg bid or 300 mg hs

PATIENT TEACHING TIPS:
- Encourage patient not to take with OTC antacids. MYLANTA II REDUCES ABSORPTION OF ZANTAC.
 • Smoking may decrease the effectiveness of Zantac.
- Teach family to observe for jaundice (an indicator of liver toxicity).

FIGURE 5-1
A poster presentation can be an effective way to provide information for staff.

Doing the Actual Teaching

Teaching is an interpersonal process that best takes place in an atmosphere of mutual trust in which the learner feels free to ask questions without feeling foolish. The teacher is responsible for establishing this atmosphere of trust. You can encourage feelings of trust by maintaining structure, setting limits, and giving appropriate, supportive feedback. Structure can be provided in the form of a road map for learning, which includes a clear statement of goals and objectives and clear identification of the responsibilities of both the teacher and the learner. Providing structure does not mean that the teacher is inflexible. Good structure provides for individual differences.

It is critical that you are able to communicate clearly and concisely the concepts you want others to learn. Use terms with which the learner is familiar or provide a definition of new terms as you teach. Provide time and an educational environment in which learners feel comfortable clarifying material that is unclear.

Feedback is extremely important during the teaching phase. It assists the learner by reinforcing appropriate behavior. If you intend to foster an environment of open inquiry, responding positively to all questions is essential. You may initially respond by saying, "That's a good question. Let's talk about it for a minute." If learners ask questions that are unrelated to the topic being discussed, you need to decide how to respond without squelching the learner's need to know. You may respond by saying, "That's a good question. Could we discuss it at the end of the session?"

Providing a comfortable physical environment is another consideration during the implementation phase. Before beginning a structured group presentation, you should think about the comfort of the seating arrangement, the temperature in the room, and other environmental factors such as noise and possible interruptions.

Timing is also important in implementation. Group learning should be scheduled when most of the staff can attend. Scheduling teaching at the beginning or the end of the shift may not be appropriate, because staff may be anxious to begin or leave work. In individual teaching, be sure to consider other tasks the individual may be trying to accomplish. Expecting the staff to learn something new when it feels rushed and overworked may lead to frustration on the part of both the teacher and the learner.

You will want to be certain that the teaching materials being used are appropriate for the given teaching setting. Nothing is more frustrating than trying to look at a handout over someone's shoulder or trying to read overhead transparencies that are poorly made and difficult to read. Be sure that there are adequate handouts for all participants and that group teaching materials can be easily seen by all participants.

Lastly, remember the old adage "That which is learned with laughter is learned well." If you can add some humor to your teaching, do so. This does not mean that you do not take the learning situation seriously; it means that you take just as seriously the responsibility of establishing an enjoyable learning situation. Use cartoons, jokes, or funny stories to illustrate your point when possible.

Evaluating Learning

The evaluation phase is extremely important and must never be overlooked. Just as there are numerous strategies for teaching, there are many ways to evaluate learning. Cognitive learning can be evaluated by using a variety of techniques, such as direct observation of behavior, questioning, and written measurements. In the example about the nursing diagnosis, the nurse who planned the teaching, after waiting a period of 2 to 3 weeks, could evaluate the effectiveness of teaching by surveying nursing care plans to determine whether the nursing diagnosis of ineffective coping was being used appropriately.

Psychomotor learning obviously should be evaluated in terms of the learner's ability to perform some new skill consistently. In the earlier example of the tracheotomy suctioning, the LPN should have been able to suction the patient correctly every time and without supervision. Affective learning is more difficult to evaluate, because it involves changes in attitudes, values and beliefs. A change in behavior does not always occur immediately after the teaching has taken place. Observing how the student responds to questions, expresses feelings, or reflects values will provide a basis for evaluating this type of learning.

Sometimes you will find it appropriate to administer a brief posttest at the end of the session or at a later date. Because tests are threatening to many individuals, every effort should be made to make this experience as nonthreatening as possible. This can be done in several ways. One might be to have participants complete the test anonymously. You might also have people grade their own quizzes. Answers could be given after the test is administered so that participants could assess their own progress. Another method is to have two or more participants complete one test as a group. This can give you an overview of what the group in general learned. Because staff members usually share their knowledge, this approach has value.

Finally, the teacher and the learner should remember that evaluation is just one more part of the cycle of learning. Evaluation provides guidelines for continued improvement, not retribution. Evaluation should be looked on as a kind of reassessment in which strengths and areas for improvements are identified.

Problems in Teaching Staff

Staff teaching, like many other management responsibilities, can present some challenges and concerns. Being aware of the more common problems will put you in a position to meet them more effectively.

FINDING TIME TO TEACH

A perpetual problem in nursing is finding time to do all the things that a nurse is expected to do. Finding time to teach is no exception. How long does the teaching process take? In the example of informal teaching of the LPN, the entire interaction described would last about 2 minutes and 15 seconds. What additional time will be needed on the part of this staff nurse? Other than supervising the practice, the nurse will actually be doing procedures he or she would be doing anyway, so the additional time needed to teach the LPN this skill is minimal.

Nurses seem to find time to do things they consider important. So one solution to the problem may lie in the nurse's assessment of the importance of different functions. The bottom line is a determination of what is best for patients. Meeting the staff members' need for learning and growth adds to their job satisfaction. More satisfied employees add significantly to the quality of life on a nursing unit and the quality of care provided. Teaching, like other aspects of nursing, becomes easier and more efficiently implemented with time and experience. To the staff nurse concerned with the need to teach, seizing the teachable moment soon becomes almost automatic.

ENCOURAGING AWARENESS OF LEARNING NEEDS

When functioning in the role of a teacher, nurses may have difficulty with situations in which a need for learning is indicated but the learner is unaware of the need. For example, assume you are a newly registered nurse and are assisting the nursing assistant in transferring a client from chair to bed. You notice that the assistant uses very poor body mechanics. This nursing assistant frequently complains of back pain.

In this situation, the need to learn to use better body mechanics is not obvious to the assistant. The role of the nurse as a facilitator of learning becomes much more important. It is the nurse's responsibility to help the learner identify the problem. How can you do this? Consider the following approaches:

Approach 1. You say to the assistant, "I noticed that you used very poor body mechanics when assisting the client back to bed. I think that could be the cause of all the back pain you've been having."

Approach 2. You say, "I noticed that when you were assisting the client back to bed, you winced several times as if you were having some pain. Are you having problems with your back when you are lifting and moving patients?"

The second approach, in which you related what you had observed to the nursing assistant and asked for validation as well as any other information the assistant may have to offer, is obviously better than the first. This approach will encourage the learner to explore some possible causes of the difficulty and may initiate a need to learn on the part of the learner. The second approach is less blame-directed and more supportive of the nursing assistant. Remember, learning occurs more easily if the learner is aware of the need to learn and if the material to be learned is directly related to improvement of the learner's work or personal life. The second approach also permits the nurse to gather more data before drawing conclusions.

Now let us consider another example. During a patient care conference, staff members complain that Mrs. C's family is "really getting in the way." One staff member says, "They try to do everything." Mrs. C has recently suffered a stroke, leaving her with left-sided paralysis. Her family plans to take her home following discharge. What type of learning is required in this situation? If you chose affective learning, you are correct. As you recall, affective learning deals with values, attitudes, and personal preferences. The staff in this situation needs to become more open to the needs of the family.

Affective learning involves several processes, the first of which is awareness. In the beginning, the learner may simply become aware of something. In the movie *Dead Poets' Society*, the teacher stands on the top of his desk (and has the students do so as well) to illustrate a technique of looking at things from a different perspective. If the charge nurse wants to increase awareness, he or she may have to arrange an incident in which the staff looks at the situation from a different angle. Consider these approaches by the nurse:

Approach 1. The nurse replies to the staff, "Come on, all of you know Mrs. C's family has been so attentive. Why don't you just let them do whatever they want to do and then you do the rest? You know they will be taking care of her when she goes home anyway."

Approach 2. The nurse replies, "I have noticed that working with Mrs. C and her family has been a problem for people. Can we schedule a patient care conference to discuss ways to deal with the family?"

Approach 3. The nurse replies, "Working with Mrs. C and her family does seem to be particularly frustrating. The family members are planning to care for her at home and she won't be going to long-term care. How does that make our role a little different?"

The first approach obviously destroys the teachable moment. The charge nurse does not respond to the needs of the staff or those of the patient and her family. The second approach is somewhat better, although no attention has been given to the need to encourage the staff's awareness nor are its feelings recognized.

The third approach is the best. First, the charge nurse acknowledges and accepts the staff's frustration. Then, without chastisement, the nurse provides an opportunity for the staff to consider Mrs. C and her family from a different angle. It also opens the door to having the staff involved in setting the goals and objectives for the conference. Other approaches include using "What if" statements. The charge nurse could say to the staff, "What if the family really does want to do everything for Mrs. C?" The charge nurse might also pose the question "What if we were Mrs. C's daughters? What would we want from the staff?"

Affective learning occurs at a rate different from cognitive and psychomotor learning. Thus, the nurse must be patient and tolerant of the need to move more slowly. The situation with Mrs. C provides an excellent opportunity to teach by example. The nurse may elect to work directly with Mrs. C's family, allowing them to take the lead in the care of the patient while personally functioning in the role of supervisor of that care. This type of teaching is referred to as role modeling.

HELPING STAFF MEMBERS WHO RESIST LEARNING

Nurses are occasionally confronted with an individual who appears to resist learning. The first step in dealing with this type of learner is, of course, assessment. The nurse should seek answers to questions such as, "Is there some reason this individual seems to resist teaching?" and "Is there something else going on in this person's life that is interfering with the ability to learn?" Because it is usual for adults to value learning, when faced with the situation of a person who does not appear to want to learn, contributing factors should be considered.

When working with the resistant learner, the nurse might explore ways to provide a feeling of success. The astute nurse will seek opportunities to provide positive feedback to the employee who seems to resist learning. In addition, the nurse will watch for clues about other factors, such as the employee's job satisfaction and perception of possibilities for advancement. Employees who see no future advancement opportunities may view learning in a very negative light.

Another factor that should be considered when facing the problem of the seemingly resistant learner is personal problems. Overwhelming personal problems may interfere with the employee's ability to learn. The determination of when a situation is overwhelming rests with the individual involved in the problem, not the onlooker. Severe anxiety also limits an individual's ability to be attentive and learn.

Previous learning experiences are also important to consider in determining possible reasons for the behavior of the resistant learner. Past learning experiences that were characteristically painful, frustrating, or embarrassing have tremendous influence on the individual's desire to seek new learning experiences. Providing a nonthreatening and supportive learning environment would be an important intervention with this particular learner.

Another factor to consider is the resistant learner's actual capacity to learn. The nurse can assess learning abilities of staff members on a day-to-day basis. If the learner has limited or nonexistent reading abilities, teaching strategies that involve reading will be seen as threatening experiences that they want to avoid. Providing other methods of learning, such as films, demonstrations, or lectures, would be more appropriate for the employee who has difficulty reading.

Critical Thinking Exercise

Develop a teaching plan for each of the following situations. Include the assessment you would need to complete clearly stated objectives, plans for the teaching itself, and a plan for evaluation. Provide the rationale for your choices.

1. A nursing student asks the charge nurse to tell her how to recognize early signs of oxygen deprivation.
2. A new nursing assistant asks a staff nurse to help her take an apical pulse.
3. A licensed practical nurse asks about the antidepressant Elavil that one of her patients is receiving.
4. The charge nurse observes a nursing assistant entering a long-term care resident's room without knocking.

■ KEY CONCEPTS

- The use of basic communication principles is essential to effective functioning in the management role and requires good interpersonal skills.
- Organizational communications are affected by a number of factors, including the structure of the organization, the many directions in which communications flow within an organization, and the various forms of organizational communications.
- Organization communications may be verbal, nonverbal, written, and group, and all have particular characteristics that will make them most effective.
- Active listening is an essential communication skill.
- Assertive communication involves both verbal and nonverbal strategies that are directed toward meeting your own needs without infringing on the rights of others. It may involve saying "no" to others.
- Confrontation requires that you directly address issues that interfere with the rights of others or that affect performance. You need to assess the situation carefully and then determine the strategies to be used in confrontation.
- An individual's needs, drives, and desires are his or her motives or motivators. A person's motivation is his or her desire "to do." It depends on the strength of his or her motives. Motives are directed toward goals. Goals are the anticipated rewards toward which motives are directed.
- According to Maslow's theory (hierarchy of needs), people have a group of needs that are arranged in a hierarchy from simple to complex; simple needs, such as the need for food and shelter, must be satisfied before more complex needs, such as the need for self-esteem, can be addressed.
- Herzberg (motivation-hygiene theory) felt that people have two different and distinct categories of needs. The first category he called hygienes, which are mostly environmental in nature and serve to prevent dissatisfaction but do not motivate. The second category of needs he called motivators, because they affect people's motivation to increase their performance.
- McClelland (affiliation–power–achievement) concentrated his research on achievement as a motivator and described the characteristics of the achievement-motivated person.
- McGregor (Theory X and Theory Y) stated that according to Theory X, people are basically lazy, are motivated by rewards, and need to be coerced to produce. According to Theory Y, which McGregor supported, people are basically anxious to do a good job and are motivated by recognition for a job well done and by being given more responsibility.
- Ideas and concepts about motivating others, team building, and coaching include establishing trust and respect, being a good listener, being a role model, taking an interest in others, supporting a competitive spirit, rewarding positive behavior, sharing goal setting and decision making, and offering constructive criticism.
- Teaching nursing personnel is a major function of all nurses and is a special responsibility for the charge nurse or unit manager.
- Teaching of staff may be formal or informal. Much of it may take place during the day-to-day routine of providing high-quality patient care.
- The teaching of staff is based on assumptions related to adult education:
  1. Adults can and will learn.
  2. Learning is an internal individual experience.
  3. Learning should relate to what is already known and should meet a felt need.

■ The process of teaching is guided by principles related to adult education:
   1. Adults learn best what they want to know and what they perceive to be personally relevant.
   2. Active participation on the part of the learner is necessary for learning to take place.
   3. Learning is easier when it is related to what the learner already knows.
   4. Learning is retained longer when it is put to immediate use. Reinforcement enhances learning.
   5. Teaching is an interpersonal process that occurs best in a climate of trust and acceptance.

■ Effective teaching requires the recognition of the many variables present in adult learners. Factors such as age, gender, ethnic and cultural background, educational level, other life experiences, and learning styles influence the individual participating in the teaching–learning process.

■ During the planning phase, the nurse and learner assess learning needs and identify goals and objectives, which provide direction for implementation and evaluation. Selection of teaching strategies is based on an understanding of three types of learning—cognitive, psychomotor, and affective—and the various learning styles of the participants.

■ Assessing for learning needs involves gathering information about what knowledge, skills, abilities, and attitudes are needed in the setting and comparing these with the competencies required by the demands of the setting.

■ Types of learning dictate methods of teaching and evaluation. A variety of teaching strategies can be used to meet identified objectives. These strategies include case presentations, posters, learning labs, self-learning modules and videos, individualized one-on-one teaching, and maintaining an adequate supply of reference books and journals on each unit.

■ Establishing an environment of trust is important during the actual teaching phase. The teacher should consider physical and emotional factors in the environment. During the implementation phase, feedback is important to enhance learning.

■ Evaluation is an integral part of the teaching process. It involves a reassessment of learning goals and objectives and is based on the type of learning.

■ Problem areas in staff teaching include increasing the learners' awareness of learning needs, finding time to teach, and working with the reticent learner.

REFERENCES

Blanchard, K., Lacinak, T., Tompkins, C. et al. (2002). *Whale Done: The Power of Positive Relationships*. New York: The Free Press.

Chandler, S. (2001). *100 Ways to Motivate Yourself*. Franklin Lakes, NJ: The Career Press.

Ellis, J. R., & Hartley, C. L. (2004) *Nursing in Today's World: Trends, Issues, and Management* (8th ed.). Philadelphia: Lippincott, Williams & Wilkins.

Herzberg, F. (1966). *Works and the Nature of Man*. New York: World Publishing Co.

Herzberg, F., Mausner, B., & Snyderman, B. B. (1959). *The Motivation to Work*. New York: John Wiley and Sons.

Joint Commission on Accreditation of Healthcare Organizations (JCAHO) (2003). *Hospital Accreditation Standards and Survey Process*. Oakbrook Terrace, IL: Author.

Juran, J. M. (1988). *Juran on Planning for Quality*. New York: The Free Press.

Knowles, M. S. (1980). *The Modern Practice of Adult Education: Revised and Updated.* Chicago: Association Press.

Lencioni, P. (2002). *The Five Dysfunctions of a Team.* San Francisco: Jossey-Bass.

Maslow, A. (1954). *Motivation and Personality.* New York: Harper & Row.

McClelland, D. (1953). *The Achievement Motive.* Norwalk, CT: Appleton-Century-Crofts.

McClelland, D. (1961). *The Achieving Society.* Princeton, NJ: Van Nostrand.

McGregor, D. (1966). *Leadership and Motivation.* Cambridge, MA: MIT Press.

McKenna, P. S. & Maister, D. H. (2002). *First Among Equals: How to Manage a Group of Professionals.* New York: Free Press.

Senge, P. M., Kleiner, A., Roberts, C. et al. (1994). *The Fifth Discipline Fieldbook: Strategies and Tools for Building a Learning Organization.* New York: Doubleday.

Sundeen, S. J., Stuart, G. W., Rankin, E. A. D. et al. (1998). *Nurse-Client Interaction: Implementing the Nursing Process.* St. Louis: Mosby.

Swansburg, R. C., & Swansburg, R. J. (2002). *Management and Leadership for Nurse Managers.* Boston: Jones and Bartlett.

Videbeck, S. L. (2001) *Psychiatric Mental Health Nursing.* Philadelphia: Lippincott Williams & Wilkins.

Whitworth, L., Kimsey-House, H., & Sandahl, P. (1998). *Co-active Coaching.* Palo Alto, CA: Davies-Black Publishing.

The Nurse as Decision Maker and Delegator

Learning Outcomes ▪ ▪ ▪ ▪ ▪

After completing this chapter, you should be able to:

1. Explain how critical thinking applies to the decision-making process.
2. Analyze your own dispositions toward critical thinking and how they will assist you in maintaining the standards of critical thinking.
3. Identify the steps in the decision-making process and relate these steps to the nursing process.
4. Discuss resources that will assist in identifying appropriate alternatives in the decision-making process.
5. Explain how identifying pros and cons, algorithms, and clinical pathways can be examples of decision making applied in the health care delivery system.
6. Describe the factors that will facilitate good group decision making and the various approaches that might be used.
7. Analyze concepts to be weighed when decision making involves ethical considerations.
8. Explain how nurses can facilitate the process of ethical decision making by patients and families.
9. Explain the role of delegation in nursing practice.
10. Describe the process of effectively delegating to others, including how the five rights can be assured.
11. Discuss situations in which tasks should not be delegated.
12. Identify common errors in delegation.
13. Discuss system supports that facilitate effective delegation.

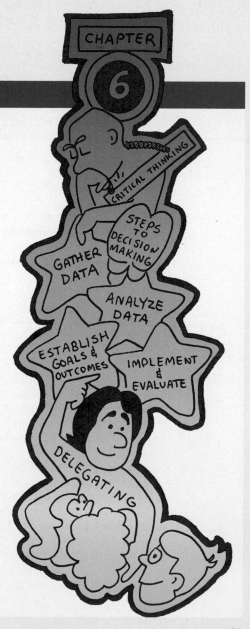

Key Terms ■ ■ ■ ■ ■

accountable	delegate/delegation	pros and cons
algorithm	delegatee	quality circles
assignment	delegator	scope of practice
autonomy	Delphi method	standards for critical
beneficence	fidelity	thinking
brainstorming	justice	strategies
clinical pathways/critical	majority rule	task force
paths	nominal group technique	thinking hats
consensus	nonmaleficence	unlicensed assistive
critical thinking	participative decision	personnel (UAP)
decision making	making	veracity

A key attribute of the registered nurse's role in modern health care is decision making. **Decision making** for nursing can be defined as a systematic cognitive process in which you must identify alternatives, evaluate those alternatives, come to a conclusion, and select an action. Registered nurses are expected to exercise judgment and make decisions based on their education and experience as well as the information at hand. Because nurses are making decisions on the behalf of patients, they are held to a high standard of effectiveness both legally and ethically. Sound decision making in nursing leads to taking action on behalf of the patient.

For nurses as managers of patient care, there are concerns beyond those for the individual patient. Nurses as managers are concerned that the actions they take are those that will result in the best outcome for the whole patient population, the most effective pattern for staffing, the most efficient process for operating a unit, or the best solution for dealing with a personnel problem. Decision making is an essential element in handling change, working with conflict, managing resources, and evaluating care and performance. Decision making is one of the major functions of the nurse manager's job. Thus, the ability to make sound decisions may be one of the most critical aspects of competent management behavior.

In the present modern health care arena, the responsibility for making sound decisions was never more critical. All nurses have management responsibilities in regard to planning patient care and may have others as well. Therefore, nurses must make effective decisions that affect groups of patients and other staff as well as their own actions. With the costs of health care rapidly increasing, the industry is becoming increasingly concerned with the economic impact of a decision as well as with client outcomes that result. Sound decisions help contain overall costs and improve productivity. They facilitate and enhance the efficient use of both human and material resources. Most importantly, they also result in improved quality of care. Effective decision making is grounded in both personal characteristics and the ability to think critically.

■ CRITICAL THINKING AND DECISION MAKING

You may have been discussing critical thinking in the context of nursing practice throughout your nursing program. We start our discussion of decision making with a review of critical thinking. Critical thinking is an essential prerequisite for making decisions. However, unlike critical thinking for some disciplines in which the intellectual process itself is the goal, in a practice discipline such as nursing, critical thinking is for the purpose of making decisions and taking action. Each attribute of the critical thinking process is important because it supports effective and appropriate actions.

According to Paul (1993, p. 20) **critical thinking** is a "systematic way to form and shape one's thinking." Paul further expands the definition as the "intellectually disciplined process of actively and skillfully conceptualizing, applying, analyzing, synthesizing, or evaluating information gathered from or generated by observation, experience, reflection, reasoning or communication." (1993, p. 110) Critical thinking, therefore, is a unique kind of purposeful thinking that is measured against certain standards. The standards require that the thinking be controlled and rigorous and involve methodical consideration of the alternatives and continual inquiry into the validity of perceptions. It requires that the strengths and limitations of our final conclusions be equally considered.

Dispositions That Support Critical Thinking

Many personal characteristics affect a nurse's ability to make effective decisions. The nurse's own philosophy, beliefs, and knowledge about nursing, human beings, and health care influence what decisions are made and how they are made. The ability of the nurse to communicate and reason also affects the decision-making process. Nurses who consistently make effective decisions develop and maintain a current knowledge base through active participation in continuing education programs, ongoing self-study, and thoughtful reflection on clinical experience.

According to Facione (1998), individuals who work at critical thinking are characterized by a common set of dispositions. Critical thinkers are *open-minded*, which means that they are open to different viewpoints, alternative interpretations of information, and willing to listen to and consider others. They try to be *systematic* in their thinking. Being systematic helps assure that you are considering all the different aspects that are important. Being *analytical* helps guide you in breaking down issues into their component parts and seeing the relationships. An *inquisitive* nature underlies constantly asking questions of both others and of yourself. An individual who is *judicious* attempts to make all judgments carefully with discretion, avoiding extremes that are difficult to justify. Further, the judicious individual attempts to be fair-minded toward others and their views. Supporting all of this is an attitude of *truthseeking*. An individual who seeks the truth is willing to give up long-held positions when evidence demonstrates them to be wrong. This often requires honesty in facing personal biases and a willingness to reconsider issues. With these characteristics, the individual with a disposition toward critical thinking will be *confident in reasoning* as an approach to problem solving and to learning. How do these characteristics relate to you? Have you considered your own willingness to engage in critical thinking? You can cultivate these attitudes in your own thinking and decision-making process (Display 6-1).

DISPLAY 6-1	Dispositions That Support Critical Thinking

Open minded
Systematic
Analytical
Inquisitive
Judicious
Truthseeking
Confident in reasoning

Standards for Critical Thinking

When we apply a critical-thinking approach to the decision-making process, we want to see certain standards consistently used. **Standards for critical thinking,** as the term is used here, is defined as a rule for the measure of quantity, extent, value, or quality of thinking. In other words, it requires that we ask ourselves questions about every aspect of the decision-making process. When you are critically thinking, you are simultaneously examining the issue before you and your own thinking process. Through monitoring your own thinking, you can improve it and the resulting decisions that you make. The standards outlined by Paul (1993) include *clarity, accuracy, precision, relevance, depth, breadth,* and *logic.* You can guide your thinking by asking yourself questions. Table 6-1 provides questions you can ask yourself as you strive to improve your critical thinking in relation to standards.

TABLE 6-1	QUESTIONS TO ANALYZE YOUR THINKING IN RELATIONSHIP TO STANDARDS
Standard	**Questions**
Clarity	Have I clearly stated the concern? Are these data clear to me? Do I understand their implications?
Accuracy	Are my facts accurate? Where did I obtain them? Can they be relied on? Do they demonstrate bias?
Precision	Am I being precise when called for rather than generalizing inappropriately? Is the level of precision appropriate to the question under consideration?
Relevance	What information is relevant to this problem? Is there other relevant information that I do not have?
Depth	Have I explored this issue in depth? Have I avoided a superficial look at a complex topic?
Breadth	Have I addressed the breadth of information needed? Is there a related topic that would shed light on this issue? Are there others who should be contacted regarding information?
Logic	Are my conclusions based on the facts that I have? Could someone else follow my line of reasoning from data to conclusion? Have I accounted for discrepancies in the data in my conclusions?

■ THE PROCESS OF DECISION MAKING

The process of decision making is the same process you have been using as the nursing process. Although the nursing process is a decision-making process for the purpose of planning patient care, the elements transfer to other situations, such as those in which you are making decisions for groups of patients, for staff, and in regard to collaboration with others. To make effective decisions, you will need to assess an entire situation through gathering appropriate data, analyze the data and come to conclusions, plan desired outcomes and actions, implement the actions, and evaluate the results. The nursing process is not a simple line from one step to another, but rather is constantly moving back and forth from one aspect to another as the situation evolves. Similarly, an effective decision-making process is active and flexible.

Data Gathering

Before you can make a decision, you must possess as complete and accurate an understanding of the situation as is possible. You will want to consider what information you must obtain and how you will go about obtaining it. In the health care environment, the information you gather will be influenced by patient and staff needs and concerns, the environment in which they exist, and the support systems available. These same factors will determine how you will obtain the information. Is the patient capable of answering questions? Should family members be involved? Which staff members should be consulted? In gathering the data, you will depend on good communication and assessment skills. You will continue to add information as it becomes available. Should relevant policies and procedures be reviewed? Are there additional resources that need to be explored?

Once you are comfortable that you have enough information with which to make a decision (or the time allowed to gather the data has ended) you are ready to move to the next step. There may be instances when you will find it necessary to make a decision in response to time constraints even when all the information you wanted is not available. In those cases, you will attempt to identify and collect the immediately available information. Failure to make decisions when they are needed results in as many or even more problems than a weak decision.

Analysis

The second step in decision making requires that you analyze the data that you have collected. Analyzing has a purpose. Through the process of analysis, we examine and study our data to determine whether they are adequate. We develop assumptions from the data, make inferences, and draw conclusions. All these intellectual activities are necessary parts of making sound decisions and should not be rushed if the situation will allow time for serious deliberation. When you are collecting data for decision making, part of the concern is identifying when you have enough data to support a conclusion. It is essential that data collection and data analysis be a constant interactive process. As data are collected, they are examined for fit with other data, for emerging patterns, for evidence of expected problems, and for discrepant findings that do not fit with what has gone before. This is where your critical-thinking skills become evident. Because nursing is a practice discipline, immersed in the "here and now" with patients, there is often limited time for data collection. However, failing to collect essential data can have very adverse consequences. In patient care, this is often clearly evident. If you failed to identify the presence of a seriously low blood pressure before deciding to administer a medication that causes vasodilatation, the consequences could be a cardiac arrest. Putting off a decision for too long in order to gather more data can have equally serious results.

EXAMPLE *Critical Thinking in Patient Care*

If a patient is exhibiting falling blood pressure and there is a protocol for initiating an intravenous (IV) line and beginning the administration of fluids in certain situations and you put off acting until you have more readings showing the rate at which the blood pressure is moving down, you may be unable to get a needle into the collapsed veins. Therefore, applying your critical thinking to the process of data collection and analysis is essential. There are times when failing to make a decision and to move forward with action will create more adverse results than to move to action with less data than would be ideal. Data needed for care of groups of patients and of managing a unit require similar approaches.

Establish Goals and Outcomes and Plan Actions

The third step, which mirrors planning in the nursing process, involves establishing desired goals and outcomes and determining alternatives for action. It requires recognizing the discrepancy between the current situation and an ideal situation and establishing a goal or outcome that will bring the situation as close to the ideal one as is possible. The desired outcome must be determined in relationship to the data that indicate the situation before the action. Goals may be both short term and long term. Identifying the desired outcome is essential to planning for action. Again, this does not stand in isolation.

The outcome also must be related to the actions being planned. Can this action achieve the desired outcome? If not, is it the outcome that is unrealistic or the action that should be changed? There is seldom a single appropriate action to achieve any particular outcome. Multiple alternatives may be identified. In the world of management, we sometimes hear alternatives referred to as **strategies.** Determining which of the alternatives to implement again requires critical thinking about the data. What do you know about the patients, the staff, the setting and how do those aspects impact the appropriate action to take? You will also want to consider such things as how much time it will take, whether needed resources are available, or whether obstacles exist to implementing the action.

When planning action, the reality is that we may have a series of alternatives that must be prioritized in the order in which they will be tried. If alternative number 1 does not work, then we try alternative number 2 (sometimes jokingly referred to as "Plan B"). For example, you may identify an approach to preventing pressure ulcers in an elderly, frail patient. However, even while planning initial measures, you are considering what else might be needed if your original actions do not appear to be working. This emphasizes the need to have a variety of good alternatives. From the alternatives, you will then choose the one that you believe is most likely to help you reach or obtain the desired outcome.

Implement the Chosen Alternative

The next logical step is to take action or implement the alternative that you have chosen. In a management role, it is possible that you will not be the person responsible for carrying out the action; your plan may be implemented by a staff nurse or another health care worker. However, you will still be **accountable** for the outcome. This means that you will answer for the outcomes that result or don't result. To assure that the desired outcomes are achieved, it is important that the plan be skillfully communicated to others and that they are adequately trained to carry out the actions. You need to be clear and specific about your decision, what you want to have done, what reports you expect to receive, and when you expect the actions to be completed. Chapter 5 gives a detailed discussion of the importance of good communications.

Evaluate Outcomes

Evaluation is the final step in the decision-making process. You will compare the actual outcomes to the goals or outcome criteria that were developed originally. You will know that the decision-making process was effective when the current situation matches the desired outcomes. Even when outcomes are met, you will find it useful to ask whether this was the best way to achieve those outcomes. You will need to examine the entire process you used as well as such factors as the use of time, energy, the impact on staff, and similar considerations. But what do we do if we find that the outcomes are not what we wanted or anticipated? Begin by reviewing the steps that we previously outlined. It is possible that one or more of the following errors occurred:

- Assessment data were inaccurate and/or incomplete, lacking necessary insight.
- Assessment data were improperly analyzed.
- Problems or concerns were not correctly or fairly identified.
- Problems or concerns were not appropriately prioritized.
- Goals were unrealistic, unclear, or imprecise.
- Decisions were reached without breadth of knowledge or the analysis of all possible alternatives and consequences.
- The strategy chosen was not reasonable or justifiable in this situation.
- The situation changed so rapidly that it was not possible to act quickly enough.
- The strategy was incorrectly implemented.
- The evaluation of responses (outcomes) was incomplete or inaccurate.

As with other skills, the more you work at decision making, the better you will become and the more effective your outcomes will be. You can learn by carefully working through the process and making decisions before asking a more experienced person for input. In this way you validate your own decision making and become more confident in your skill.

∪ Resources for Decision Making

Determining what data need to be collected and possible alternative actions for problems identified are both critical to the success of decision making. If we do not know what data are needed or whether the alternatives that we outline do not adequately allow us to work with the problem, there is little hope for resolution. Determining the data that would be important to gather may be complex; it may require collaboration with others on the health team and may require effective communication skills. What techniques are available to us to assure that we are outlining relevant, logical, realistic, appropriate, reasonable, and justifiable alternatives?

TEXTBOOKS, LIBRARIES, AND INFORMATIONAL RESOURCES

As a nursing student, one of the first resources you consult is your nursing textbook. A text provides you with a discussion of which approaches to use, why, and under what circumstances each should be considered. If you feel you need a broader review of the topic, your search may include specialty texts and professional journals. These same resources are available to you as a registered nurse. Most large medical centers have a medical library. Some journals or excerpts from journals are available on the Internet. Even when the articles themselves are not available on the Internet, the resource can be used to identify appropriate references that may be requested from a library. Relevant journal articles may be copied and placed on a staff bulletin board or even tucked in with the patient record in order for everyone caring for the patient to have information in greater depth. (See Chapter 13 for a detailed discussion of this topic).

POLICY AND PROCEDURE MANUALS

Other resources that you might consider using are the hospital policy and procedure manuals. If kept up-to-date, these manuals will provide you with information about the latest protocols for working with a wide variety of conditions and situations. They also provide the best source with regard to the approach that a particular facility has developed for working with the risk management aspects of patient care. This is particularly true in situations relating to certain trauma situations such as gunshot wounds, animal bites, and stab wounds, which are conditions often first seen in the emergency department.

EXPERIENCED COLLEAGUES

A third valuable resource can be found in your experienced colleagues. As a new graduate, this is a resource you will call on many times. Because their backgrounds include more practice, training, or education, experienced nurses can quickly identify factors that you will want to consider, implement, or further research. If you are respectful in your approach and questions, you will find colleagues are very willing to provide assistance. It is also important that as you move from your role as a novice to one of an expert in an area, you remember what it was like when you were just beginning your nursing practice and had many questions about the best ways to proceed. One of our professional obligations is to assist those who are just beginning their careers in nursing. In larger facilities, there may be expert clinical nurse spe-cialists whose role is to assist with planning for complex situations and to provide ed-ucation and guidance to the staff.

Decision-making Tools   *Aids to decision making*

Another equally important part of the decision-making process is that of choosing the best alternative from among all those that should be considered. This often involves prioritizing alternatives or using an "if this, then that" or an "if not this, then that" type of technique. A number of different approaches can be employed. Some of these are well adapted to individual use in situations in which decisions must be made rap-idly. These are discussed here in the narrative. Others are be used in more formal sit-uations in which decisions will be made over a longer period of time. These are pre-sented in Table 6-2. Further information on all these decision-making tools and references for more detailed background is available online at www.mindtools.com (MindTools, 2003).

Most of these approaches can be employed either as an individual or as a mem-ber of a group responsible for making the decision. Note that these approaches do not remove the burden of making a decision. Rather, they are aids to support an effective process.

Critical Thinking Exercise

You are thinking about making a change in your job. Using one of the decision-making tools described in the text, work through the process of making the deci-sion. What are the factors that you need to consider? What issues will weigh in the decision? Which decision-making tool did you decide to use and why?

LISTING PROS AND CONS

From past experience, everyone is familiar with the process of identifying **pros and cons** (those factors that support a particular decision and those that oppose that de-cision). These may be listed quickly in one's mind or may be listed in writing in a more formal approach. Typically, the strategy chosen for implementation is that with the longest list of pros and the shortest list of cons. The alternatives might also be evaluated from the perspective of which is most beneficial or least harmful. The im-plications of each pro or con might be noted. For example, a pro for a particular ac-tion might be decreased costs—the implication being that there would be funds avail-able for another needed purpose.

The advantages of listing pros and cons are that the method is simple and direct and can be done quickly and inexpensively. The main disadvantage is that it is diffi-cult to know all the possible alternative strategies and their various pros and cons in a typically brief time. In addition, there may be overreliance on both the subjective aspects of each pro or con and the number of pros versus the number of cons. Un-fortunately, no method will allow you to compare and contrast the various alterna-tives in an objective manner. Nurses frequently use this approach for problems re-quiring an immediate decision and in situations in which the focus is short term.

TABLE 6-2	FORMAL DECISION-MAKING TOOLS
Tool	**Description**
Decision trees	The decision tree helps you to decide between several courses of action. A decision tree may be simple or complex, but provides a visual representation of the possible options and outcomes. The decision is written in a box on the left side of a paper. Each possible strategy is written on a line drawn out from that box. At the end of each line, positive and negative effects of that strategy are written in different circles. If other decisions are needed along the branches, then these are drawn in boxes. When the tree is completed, it assists in seeing the whole scope of alternatives.
Force-field analysis	Force-field analysis is used to identify the driving forces behind a change or action and the restraining forces that will inhibit change or action. The plan is placed in the center of the page and then the forces are written on arrows with the forces for change on one side and the forces against change on the other. This visual representation again presents a whole framework and encourages addressing each aspect or adding driving forces if needed in order to create change.
Grid analysis	The matrix or decision grid is a visual grid that allows us to compare alternative strategies for attacking an actual or potential problem. Various factors relevant to the decision, such as cost, time, and resources, are written across the top of the grid. The alternative strategies are listed down the side of the grid. *Narrative style:* Where the boxes intersect, you identify factors that relate to both areas to be considered in reaching a decision. The various alternatives are easily compared. *Numerical scoring:* Each strategy is identified, and the various qualities of that strategy are assigned a numerical value ranging, for example, from 1 to 10, with a score of 10 being the highest. Scores may be assigned for desirability, probability of success, and other factors such as cost and time. These are then totaled, and a decision is reached based on the highest earned score.
Paired comparison analysis	Paired comparison is another grid technique for examining a larger number of options. Each option is assigned a letter (example A–E). On the grid, A–E become both the row titles and the column headers. Then, the square in which the column intersects with itself is blocked off. You are left with two squares that show the intersection of each pair. Block one of those off. In the remaining squares, look at the two options represented. Identify the preferred one. Put that letter in the square. Then add a numerical rating of how much better. Do this with each pair. Then add the scores for each option. The highest score is the preferred option.
Pareto analysis	This strategy focuses on deciding what to change in order to solve a problem. The basic premise is that doing 20% of any job generates 80% of the result. The problem is identified and then factors that contribute to that problem are listed. Each is assigned a numerical value. (This might relate to cost, customer complaints, or number of errors.) Then the list is reviewed and the efforts at change are directed at the contributing factor that has the highest numerical score.

ALGORITHMS

An **algorithm** is a precise set of processes that leads to specific outcome. The term originates from the algorithms in mathematical formulas. In health care, we see algorithms as a series of questions to ask that can be answered "yes" or "no" and then a set of actions or additional questions that are based on which answer was chosen. Algorithms are designed to provide a consistent approach to decision making. They can be used for many different types of decisions. In health care, we often see them designed for emergency or critical care decisions. Basic cardiopulmonary resuscitation (CPR) is an algorithm in which the first question is "Does the person respond to shaking and shouting?" If yes, CPR not needed. If no, check for breathing?" Each question requires assessment in order to determine the answer. The process continues as the responder is guided to the correct action or next needed assessment by the answer to a question. The assessment made by the nurse must be accurate for the algorithm to work. An algorithm is frequently pictured in a branching diagram.

Algorithms for critical care situations such as advanced cardiac life support (ACLS) and pediatric advanced life support (PALS) are memorized by nurses in order to facilitate their immediate and smooth implementation in the face of an emergency. Other algorithms are not designed for emergency situations and might be followed through a written plan. For example, there might be an algorithm to guide the determination of the person who can consent to medical treatment for a person who was admitted in an unconscious state. The basis of this algorithm would be the state laws regarding consent, but the algorithm simplifies the process and assures that all the correct steps are taken and documented.

CLINICAL PATHWAYS

Clinical pathways, sometimes referred to as **critical paths,** are another approach to decision making developed for use in hospitals and in home health situations. Clinical pathways spell out interventions, activities to be taken, and short-term outcomes relevant to specific diagnoses along a given timeline. They represent standardized plans for achieving desired outcomes and are an outgrowth of nursing care plans. Again, the use of clinical pathways requires ongoing assessment that must be correct. They have the benefit of being multidisciplinary and also can be used by the patient or the family. Clinical pathways establish the standard of care for each diagnosis and the outcome that should be anticipated. If adverse outcomes occur, alternative pathways may be taken.

THINKING HATS

The **thinking hats** strategy encourages you to look at a situation from multiple perspectives. You might look at all those who will be affected by a decision and consider it from each of their viewpoints. This might include the patient, the family, the physician, and the pharmacist when the decision relates to a problem with medication. You would try to consider "What would be the patient's view of this situation?" You would proceed through each person. Each decision could have a different set of people affected.

De Bono (2000) suggested a set of hats that help address different attitudes or approaches to the problem. He designated them with different colors. The white hat viewpoint considers facts and data. The yellow hat viewpoint looks at the positive ideas and takes the optimistic viewpoint. The black hat viewpoint is the pessimist and looks at all the problems and considers what you might have to do in relationship to those problems. The red hat position tries to examine the feelings and gut reactions associated with the situation. The green hat viewpoint is the creative one. From a green hat perspective you try to think of creative and new approaches. The blue hat is for the leader of a group who tries to get each of the other viewpoints on the table. The value of this approach is that it broadens your understanding and encourages you to address significant points of view that you might overlook.

■ GROUP DECISION MAKING

With the advent of approaches to management that were less authoritarian, and with shared governance becoming more and more popular, participative techniques of decision making have received more attention. **Participative decision making** means a group of individuals make the decision rather than a single individual. Group decision making can be particularly effective if the decision will have an effect on the employees making the decision. The acceptance of and commitment to the decision can be greatly enhanced when those to be affected by the decision participate in it.

Factors Resulting in Good Group Decision Making

Although group decision making has become popular, it may not always be the best approach. How will you know when to use it? When should a decision be a group decision and when should it be made by an individual? The following have been identified as important considerations in the process.

First, you should ascertain whether the group has adequate knowledge of the subject or situation. Such knowledge can be the strength of group decisions; lack of knowledge may be its downfall. If you are in the position of determining who will make the decision, you will want to be assured that those involved with the process have sufficient information and insight to produce a decision that will be effective.

Second, you will want to be assured that there is time for group decision making. Participative decision making is not appropriate for problems needing an immediate solution. Often, priorities relating to time or expense will not allow five or six persons to meet for 3 or 4 hours to reach a decision that could have been made by an individual in 15 minutes. As a third consideration, you will want to determine that the group possesses sufficient maturity to reverse the decision if it is found to be ineffective or otherwise unacceptable. A mature group also is composed of individuals who can cooperate, tolerate conflict, allow for individual differences, and support diversity and group process. The group should not be dominated by one or two individuals for whom winning is as important as the goal to be attained.

Finally, you will want to be certain that management will support the group's decision. If the members of a group believe they have the decision-making power, only to learn that someone higher up in the organization has reversed the decision, a great deal of damage can be done. Morale, productivity, and job satisfaction may all decrease.

Types of Participative Decision Making

Several different group decision-making processes are currently being used. We discuss some of the more common approaches. The advantages and disadvantages of group decision-making approaches are reflected in Display 6-2.

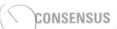

CONSENSUS

A **consensus** is a general agreement that the members of the group will support a specific strategy even if was not their most preferred strategy. Reaching decisions through a consensus requires that people thoroughly discuss their differences and be willing

DISPLAY 6-2	**Advantages and Disadvantages of Group Decision-Making Approaches**

TYPE OF PROCESS	ADVANTAGES	DISADVANTAGES
Task force	■ Uses the expertise of appointed members.	■ Members with dominant personalities may influence the group. ■ May leave members dissatisfied because the group dissolves after making recommendation.
Quality circles	■ Uses the expertise of volunteer members who share a common concern.	■ Time consuming. ■ Because of voluntary membership, may not get the best input. ■ Productivity relies on the ability of the group to work together effectively.
Brainstorming	■ Generates a large number of creative approaches.	■ Because focus is on generating a number of solutions, quality may be lacking. ■ Process can be stifled by premature critique of solutions posed.
Nominal group technique	■ Allows for consideration of a large number of alternatives. ■ Group members are not pressured toward a particular solution.	■ Time consuming. ■ Requires advance planning. ■ Members may not realize much satisfaction in the process.
Delphi method	■ Generates many alternatives. ■ Can involve a large number of participants, because they do not have to come together. ■ Because participants do not meet together, one cannot influence another.	■ Requires much time from start to finish. ■ Requires advance planning. ■ Participants may have a low sense of accomplishment.

to figure out compromises where they differ. Most often, this requires that the original proposal or alternative be revised, a process that also involves the group. The chief disadvantage of this technique is that it requires considerable time and all persons involved must be present for the discussion. However, typically it facilitates the implementation of a decision, because it has already been accepted and results in high-quality decisions. Many people responsible for providing leadership to groups like to make decisions through the process of a consensus. Consensus is particularly well suited to groups of professionals who have the same goals and work well together.

MAJORITY RULE

Another approach to decision making involves **majority rule.** A simple vote is taken and the strategy preferred by the majority is adopted. It is the system of decision making by which we elect most public officials as well as that set forth by Robert's Rules of Order used by many organizations. Making decisions by majority rule has the advantage of quick implementation and provides a way to move forward if there is not time for consensus building or if a consensus cannot be reached. Typically, the majority is considered one over half, but in certain circumstances a two-thirds majority may be required, meaning that two thirds of those voting must have supported the proposal for it to be accepted.

Majority rule means (unless there was a unanimous vote) that some persons win and others lose (see Chapter 9). The potential of a significant group in opposition to the decision is the biggest drawback to majority rule. On occasion in such situations, certain group members will form coalitions to support their position and block the action of the group. Individuals who were opposed to the decision may refuse to follow the plan. This can be damaging to the organization.

BRAINSTORMING

Brainstorming is a way to gather as many alternatives as possible. In its classical form, brainstorming is a fairly expensive process because of the personnel time involved. The manager plans a retreat away from the work environment at which participants think freely of all possible strategies. It is believed that when the participants are away from the constraints of the work environment, such as telephone interruptions and other activities, better ideas will be generated. A key aspect of brainstorming is that no ideas are critiqued as they are proposed. Everything is written down for future consideration. A good brainstorming session may last 2 or 3 days. Later, a group will sit down and begin to identify the feasibility and usefulness of the various ideas. Sometimes, the first part of the retreat involves brainstorming and the second part involves consideration of the ideas generated.

Brainstorming in a simpler format is also used as a method of solving problems in the work environment. A manager, when meeting with the staff, will say, "Let's brainstorm that problem for a while." Brainstorming in this context provides an opportunity for a manager to seek multiple ideas or strategies and it encourages others not to be critical of their own or others' contributions. This leads to sharing of ideas and may result in an increased number of strategies from which to choose. The process may not accomplish the same level of creativity as a classic brainstorming session, but it may offer a reasonable alternative to the time commitment and cost of classic brainstorming.

THE TASK FORCE

A **task force** is a group formed specifically to address a single problem or concern. This process begins with the selection of the individuals to participate in the group. They may be appointed by a manager (or several managers) or may be elected by groups within the organization The task force works best if it includes someone representing each group that will be affected by the decisions. You can see that one of the major attributes of this process is its ability to capitalize on the expertise of members of the task force. They collect information, analyze it, outline alternatives, make a recommendation, and send the recommendation to the decision maker. This might be a manager or a council of managers. After completing their work, the task force is disbanded.

QUALITY CIRCLES

Quality circles bring together persons who are working in the same area and have common concerns. They meet on a regular basis to creatively address day-to-day problems that inhibit the ability to meet their goals in a time and cost-effective manner. They also identify new strategies that would improve performance in their departments. The effectiveness of the group's decision making relies on the ability of the group to work together. In organizations that use some forms of quality management (see Chapter 4), quality circles are often empowered to implement their ideas. In other organizations, strategies that are developed are referred to a manager for permission to implement.

NOMINAL GROUP TECHNIQUE

The **nominal group technique** involves seven to ten individuals selected by the manager. The manager presents the problem to the group, and each participant writes down what he or she sees as the best solution without discussing it with others. The leader then shares the ideas with the group and writes them on a chalkboard or flip chart. There is no discussion until all ideas are written down. Then each solution is analyzed. Participants are asked to rank the solutions privately and individually from most acceptable to least acceptable. The solution that receives the highest overall ranking is then presented as the first alternative. This process allows for consideration of a number of approaches without the members of the group being pressured toward a particular approach.

THE DELPHI METHOD

The **Delphi method** is similar to the nominal group technique. The person initiating the Delphi process chooses participants. Participants may be polled for suggested alternatives, which are then compiled and distributed to the participants. The manager may add alternatives to the list. Participants then select their preferred alternative and return the written information to the organizer. The membership of the group is anonymous, with only the manager knowing to whom he or she has sent information and/or questionnaires. The fact that the participants do not meet together prevents one person from influencing the decision of another. Because the participants are never identified by name, they are free to approach the problem and suggested solutions creatively and objectively without fear of repercussions.

Critical Thinking Exercise

As a new assistant charge nurse, you have been assigned responsibility for scheduling the hours of the employees assigned to your unit. This is a task that has always been done by one individual without consultation from others. You would like to try a group decision-making process. What factors need to be considered in moving to this process? What will be the benefits? What will be the drawbacks? If you decide to proceed with your plan, how will you structure it?

■ ETHICAL DECISION MAKING

Ethics deals with concerns about right and wrong or good and evil. A certain number of those issues have clear-cut answers, at least in Western society, and are supported by laws that have been enacted through our legal system. Because of the tremendous changes that have occurred in the health care delivery system, including such areas as advances in technology, life-support systems, patients' rights, diseases for which we have yet to find a cure, and a host of treatment modalities, ethical concerns with less clear answers impinge on us daily. Whereas some of those ethical concerns require nurses to make ethical decisions, the majority of the ethical decisions in health care are made by patients and their families.

Identifying Ethical Questions

When questions arise around health care, they often arise in the context of decisions to be made about quality of life and choices around dying. These decisions have many ethical implications but are clearly patient and family decisions. Other decisions involve your personal ethical framework and the actions you will take in relationship to personal actions.

Sources of Ethical Guidance

Numerous workshops and conferences have been held to assist health care professionals in seeking personal answers to the many questions that arise. Exercises in values clarification, which encourage individuals to assess, explore, and determine their own value system, are included in most current nursing education programs. Documents such as the "Code for Nurses" developed by the American Nurses Association and the "The Patient Care Partnership: Understanding Expectations, Rights and Responsibilities" published by the American Hospital Association help provide a framework for consideration of ethical issues. All of us need to become aware of our own attitudes, beliefs, and values so that we might provide the best possible care to our clients, free of personal biases and prejudices. Ethicists also have provided us with basic ethical concepts that can be used to reach decisions. You may have been exposed to some of these precepts in humanities classes that you have taken as part of your nursing education program.

BENEFICENCE

Beneficence refers to the commitment to do or bring about good. Similar to this term is **nonmaleficence,** which means to do no harm. These two concepts are linked in the Hippocratic Oath, a code of ethics for physicians that has been administered to those about to receive a medical degree since the times of ancient Greece. We struggle with the implications of these two principles. What about treatments such as radiation and chemotherapy that bring suffering and distress? When does the potential good outweigh the known harm? Who decides what is good or bad for the individual? In the past, those in the health care system made this decision for patients out of a belief that those who understood disease, illness, and treatment were best qualified to make this decision. This is no longer true; changes in society have brought about a greater attention to the next principle.

AUTONOMY

Autonomy refers to the right of each individual to make personal decisions about those things that affect themselves. We hear a great deal about individual autonomy in discussions of consumers' rights, informed consent, right to choose, right to know, and similar applications of the concept. As health care providers, we also have autonomy and the right to make certain decisions about our personal ethics and actions. In U.S. society, autonomy is often identified as the highest value. There may be times when this is not seen as true. In some families, the highest value is their family as a whole, not the individual, and this will be reflected in the way decisions are made. The right to autonomy is difficult for us when our clients choose alternatives that are in conflict with our own value system. We also must recognize that individuals are not free to make decisions that infringe on others. For example, even if a patient decides to commit suicide, the responsible health care professional not only does not assist but also initiates action to prevent this from happening. (In Oregon, where assisted suicide is legal, there are still multiple constraints within the process and no health professional is obligated to participate.) Thus autonomy is always tempered by other ethical values.

JUSTICE

Justice relates to the obligation we have to be fair to all people. Laws in regard to nondiscrimination are based on the belief that all individuals should be treated fairly regardless of age, condition, race, religion, or sexual orientation. We challenge ourselves to define what is "fair." Justice may not mean that every person receives the same thing or the same time, but may mean that each person receives what is essential to his or her care. Where do one person's rights end and another's begin? How does justice relate to the problems of scarce medical resources? All of society struggles with how justice can be worked out within the context of social and economic realities.

FIDELITY

Fidelity refers to the obligation to carry out the agreements and responsibilities one has undertaken. We value our commitment to the patient and consider leaving a patient without handing care over to someone else as patient abandonment. Fulfilling our responsibilities is critical to assuring that the standards of good nursing are met. As professional nurses, we often struggle with the ambivalence we feel when asked to assist in an area that is understaffed (such as the labor and delivery room) when we realize we have minimal skills to provide appropriate care in that area. Although the advisable (and often only) decision is to refuse to accept an assignment in an area in which our knowledge is lacking, emotionally we may wish to help out because of our commitment to fidelity to the patient. Similar emotions are experienced by nurses when a collective bargaining unit calls a strike or takes a tough approach to improving working conditions and salaries. We also struggle with concepts of fidelity and veracity when we observe a colleague whose practice is impaired because of chemical abuse. Although some states' nurse practice acts contain regulations that clearly spell out the approach we must take to chemical abuse, this is not true in all states. To whom must we be faithful—the client, the state, or our colleague and friend?

VERACITY

Veracity refers to the obligation to tell the truth. Health care providers have obligations for veracity in the performance of their jobs. They must be honest about mistakes and not cover them up. They must be honest about any substandard practice of others and report that to the appropriate person. Patients deserve honest answers about their diagnosis and treatment. Although in the abstract this seems quite clear, there are instances in which the issue is cloudy. For example, the family of the patient with a head injury asks whether you have ever seen someone so seriously injured return to full function. You have not ever seen this happen. A simple "no" would be a true answer but may destroy hope and create great pain. Another answer that acknowledges their pain and fear and the uncertainty they face and does not directly answer their question may be far more helpful that the simple truthful word. Some would suggest that this is avoiding the issue and is therefore not acceptable. Bok, an ethical philosopher who addressed lying as a moral choice, identified that there may be situations in which telling the simple truth is not the appropriate action (Bok, 1978). The difficult task is to determine where the line lies. She suggests that recognizing the seriousness of such a decision and carefully identifying your rationale will help you to make the best choice. Talking it over with others may keep you from making such a decision without weighing the consequences. As is true for all moral decisions, you are never assured that your decision is best, but only that you did your best to make that decision responsibly.

Critical Thinking Exercise

A family, acting on its knowledge of an 89-year-old aunt, decided to discontinue the tube feedings that were maintaining the life of the woman who was in a persistent vegetative state after a massive stroke. She had been a resident of a long-term care facility for 6 years before this. The actual carrying out of this order and the expected demise of the patient were so emotionally painful to the staff who had cared for her for years that she was transferred to another facility in order to take this action. What ethical principles were upheld by the action of the family? By the actions of the staff? What ethical principles were not supported by the family's action? By the staff's action? How might you have responded?

Personal Decision Making Within an Ethical Framework

Each of us will establish our personal framework for ethical decision making. Some of these decisions will relate to everyday issues that reflect on your honesty, trustworthiness, and fidelity. Others might address your personal involvement in a specific type of care or a decision you might make to withdraw from participation in care. In addition, you will need resources as you seek to help patients and families in their decision making.

As you struggle with reaching decisions regarding ethical concerns, you will find that the decision-making steps we discussed earlier in this chapter can be applied to ethical situations. First, you will want to assess the situation and clearly identify the problem that is concerning you. Why is it bothering you? What ethical principles might be involved? Are conflicting values present? Which people are involved in the problem? Who should be involved in the decision? Next, you will gather data. As before, you will want to have as much accurate information as possible to guide your decision making. In situations involving ethical issues, it is sometimes helpful to seek other viewpoints to gain as clear a perspective as possible. You must carefully analyze the data that you have.

You will follow with the next step—identifying options or alternatives. In ethical dilemmas, often many possible alternatives exist and it is difficult to determine how one might be better than another. One of the characteristics of a dilemma is that there may be no good answer. In these instances, it is helpful to identify as many alternatives as possible. You will then have more options from which to choose.

Making a decision is not always easy. There are times when it is even painful. Likewise, accepting a decision that has been made can also be difficult. There are times when another's rights, such as autonomy, come in direct conflict with our own values. Because many of these issues are emotionally laden, you may wish to share your thoughts and concerns with others. If the decision affects employees on the unit on which you work, you may want to make arrangements for a ward conference, perhaps guided by an expert in the area creating the concern. Attorneys, ethicists, clergy, physicians, and other professionals are often willing to participate in such discussions. An agency ethics committee may be a valuable resource for decision making.

Critical Thinking Exercise

You are employed as the evening charge nurse on a postanesthesia unit. You have always believed that each nurse is responsible and accountable for the care he or she gives. You also believe that nurses should be supportive of one another, but now you are concerned that one of the older nurses who has been employed in the unit for a number of years is abusing drugs. What standards of critical thinking will you employ to gather data that will either support or dissolve your apprehensions? Are there some data that are more important than others? Why? What are your responsibilities in this situation?

Supporting Ethical Decision Making by Patients and Families

Many of the ethical decisions in health care are made by patients and families or surrogate decision makers. It is they who decide about life-sustaining treatment or its withdrawal. It is they who decide about genetic testing and abortion. What is the nurse's role in these situations? How can nurses act as advocates of patients and families and not infringe on their decision making? Shannon (1992) suggests that nurses can best help patients and families by seeing the nursing role as one of assuring that the processes used are appropriate and involve all the relevant persons. She suggests that this can be done through knowing, facilitating, and guiding.

KNOWING

Knowing refers to the nurse's own knowledge base surrounding the issue. This includes striving to know the patient better, the patient's feelings and thoughts, as well as the patient's physical condition. The nurse uses assessment skills to discover what is important to the patient, how the patient views what is currently happening, and who is significant in the patient's life. Questions of concern are "Who does the patient want for companionship?" and, conversely, "Are there those that the patient does not want involved in any decision making?" Another thing to ascertain is whether the patient is cognitively able to understand what is happening. The nurse also needs to get to know family, loved ones, and whoever may a surrogate decision maker. What are the views and concerns of these individuals? How do they fit into the overall picture of this person's care? What part will they play in any decision making?

The nurse's knowledge base must encompass the physical illness, the physician's plans for medical care, the prognosis, if one has been established. The nurse needs to understand the position of the primary provider as regards decisions. What is the ethical basis for decisions that person is making? Recognizing that those who have cared for someone for a long period of time may have feelings regarding the situation even when they have no voice in decisions helps the nurse to understand the responses of other health care providers. Above all, the nurse needs to do a self-assessment and identify personal issues, concerns, and feelings so that they do not cloud the ability to be helpful to the patient and loved ones.

FACILITATING

An important aspect of the nursing role is facilitating the acquisition of information by patients, families, and others who may be significant. Patients and families often need facts and background on which to make ethical decisions. They may need explanations of the complex language that has been used in providing information to them. For example, families may be told that the conference will discuss the patient's prognosis. Do they know what a prognosis is? Do they know what palliative care means? Patients and families also need information about resources, to whom to talk with talk about their concerns.

Another aspect is facilitating communication between and among others. Nurses have many skills to offer patients and families in facilitating communication. The nurse may identify that family members have differing perceptions of the situation and really need to talk with one another. This is often helped by having another person there to reflect on what was said or assist nonassertive family members to state their views. Sometimes the nurse may suggest that someone else be brought into the conversation: "You have mentioned how much you rely on your daughter. Would it be helpful if we arrange for her to be here as you discuss this concern?" Sometimes facilitating requires that the nurse arrange a place for family members to meet together to talk about concerns.

Facilitating communication with the medical provider is essential. It is the medical provider who will determine the medications that may be used, whether the patient is referred to hospice, whether a do-not-resuscitate order is written. The nurse is often in a position to help focus on the need for communication with the physician. "It sounds as if you have questions for the doctor. Would you like me to arrange a time for you to meet with her together?"

GUIDING

Guiding involves assisting patients and families to work toward and through the decisions they must make. Nurses can raise points that the patient and family may not have considered: "Have you thought about. . . ?" or "Have you considered. . . ?" Clarifying such as "It sounds to me as if John is saying he cannot physically manage your care at home. John, is that correct?" Sometimes guiding involves helping families to identify what is happening to themselves in the midst of the crisis, such as "Mary, you have been here for 24 hours straight. I know that you want to be here to support your mother but unless you get some rest you will not be able to do that." Guiding might include giving people "permission" to fulfill their own roles in life in the midst of an ongoing crisis. This might happen through the nurse assuring people that they can leave to take care of children and that the staff will be alert and contact them if they are needed. Sometimes the most important part is simply the presence of the nurse when difficult decisions must be made. Staying alongside provides emotional support without words.

EXAMPLE *Supporting Patient Decision Making*

A 74-year-old man who had been diagnosed with extensive lung cancer decided that he was not going to try further treatment after the initial radiation and chemotherapy were unsuccessful. He had talked with his physician and decided he wanted to leave the hospital and go home. When this man's adult son talked with a nurse about his care at home, the nurse inquired, "Did the doctor talk with you about hospice?" The son replied "Oh no! My dad's a fighter. He won't give up! He can beat this!" Clearly, the son understood neither the implications of his father's decision nor what care and support hospice might provide. The nurse replied, "I really think that you need to sit down with your father and talk about his plans and what he sees as happening during the next period of time after he is discharged. Then it will be possible to plan more effectively in relationship to his needs. He has been resting but I think it is a good time for you to talk with him. I would be glad to go in with you to answer any questions either of you might have." When this conversation occurred, the father explained that he knew not having the treatment meant that he would not survive this lung cancer, but no one could give him any assurance that more treatment would help. He helped his son face the reality that they were discussing end-of-life care. Because the nurse recognized the need for communication between those involved, this family began a conversation that was to continue over the coming months.

■ DELEGATION

Delegation occurs when you authorize a competent person to act for you or in your stead. In 1987, the National Council of State Boards of Nursing, Inc. (NCSBN) became concerned about the ability of nurses to delegate. This concern continued from 1990 to 1995 when this organization developed conceptual and historical papers on delegation. The NCSBN defines delegation as "transferring to a competent individual the authority to perform a selected nursing task in a selected situation. The nurse retains accountability for the delegation" (NCSBN, 1995, p. 2). Since that time, delegation is included in the skills that are tested within the National Council Licensure Examination for Registered Nurses (NCLEX-RN) framework.

In Chapter 1 we discussed that effective leadership and management require working with and through others to accomplish a given task. This goal requires an ability to guide, teach, and direct others. Directing others requires the ability to delegate. The degree of success a person achieves in the leadership role may well relate to his or her ability to delegate. Without delegation skills, nurses caring for patients in today's health care environment will not be able to complete their duties, tasks, and responsibilities and will find that they are stressed and exhausted by the many activities associated with their role. This can result in anger, aggression, feelings of inadequacy, frustration, depression, or lack of control. Effective delegation, like many other skills, can be learned. Once the skills of delegating are mastered, the nurse will be more productive. In addition, the nurse often will find the job and the interpersonal relationships associated with the responsibilities of the job more enjoyable.

The person who is giving the direction, that is, doing the delegating, is called the **delegator.** Although at one time in nursing, this was most likely the supervisor, head nurse, or team leader, today most registered nurses are required to delegate some aspects of nursing care. The individual to whom the tasks are assigned is referred to as the **delegatee** and is almost always an individual with less educational preparation, frequently unlicensed assistive personnel, clerks, or assistants. Both the delegator and delegatee play an important role in effective delegation.

Assignment

In many settings, the terms *delegation* and *assignment* are used interchangeably. However, **assignment** most commonly is used to describe the entire set of tasks and responsibilities given to an individual. When making daily assignments for care, this is often seen as "dividing up" the patients among the caregivers available. If you fail to take into consideration that there are many complex issues involved and not all staff members are equally appropriate to all aspects of care, you are failing in your responsibilities for managing patient care effectively. When your team contains other registered nurses, you may assign complete responsibility for patients to them. Their own scope of practice includes the expectation that they will be responsible and accountable for care. A licensed practical (vocational) nurse might be assigned to give all medications on a long-term care unit. That role lies completely within the legal scope of practice for the LPN and that individual would be accountable for giving medications appropriately. When unlicensed assistive personnel are given roles in facilities, we often speak informally of their assignment. However, they do not have a legal scope of practice and are not accountable for nursing care. They may do some tasks of care, but the oversight and accountability remain with the nurse. Thus it is sometimes helpful to distinguish that they are being delegated specific aspects of patient care and are not assigned to the patient in any comprehensive manner.

Reasons to Delegate

There are a number of reasons why it is important to delegate tasks to others. The health care industry has seen a number of changes in the last two decades. Today, as we look at the utilization of caregivers who have been educationally prepared at several levels and in a variety of programs, the importance of effectively delegating takes on new meaning and importance. As nurses strive to meet the need for quality care for all, appropriate delegation of responsibilities and tasks is critical.

COST CONTAINMENT AND THE USE OF UNLICENSED ASSISTIVE PERSONNEL

As the control of reimbursement shifts from the client to the insurance provider in capitated payment, most health care agencies providing care to the public have had to look at ways to decrease the cost of that care in order to cover operating expenses. To accomplish reduction in cost, most agencies are moving toward some type of managed care and are seeking ways to reduce costs of supplies, staffing, and overhead. (See Chapter 3 on managing resources responsibly.) This has resulted in the downsizing and restructuring of facilities providing health care.

Restructuring has included changing what is referred to as the skill mix of employees that provide care. In other words, rather than operating with a staff composed primarily of registered nurses, the new staffing patterns also include the use of caregivers prepared for these roles with varying degrees of education. Of concern to some nurses is the use of **unlicensed assistive personnel (UAP)** who are performing tasks once done by nurses. The National Council of State Board of Nursing (1995) defines UAP as "any unlicensed personnel, regardless of title, to whom nursing tasks are delegated." In health care facilities, the category of worker identified as a UAP typically includes positions with job titles as nurse aides, certified nurse assistants, nurse technicians, patient care technicians, personal care attendant, and unit assistants.

The use of UAP is based on the assumption that there are routine tasks that can be done as effectively by persons with less educational preparation and fewer other responsibilities than the individual responsible for managing nursing care. These routine tasks would be assigned (delegated) to the UAP, leaving the nurse manager to concentrate on tasks that cannot or should not be delegated to others. Because the health care facility can hire UAP for lower wages than professional nurses, it is reasoned that there is a cost saving.

Critical Thinking Exercise

You will be the team leader for a team composed of four staff members. On your team are one licensed practical nurse, two nursing assistants, and one nursing student in her final semester. As a team, you have 22 patients. Of these patients, five had abdominal hysterectomies yesterday afternoon. Four patients are scheduled for surgery this morning. Four patients are scheduled for discharge if their progress is as expected and need discharge teaching. One patient is still seriously ill with major dressings, total parenteral nutrition, and patient-controlled analgesia with morphine. Three patients are second day post-op and five are third day post-op. As you plan the assignments for your team, what activities will you delegate? To whom? Why did you make these choices?

TIME MANAGEMENT

Another reason for delegating relates to effective time management. This is an extension of the thinking that has resulted in changes in the skill mix at health care facilities. The assumption exists that many tasks occurring on a nursing unit do not require the skills of a registered nurse. Delivery services, housekeeping tasks, and clerical responsibilities have been assigned to others for many years. Now many basic nursing skills, such as checking vital signs, ambulating and transporting patients, and performing basic treatments, are being shifted to caregivers who have less educational preparation. This can result in making better use of the registered nurse's time, which is focused on assessing, coordinating, directing, and teaching, for example.

Critical Thinking Exercise

You constantly find yourself unable to complete your patient care assignments in the time available. As a new graduate, you know that this situation could become better if you were more comfortable delegating some of your responsibilities to the nursing assistants on your team. How will you go about moving yourself toward delegation? Where will you gain support? What information will you need? Where is that information available?

TEAM BUILDING

A third reason for delegating responsibilities relates to the positive effect such activity can have on building team spirit. People to whom tasks are appropriately delegated receive a sense of satisfaction and improved self-esteem when they are recognized for doing a task well. Teams function more effectively. As employees learn to handle basic skills, they are often motivated to continue their education. Delegating tasks also results in personal growth of the nurse manager, who becomes more accomplished in the skills needed to coach a team and orchestrate accountable nursing care. As outlined, delegation can be a win–win approach to patient care when carried out correctly.

Accountability and Delegation

You remain **accountable** (legally responsible for) the tasks that you delegate to others. When you delegate a task to another worker, you are freed of the time that it would take you to carry out those responsibilities, but you remain answerable (accountable) for ensuring that the task is completed properly. Once completed, appropriate communication associated with the tasks that have been delegated must also occur. Patient care must be documented and the response to treatments communicated to others. The NCSBN (1995, p. 3) states, "The delegating nurse is responsible for an individualized assessment of the patient and situational circumstances, and for ascertaining the competence of the delegatee before delegating any task. The practice-pervasive functions of assessment, evaluation and nursing judgment must not be delegated." This requires knowledge and judgment on the part of the nurse.

Some nurses become concerned about delegation because they believe that another person is "working on their license." This is a misunderstanding of the meaning of accountability. The nurse is accountable for delegating appropriately according to the five rights of delegation discussed later. If the nurse knows that the individual has received training on a particular aspect of care and has been authorized by the agency to perform that care, and is legally allowed to perform that care, then the nurse can delegate the task and the individual will be responsible for doing it correctly. The nurse will not find him or herself in legal jeopardy if the delegatee made an error. However, if the nurse fails to assure that the person to whom a task is delegated has the necessary skill, then the nurse will be legally liable for having delegated inappropriately. There is legal responsibility in delegation.

Legal liability aside, the nurse is responsible for the overall nursing process in relation to the patient's care. The responsible nurse oversees the patient's care in order that the desired outcomes are met. Failure to follow through on appropriate oversight might not result in an error but might result in plans of care not being revised when needed or early signs of problems not being noted.

Characteristics of Successful Delegation

 A number of factors can result in delegation either working successfully or compromising patient care. As with all new experiences, the individual who is new to the delegation process may need assistance and may need to revise plans more frequently. The person new to delegation may need more time to make decisions about appropriate delegation. An experienced mentor can assist you in becoming a more skilled delegator.

The NCSBN has identified the five rights of delegation (NCSBN, 1995):

1. Right task
2. Right circumstances
3. Right person
4. Right direction/communication
5. Right supervision/evaluation

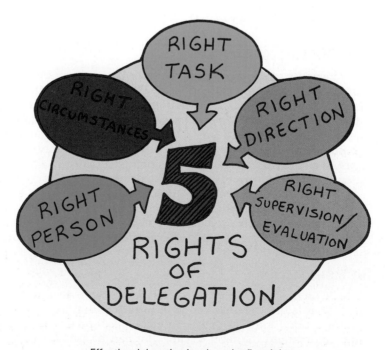

Effective delegation involves the five rights.

Achieving these five rights requires the collaborative effort of both the nursing service administrator and the staff nurse. The nursing service administrator is responsible for such items as job descriptions; role delineation; development of organizational policies, procedures, and standards; and assurance of adequate human resources. The staff nurse is responsible for assessing the client, delegating appropriately, communicating clearly, providing monitoring and supervision, and other "do" aspects of delegation. You can see how the two roles are important and work together to assure good patient care.

To assure that the five rights are carried out appropriately, you may wish to follow steps we just discussed in relation to decision making for decisions related to delegation.

Assessment and Analysis in Regard to Delegation

Before you delegate responsibilities to others, you need to thoroughly assess in regard to the first three of the five rights of delegation. Delegation can only occur when there is a match between the patient's needs that will be met by the delegatee and the delegatee's level of competence and understanding. This means that tasks that are beyond the ability of the delegatee (regardless of that individual's title within the organization) will not be delegated to that person.

ASSURING THE RIGHT TASK

What task or tasks need to be done? Is this a task that requires skilled nursing for either assessment or to carry out the task? Is this a task that is restricted by law in regard the person who can carry out this task? The tasks being delegated must not require the use of nursing judgment while being carried out. This means that the tasks are routine in nature and that they can be performed according to exact, unchanging directions.

ASSURING THE RIGHT CIRCUMSTANCES

What are the circumstances of the patient at this time? Has there been an appropriate assessment of the patient? Is the patient stable? Is the patient at high risk? What is the plan for patient care? What are the outcomes desired for this patient? Is there teaching that must be done simultaneously? Exactly what is needed at this time? An assessment of the client's needs must have been completed by a registered nurse and communicated to others for any client for whom you intend to delegate any aspect of care. If a complete assessment has not been done, specific needs may not have been identified that may not be noticed by persons with lesser educational preparation.

You will want to be assured that the client's condition is relatively stable and that there is not much potential for change. The results of the care that is being delegated should be reasonably predictable. For example, if the UAP is assigned the task of ambulating a client, the client is expected to be able to ambulate with assistance.

ASSURING THE RIGHT PERSON

Who is on my team? What does each person's job description or license allow them to do? What is this person's **scope of practice;** that is, what are they legally allowed to do? What do I know of their training, skills, and abilities? The delegator must know and understand the level of care that can be performed by the delegatee. In other words, the nurse making the assignment is aware of the competency level of the individual to whom care is being assigned. You will need to know how often the delegatee has completed certain tasks and/or what his or her level of preparation for such an assignment has been. You can learn to be more comfortable when delegating tasks to others if you understand their job descriptions and personal abilities and limitations.

When you have registered nurses on your team, you are most likely aware of their capabilities. You are at least familiar with their scope of practice. However, some of you may not have worked with licensed practical (vocational) nurses. What they may do in regard to patient care varies from state to state because of differences in licensing laws. You will need to investigate what your state outlines as the scope of practice for the LPN. Within these legal constraints, you will also need to learn the agency policy regarding the role of LPNs and what protocols they can carry out. Beyond this and as stated earlier, you will also want to consider what you know of the individual's strengths and weaknesses. What skills were taught to the individual in orientation? Where has that individual been working? How long has the individual been working? What are his or her unique strengths and weaknesses? What type of client has the individual been working with? What are the requirements of the task? What is the level of skill required? What experience has the delegatee had with those expectations? How long will it take this person to complete the assignment? What has already been assigned to that individual? How do I know the individual is capable of handling the responsibility?

Planning for Delegation

With the information you have gathered, you will plan specifically what tasks or responsibilities you will delegate to those on your team. To do this, you will need to ask yourself questions about matching the person with the tasks. Finding the answers to questions such as these will help assure that you are delegating the right task to the right person, that you are matching the complexity of the task with the skills of the worker. You will consider these things as you determine the assignments of all the various members of your team. This will help assure that the individuals to whom you are delegating the tasks have the necessary knowledge and skill to carry out your requests and that sufficient time is available for them to complete the assignments. When you are a charge nurse, this may include delegating the specific roles and responsibilities to a variety of individuals, such as licensed practical (vocational) nurses and unlicensed assistive personnel, in order to assure appropriate care for the group of clients for whom you are responsible.

You want an outcome of your planning to result in assigning the right task to the right person. The unlicensed care providers on your team are much more limited in their scope of practice. Sometimes unlicensed care providers do not clearly understand their own roles or may not appreciate that there are differences in level of responsibility. In these situations, you will be educating the individuals as well as assigning them to care.

Planning ahead helps prevent problems before they occur and helps assure that the circumstances surrounding the delegation are right. This involves identifying, in your mind, the persons who can best handle the tasks that you wish to delegate. Typically, this includes tasks that are routine in nature for which there are established protocols and outcomes. Such tasks usually require little decision making or critical thinking. Adequate time and personnel are available to provide the needed supervision. All delegated activities need supervision and follow-up. When either the time or the personnel to provide this is lacking, problems may result.

 ## Implementing Your Plan for Delegation

Once you have decided on the basis of your assessment and planning, what tasks to assign to which workers, it is important that you communicate your expectations clearly. This is the point of right communication in the NCSBN list. Clear communications ensure that others know what is expected of them. This should be done on a client-specific and delegatee-specific basis. Delegatees need to know specifically what you expect them to do and when you expect the task to be completed. They need to know the specific activities to be performed and any specific client instructions and limitations. With this knowledge, they are more able to follow through on the tasks that have been assigned. It is helpful to the delegatee if you briefly explain the purpose or reasons for what you have asked them to do. While quickly explaining the reasons, it would also be appropriate to include any limitations or restrictions that must be considered. For example, you instruct the nursing assistant to help transfer a patient from her bed to the wheelchair. "Mary, please assist Mrs. Jones to move from her bed to the wheelchair before lunch is delivered. She lacks the strength to move herself but needs to get up. Her left side is weak because of her stroke so be sure she is adequately supported on the left side." Thus, in a very short period of time you have indicated what you want to have done, why it is necessary to do it, the limitations that must be considered, and the time during which you expect it to be done.

You want to be certain to allot sufficient time to ensure clear guidance and direction. You should anticipate how you will assure that the instructions are understood and able to be followed correctly. This becomes even more critical if you are working with people from another culture, for whom the communication process may be different from your own or if the assistive person is using English as a second language. (See Chapter 5 on communication). This can be assured by allowing the delegatee opportunity for feedback or questions. Allowing for feedback is especially important when working with individuals who speak English as a second language. In the previous situation, you might be more certain she understands what you expect the delegatee to do by asking, "Do you have any questions about getting Mrs. Jones up?" Mary's response will indicate her understanding of your expectations. It is important that you let assistants know what things you expect to have reported back to you and when you want them reported. Can it wait until toward the end of the shift? Should you know immediately? You also need to indicate which actions you see as possessing a critical timeline for accomplishment. This means that you help the assistive personnel establish priorities for care.

When a task is delegated, it is critical that you provide the autonomy for the delegatees to decide how to accomplish their work. If you look over their shoulder or supervise their activities too closely, you will communicate that you lack confidence in their ability. This further robs them of self-esteem. Following too closely will also consume the time you need to do those tasks that cannot be delegated. This is one of the most difficult aspects of delegating for the person who is new to such skills. The novice to the art of delegating is anxious to assure that care is given properly and in a timely manner. As a student, you may have learned that the best way to assure that care was given properly was by doing all of the task yourself. Initially, most people

DISPLAY 6-3	**Common Errors in Delegation**

Failure to delegate
Failure to release control
Inadequate or unclear directions
Lack of follow-up or supervision

have difficulty letting go of these learned behaviors and becoming comfortable as-signing some tasks to others. See Display 6-3 for a summary of the common errors in delegation.

Evaluation of Delegated Duties

When you are working with and through others, you can assure that care is provided to appropriate standards by providing the right supervision and evaluation. This is the right supervision aspect of the characteristics of effective delegation. Supervision is the "provision of guidance or direction, evaluation and follow-up by the licensed nurse for accomplishment of a nursing task delegated to unlicensed assistive per-sonnel" (NCSBN, 1995). You might monitor the quality of the work by visiting selected patient rooms to ascertain that the environment has been appropriately maintained. You may double-check selected patient records to be sure that documentation is be-ing done according to standards. You will ask for and obtain feedback on the care given and the basic status of the client. When others are to provide assessment data for you, you may need to specifically ask for the data to be reported, and follow-up may be necessary. You will want to check back with the individuals to whom you have assigned tasks to determine that the responsibilities were completed without problems, to learn any other facts pertinent to care that may have emerged, and to provide reinforcement to the delegatee for a job well done. This can be easily accom-plished without seeming to check-up on the activities of the delegatee or creating the impression that you are not certain the task will be done correctly. Observing the del-egatee as you move about your own tasks allows for much assessment. How is the person working? Do the patients who were assigned to this person's care look com-fortable? Are the rooms neat? Do the tasks appear to have been completed in a timely manner? Does the patient or the patient's family seem satisfied with the care?

Asking for the delegatee's input or impressions is a good method of receiving feedback. Questions such as "Did Mrs. Jones seem to appreciate getting out of her bed?", "Did you have any difficulty getting Mrs. Jones into the wheelchair?", or "How did Mrs. Jones respond to getting out of her bed?" might be appropriate openings to discussion of the delegated task we discussed earlier. At this time, it is also important that you provide positive comments regarding activities that were done well. Positive feedback is a powerful motivator (see Chapter 7 on providing evaluation and feed-back). You need to look at your own schedule and determine that you will be avail-able to provide adequate supervision and assistance if needed.

Supervision includes checking with individuals throughout the day to determine whether they are completing tasks. For example, you might monitor a nursing assistant by checking with him or her every 2 hours to find out what tasks have been accomplished and what is yet to be done. If care is not progressing quickly enough, you will need to examine the environment and the situation to determine what needs to be modified. It may be that someone else needs to provide assistance. You may need to help this individual with setting priorities. However, employees should be encouraged to attempt to solve problems themselves and should be encouraged to ask questions or seek clarification about the task anytime before its completion. This means that you must be available to the employee to whom you have delegated responsibilities.

This emphasizes the point that asking others to do a task does not absolve you of any further follow-through. As stated earlier (and it bears repeating), when you are the registered nurse delegating tasks to others, you remain accountable for the accomplishment of those tasks. You will need to supervise patient care to assure that it is provided appropriately. Supervising care means that you know what is happening with the patients and with the staff, what has been accomplished, and whether any problems are occurring. When you are supervising the accomplishment of the assignments you have given to others, it is important to communicate a feeling of being helpful rather than critical. You also need to leave the responsibility for the task with the delegatee as opposed to taking back the responsibility for seeing that it is accomplished. We will discuss that in more detail later. You can gain information about the status of care by asking such questions as "How are you doing with your tasks?" "Is there anything with which you need assistance?" "What problems have you encountered this morning?" "Do you have any questions?" or "How are things going?" If you notice that the individual seems flustered or frustrated, statements such as "You seem to be bothered by something" may encourage the individual to share with you concerns that might otherwise be overlooked.

If you are working effectively as a manager of care, you will want to be certain that all patients have been adequately evaluated and that their needs have been anticipated as early as possible. You will also want to be certain that the right services have been provided and the needs that relate to quality outcomes have been addressed (See Display 6-4 for successful delegation tips.)

DISPLAY 6-4	**Tips for Delegating Successfully**

■ Know the abilities of team members, including their scope of practice and educational preparation.
■ Plan ahead to prevent problems.
■ Match the tasks to be accomplished with the skill level of the person to whom the tasks are being delegated.
■ Communicate your expectations clearly; ask for feedback.
■ Provide needed authority for accomplishing the task to the person to whom the task is delegated. Don't take back tasks.
■ Monitor how the task is being accomplished.
■ Assess results.
■ Provide positive feedback as is appropriate.

Critical Thinking Exercise

The following events are occurring at 6:30 p.m. on the surgical unit. As the charge nurse, consider what action is a priority and what actions can be delegated to others if they are available.

a. A family member is at the desk complaining about care and demanding to see the nurse in charge.

b. A physician is waiting in a patient's room for assistance in performing a difficult and complex dressing change.

c. The unit secretary tells you that a patient has called and asked for his pain medication.

d. The admitting department has called and stated that they have a patient ready to send to your unit for admission.

e. You have not had time to take your dinner break, and the hospital cafeteria stops serving dinner in half an hour.

■ DETERMINING WHEN NOT TO DELEGATE

Just as it is important to delegate some tasks, some situations occur in which a nurse should not delegate. It is important that you recognize these situations and retain authority and responsibility for the nursing actions.

Legal Limitations

The most obvious of the times you should not delegate is represented by activities that are not within the scope of practice of the individual to whom you might delegate the task. The scope of practice for registered nurses and for licensed practical/vocational nurses is outlined in state practice acts and may vary from state to state. Some states also license nursing assistants. You need a clear understanding of the scope of practice outlined in the practice act. You cannot delegate something that the delegatee is not allowed to do. When working with individuals who are unlicensed, it is important that you have a good understanding of the job descriptions or specific competency certification operative in the agency or facility in which you are working.

Jobs Requiring Specialized Skill, Knowledge, or Position

It is not appropriate to delegate jobs that require specialized skill and knowledge or those that are specifically associated with your role as a registered nurse. For example, completing a neurologic assessment should not be delegated. Even nonspecialized tasks may be inappropriate to delegate if the delegatee lacks specific knowledge. Asking a nursing assistant to secure an unusual piece of technical equipment that is needed for an examination later in the day may result in frustration and wasted time, because the UAP may not understand the equipment well enough to be able to efficiently locate the equipment you are requesting.

Similarly, if you are working in the capacity of charge nurse in a long-term care facility and one aspect of your job description includes evaluating the performance of the certified nursing assistants working on the unit, this is not a task to be delegated. When you delegate tasks that are clearly a part of your role, you not only erode that role, but you also deny yourself the opportunity to build confidence and trust with your staff, to enhance morale, and to maintain overall control.

Tasks requiring nursing judgment should not be delegated to those without formal nursing education. Questions that you should ask yourself are, "Does this caregiver have the ability to carry out this responsibility?" "Are the expected results predictable?" "Can the task be completed without additional directions and without complex observations?", "Does the task involve critical decision making?" "Does the task require ongoing nursing assessment?" and "If the individual needs assistance, am I available to help?" Quickly thinking about these answers will help you determine which tasks should be delegated and which you would be wiser to perform yourself.

■ COMMON ERRORS OCCURRING IN DELEGATION

As we stated earlier, delegation is a skill that can be learned. Those who do not approach it thoughtfully may make some errors in the process. Some of the more common errors are discussed next.

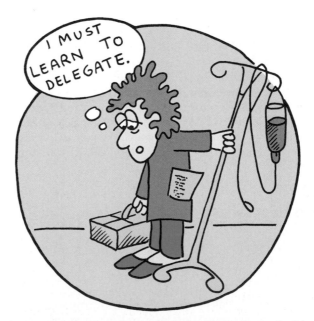

New graduates may overload themselves in an effort to be fair.

Overloading Yourself

A common error of newly registered nurses is overloading themselves in an effort to be fair. For example, if there are many patients who need IV medications and high levels of assessment skills, you should not assign all the patients to your own care and give lesser prepared staff total responsibility for the remaining patients. You may need to work in partnership with a nursing assistant, who can provide for standard-ized needs and routine care, so that you have the time to focus on priorities of care that only you are educated and licensed to provide.

Adapting to Old Patterns of Behavior

Another problem for beginning nurses arises when staff members have a previous pattern of assignment with which you disagree. The "We've always done it this way" argument may seem overwhelming. Use your knowledge of management styles and your communication skills to work with your team to achieve an assignment pat-tern that everyone supports. Perhaps there are strengths to their pattern that you do not understand. Perhaps they have not considered alternatives to solve prob-lems they encounter. Working collaboratively with the staff and demonstrating re-spect for their experience will help you achieve higher-quality care and better inter-personal relationships.

Unclear Communications

We have already provided considerable discussion regarding the importance of clear communication. However, we need to indicate that unclear communication is one of the common errors of the person new to delegation. After assignments are deter-mined, you should concentrate on giving clear instructions to others. If you are not certain that an assignment you have made is clearly understood, ask the person to repeat the instructions. Be thorough; define what you expect the outcomes of the as-signment will be. You may feel at times as if you are spending a lot of time coaching, but remember that coaching is a critical part of managing a team. (See Chapter 12 for more discussion of the coaching role.)

Failing to Release Control

Many things interfere with our ability to delegate. One may be our need for control. An inability to delegate may be a result of the feeling, "If I want it done correctly, I'd better do it myself." It may also reflect an anxiety about mistakes: "What if she makes a mistake and I am accountable for the patient's care?" These responses may be re-lated to lack of confidence in the ability of others, to a fear of losing control, or to con-cern that someone else may do the job better. When you feel reluctant to delegate, ex-amine the situation closely. Are there real barriers, such as inadequately prepared assistive personnel, or are the barriers within you?

Under normal circumstances, once the task is delegated the delegator should not take it back. You must give the person to whom you have delegated the responsibility the authority to carry the task forward. Having authority means that staff members can obtain adequate resources, assistance, and information. It also means that you will check with them regarding progress on the task but will not step in and take over unless absolutely necessary. If the task is not completed in a timely manner, you should be certain that your instructions included expectations regarding timelines. When you delegate a task and then perform it yourself, you communicate to delegatees that you lack confidence in their ability to carry out what you have requested. It implies dissatisfaction with their performance.

Yielding to the Pressure to Delegate Inappropriately

Situations may occur in the work environment in which you are pressured to delegate inappropriately. The most common of these situations occurs when there is just so much work to be accomplished that you cannot see how it can all be managed. You feel so overloaded with responsibilities that you have a tremendous need to get all tasks accomplished. You then ask others to carry out responsibilities that are not appropriate for their level of education or training.

For example, assume you are working in a long-term care facility. You may find that you are overloaded with treatments and administering medication, and the doctor has just arrived on the unit and wants you to make rounds with him. At the same time, you are notified that a new patient is arriving on the unit. You ask the licensed vocational nurse who is working with you to do the admission. Although this may safely get the patient into bed, it results in an incomplete assessment of the patient. Specific data need to be gathered by the registered nurse that will be used in planning care that cannot be gathered by others. The chaotic nature of the unit has pushed you into inappropriate delegation.

At other times, nurses feel pushed into delegating by their superiors who may be encouraging the delegation in an effort to reduce your load. You need to remain in control of your own practice, making the critical decisions about what you will do and what you can safely delegate to another. If you believe that you are being asked to delegate a responsibility that you need to complete yourself, you will need to assume an advocacy-type role. Diplomatically pointing out the reasons that you believe you should do the task, while remaining respectful of your supervisor's role, is usually adequate in such circumstances.

■ SUPPORT FOR EFFECTIVE DELEGATION

Although the changes that have occurred in the delivery of health care seem to mandate that all nurses be skilled in the art of delegation, supports are needed within the system to facilitate effective delegation.

Job Descriptions

As new and different jobs are created in the health care delivery system, it is important that the tasks associated with these jobs be analyzed and that job descriptions be developed for them. Task analysis involves looking at the what, how, how often, and why of activities. After the analysis is completed, tasks need to be bundled; that is, the tasks need to be assigned to a particular job description (Minnick & Pischke-Winn, 1996). Things that need to be considered include the examination of the predictability and the frequency or timing of the tasks, the preparation that is needed to carry out the task, and the worker's motivation for completing the task. Too often, new positions are created or new workers are brought into the care environment without the adequate development of job descriptions. In other instances, the job descriptions have been developed but have not been adequately communicated to the individuals who need to be knowledgeable about them. At times, the individual responsible for delegating assignments is working without adequate information about the job of the person to whom tasks are delegated. When a clear understanding of the role to be played by all individuals working in a given situation is lacking, role confusion results. This often leads to conflict in the work environment. (See Chapter 9 for content related to managing conflict.)

Recruitment and Selection

Once job descriptions are developed, realistic timetables for recruiting and selecting workers must be put into place. This includes job postings, testing for competencies or aptitudes, background investigations, interviewing, health screenings, and salary negotiations. If any parts of this process are hurried or overlooked, the best-qualified individuals will not be brought into new positions. High turnover among staff may result. Problems result for the nurse in settings in which turnover is high. The demands of delegation may mean that the registered nurse is not gaining time for higher-level tasks. The nurse may find that he or she simply trades time with patients for time with UAP who need much help and assistance in the initial stages of their employment. High turnover results in persons never getting beyond the initial stages.

Providing Time for Delegation

Nurses need time for assessment of patients, planning of care, and the teaching and communicating, which are essential attributes of the nurse's role. Time taken from direct patient care for supervising and teaching lesser-prepared workers may be resented by nurses if they feel that there is not enough time to fulfill nursing responsibilities. Therefore, the use of assistive personnel must be balanced with the needs of the patients for care by a registered nurse. A system design that recognizes the essential role of the nurse and includes this in planning for staff mix supports effective patient care and the time for delegation.

Effective Training

All individuals who are involved in patient care and its delegation should have adequate training and preparation for their roles. The training that is required can be of two types. The first type of training to be considered is that which occurs with the new employee. This can range anywhere from a formal orientation to the facility to actual on-the-job type of skill preparation. The training provided should be aligned with the job description for the position the employee will fill. It also should be geared to their previous level of understanding or preparation. (See Chapter 5 for content on teaching staff.) The use of assistive personnel and the high rate of turnover that occurs among assistive personnel often create the demand for ongoing teaching by the registered nurse. If assistive personnel are not well trained, then the nurse may end up redoing work that was not done correctly or patient care is negatively impacted.

The second type of training that needs to occur is the preparation of individuals who will be responsible for supervising the new workers. They need to be aware of the level of ability of the worker, the jobs they are expected to fulfill, and any limitations that need to be taken into consideration. If the positions involve a defined scope of practice, this information should also be shared with the supervisor.

Critical Thinking Exercise

From your reading, identify those aspects of delegation that you believe to be the most important. Talk with a classmate and see if that person views the situation similarly. Discuss why you have both chosen similar approaches or discuss the reason for your differences of opinion. Did either of you change your point of view after the discussion?

■ KEY CONCEPTS

- Decision making in nursing is a systematic process involving judgments. The nurse's prior knowledge about health care, clinical experience, and practice in decision making is critical.
- Critical thinking, based on standards of clarity, accuracy, precision, relevance, depth, breadth, and logic, is the basis for effective decision making. The effective nurse cultivates a disposition toward critical thinking by trying to be open minded, systematic, analytical, inquisitive, judicious, truthseeking, and confident in reasoning.
- The process of decision making is similar to the nursing process and involves gathering data, analyzing the data, establishing outcomes and action plans, implementing the chosen alternative, and evaluating the outcomes. These aspects are not linear steps but constantly reflect back and forth.
- There are a wide variety of resources available to assist in decision making. These include textbooks, libraries, and informational resources; policy and procedure manuals; and experienced colleagues.
- A number of decision-making tools are available to assist with the process. Simple tools include listing pros and cons, following algorithms, using clinical pathways, and striving to view the situation from multiple perspectives. More formal decision-making tools include using a decision tree, force-field analysis, grid analysis, paired-comparison analysis, and Pareto analysis.
- Participatory (group) decision making may be employed, depending on the time available, the knowledge and maturity of the group, and support of management.

■ Participatory decision making is commonly employed in today's society. Participative decisions may be made by consensus, majority rule, brainstorming, the task force, quality circles, nominal group techniques, and the Delphi method.

■ Reviewing guidelines for decision making may help assure that the outcomes are positive. This includes considering the time allowed and the situation, acting promptly once the decision is reached and using good communication skills to assure that the decision is appropriately implemented and evaluated.

■ When problems occur in the decision-making process, they should be reviewed to identify errors in the process. The more the decision-making process is critically applied, the better one is able to use it skillfully.

■ Many times, the decisions made by a nurse involve ethical issues. Several basic ethical concepts can guide us in this process. These include the concepts of beneficence, nonmaleficence, autonomy, justice, fidelity, and veracity.

■ Nurses assist patients, families, and others in the ethical decision-making process through knowing, facilitating, and guiding.

■ Delegation is the art of transferring to a competent individual the authority to perform a selected nursing task in a given situation. The nurse retains accountability for the delegation.

■ Skillful delegation allows the nurse responsible for managing care to make good use of professional knowledge and to more effectively manage time.

■ The NCSBN has identified five rights associated with delegation: right task, right circumstances, right person, right direction/communication, and right supervision/evaluation.

■ To determine which tasks can be delegated and which should not, factors that you will want to consider include legal ramifications such as scope of practice, skill level of the delegatee, whether the task requires nursing judgment, whether the results are predictable and the task can be performed without further instruction, whether the task requires critical judgment, and whether the task requires ongoing nursing assessment.

■ Effective delegation can be completed by using a nursing process format that requires assessing the situation, analyzing the data, planning outcomes and actions, implementing the planned actions, and providing evaluation through follow-up.

■ Being able to communicate effectively is critical to the ability to delegate.

■ Individuals new to the art of delegating may make common errors, such as overloading themselves, trying to be too fair, following old established behaviors, and failing to release control of the situation.

■ Work environments that support effective delegation include current job descriptions, effective timelines for recruiting and selecting employees, adequate training of the new employee and/or their supervisor, and recognition of the teaching role required for delegation.

REFERENCES

Bok, S. (1978). *Lying: Moral Choice in Public and Private Life.* New York: Random House.

De Bono, E. (2000). *Six Thinking Hats* (rev. ed.). London: Penguin Books.

Facione, P. (1998). *Critical Thinking: What It Is and Why It Counts* [Online]. Available from California Academic Press at http://www.insightassessment.com/pdf_files/what&why98.pdf. Accessed May 11, 2004.

MindTools. (2003). *Techniques for Effective Decision Making* [Online]. Available at http://www.mindtools.com/pages/main/newMN_TED.htm. Accessed August 3, 2003.

Minnick, A., & Pischke-Winn, K. (1996). Work redesign: Making it a reality. *Nursing Management*

National Council of State Boards of Nursing (NCSBN). (1995). *Delegation: Concepts and Decision-Making Process.* Chicago: National Council of State Boards of Nursing.

Paul, R. W. (1993). *Critical Thinking: How to Prepare Students for a Rapidly Changing World.* Santa Rosa, CA: Foundation for Critical Thinking.

Shannon, S. (1992) *Caring for the Critically Ill Patient Receiving Life-Sustaining Therapy: Combining Descriptive and Normative Research in Ethics.* Unpublished Dissertation, University of Washington, as adapted in Wilkie, D. J. (2001) *T-NEEL (Toolkit for Nursing Excellence at End of Life Transition).* Seattle: University of Washington. Available as CD-ROM.

7 The Nurse as Supervisor and Evaluator

Learning Outcomes ■ ■ ■ ■ ■

After completing this chapter, you should be able to:

1. Describe the essential elements of effective supervision.
2. Discuss the purposes of evaluation and feedback.
3. Identify standards on which evaluation should be based.
4. List at least five guidelines to be observed when providing both positive and negative feedback.
5. Discuss the purposes of performance appraisal from the perspectives of both the employee and the organization.
6. Identify three characteristics of an effective performance evaluation system.
7. Explain the advantages and disadvantages of using narrative techniques, rating scales, checklists, and management by objectives as evaluation tools.
8. Explain how the timing of a performance appraisal interview and the place in which it is conducted may affect the outcome.
9. Discuss how peer evaluation may be used to enhance nursing practice.
10. Explain the process of progressive discipline.
11. Develop a personal strategy for responding effectively to personal feedback and performance appraisal.

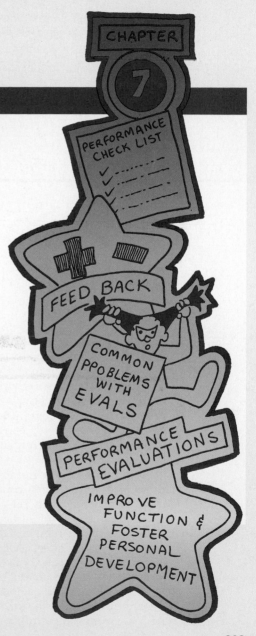

CHAPTER 7

PERFORMANCE CHECK LIST

FEED BACK

COMMON PROBLEMS WITH EVALS

PERFORMANCE EVALUATIONS

IMPROVE FUNCTION & FOSTER PERSONAL DEVELOPMENT

Key Terms ■ ■ ■ ■ ■

checklists	management by objectives	progressive discipline
coach	mentee	rater bias
coaching	mentor	rating scales
coaching role	mentoring	self-evaluation
critical-incident technique	narrative or essay technique	second reprimand
disciplinary procedures		standards of care
due process	negative feedback	standards of nursing practice
employee performance evaluation	peer evaluation	
	performance appraisal	supervisor
field review	performance feedback	supervisory role
first reprimand	performance standards	suspension
interview	positive feedback	termination
job descriptions	positive performance	written reprimand

W hat do we mean when we speak of the nurse as supervisor? Federal labor law contains a definition of **supervisor** that governs collective bargaining. This federal definition relates to having the authority to hire and fire or make the recommendations that can result in those actions. Based on this definition, nurse unit managers are legally supervisors. However, in every nursing workplace, nurses are responsible for the nursing care provided to clients or patients in that environment. As we mentioned when discussing delegation, registered nurses retain this responsibility regardless of whether someone else is providing part of that care. This places the nurse in a supervisory role in relationship to other caregivers although the focus is on the supervision of care.

Additionally, the nurse is often called on to provide performance feedback to these individuals. **Performance feedback** provides individuals with information on their own behavior in relationship to expectations and standards. Informal feedback works best when it is immediate and not delayed. In Chapter 5, we discussed aspects of motivation, and one of the factors that motivates people is receiving feedback on performance. Evaluation of personal performance, accompanied by well-structured feedback, can be key to an individual's improvement and continued growth. It is also essential to the provision of high-quality patient care.

This chapter focuses on developing clear standards and methods for performance supervision and evaluation and various methods, both informal and formal, for communicating the information to others. These approaches to evaluation

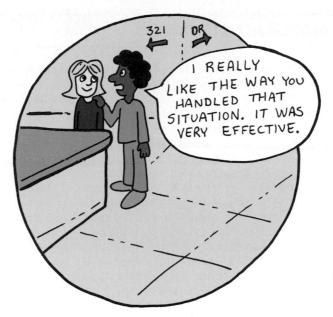

Informal feedback gives the employee day-to-day and hour-to-hour information about their performance.

help you to overcome personal bias and enable you to provide objective, useful feedback to others. We examine the day-to-day feedback that is often termed *coaching* as well as the formal performance appraisal. Characteristics of a good performance appraisal system are presented, and different tools that can be used in the process discussed briefly. We also review some of the pitfalls encountered in the process.

Communication skills create the essential foundation for providing feedback appropriately. As discussed in Chapter 5, you will need to be aware of your own nonverbal as well as verbal messages. You will need to be skilled in assertive communication and able to confront others when appropriate. Basic interpersonal relationships that include trust and genuineness will make your feedback to others less threatening and more useful.

■ THE RELATIONSHIP BETWEEN SUPERVISION AND EVALUATION

Supervision involves the total oversight of someone else's work. It includes assuring that he or she understands the expectations, that the work is assigned and structured appropriately, that the work is observed, and that performance is evaluated against the expectations. Therefore, we discuss supervision and evaluation together, because one cannot happen effectively without the other. While overseeing an individual's performance in order to assure appropriate care, simultaneously you must evaluate both the outcome for the patient and the performance.

■ **PERFORMANCE STANDARDS**

Whether your evaluation is informal or formal, you should strive to base it on appropriate **performance standards.** What are those standards? How do you articulate them? Does the person being evaluated know what those standards are? Are they aware of the expectations of the job?

Some of the standards that may be used for evaluation include job descriptions, policies and procedures, and standards of practice (see Chapter 2). A good evaluation system includes standards for attitude and interpersonal skills along with specific job-related clinical skills. These are often referred to in business as soft skills.

You will be comparing specific behaviors of the individual with standards. When they match or exceed the standard, positive feedback is important. When they fail to meet the standard, then you have objective data regarding the behavioral discrepancy to communicate to the individual.

Use of clear standards can help protect against bias in evaluation. Many types of bias may occur without the individual's self-awareness. For example, the person who is outgoing and friendly may create a positive impact even when skills are very ordinary. Of course, attitudes are also important but must not be confused with other expected skills. Attractive personal appearance creates bias in favor of an individual (Drogosz & Levy, 1996). Bias based on gender or racial and ethnic background is illegal as well as poor practice.

Job Descriptions

As discussed in Chapter 2, each organization has many job descriptions that, when reviewed in total, provide a great deal of information about the structure of the organization. **Job descriptions** should contain statements that describe the duties for which the employee is responsible. They should include only those characteristics that are important and necessary for successful performance. Good job descriptions are kept up-to-date and are clearly written so as to avoid differing interpretation. The best employee evaluation systems evolve from job descriptions. In other words, an individual would be evaluated on the basis of what that person is expected to accomplish within the organization.

As discussed in Chapter 2, nursing job descriptions are based on the purpose, philosophy, and objectives of the nursing department. They include the performance standards for the nursing role. For example, if the department expects all registered nurses to be responsible for ensuring that nursing care plans for the patients assigned to their care are up-to-date, then the job description should state, "Maintains current nursing care plans for all patients." It may seem that developing this degree of specificity about each position in an organization would be a never-ending job, but it actually saves time and misunderstanding once it is done. People understand what is to be done and who is to do it.

When you are evaluating someone, ask yourself, "What is the job description for this individual?" or "Is this person expected to be performing this task?" Your familiarity with job descriptions will make evaluation more specific and objective. However, job descriptions alone do not fully describe what an individual does. These documents must always be somewhat general and open ended to possess the flexibility required to meet the changing needs of the patients and of the organization.

Policies and Procedures

As pointed out in Chapter 2, each health care agency has specific policies and procedures that describe when and how actions are to be carried out. Most institutions provide instruction in regard to policies and procedures as part of employee orientation processes. Most policies relate to patient care activities. Policies may also relate to timeliness, absenteeism, and participation in agency committees. Important policies may be reinforced by discussions at intershift report, posted signs, and frequent staff education classes.

Some policies are so important to an organization that every person is expected to know the policies and adhere to them always. An example might be a policy in a long-term care facility that states, "All staff will knock on the resident's door and wait for acknowledgment before entering the room." Regulatory authorities require that residents in long-term care have privacy.

However, from a realistic point of view, other policies are not used often. For example, there may be a policy that specifies what the nurse is to do when a patient states that he or she wishes to leave the facility against medical advice. Because this happens rarely, the nurse may not be certain of the appropriate actions when encountering this behavior and would be expected to consult the policy manual. Planning an employee evaluation system includes identifying which policies the individual is expected to know and which the individual would be expected to verify by checking in a manual when the policies are needed.

A well-thought-out evaluation includes the individual's proficiency with skills required for the specific position. Some skills may be universal, such as those required for cardiopulmonary resuscitation (CPR). Other needed skills may differ between units. This may include use of specific equipment and supplies. Agency procedure manuals attempt to systematize the approach to common procedures to help assure standard outcomes. Many health care agencies have a standard plan for checking the competencies of staff in regard to essential skills in their particular unit. These competency checks are often done in a workshop fashion, where staff members move between stations, with each station set up for a particular skill. If an individual fails the competency test, then remedial teaching is provided and the person retests to demonstrate the expected competency. When you are observing an individual, you must be familiar with the standards for procedures in use at the facility in order to evaluate performance. For example, in a long-term care facility, a transfer procedure may require the application of a gait belt before beginning. That step may be absent from the procedure in an acute care facility.

The Joint Commission on Accreditation of Healthcare Organizations (JCAHO), often referred to simply as the Joint Commission, requires that institutions assure that employees are competent to perform their assigned duties. Competency testing for technical skills provides a consistent, clear approach to evaluation that is easily implemented. Competency testing for critical thinking and problem solving is much more difficult to accomplish. Some institutions are using scenarios to check decision-making competence. Direct observation of an individual problem solving in real patient care situations remains the best method of determining competence in these high-level skills.

Standards of Nursing Practice

There are general **standards of nursing practice** that specify expected behaviors of the registered nurse. These can be used as a basis for measuring the performance of registered nurses. The American Nurses Association (ANA) has developed both generic standards for nursing practice and specialized standards of nursing practice that pertain to specialty areas of nursing practice. These standards are less specific than agency standards but may speak to broad conceptual issues such as the nurse acting as an advocate for the patient. Standards of nursing practice have also been developed by specialty organizations, such as the Infusion Nurses Society.

Standards of Care

Standards of care identify specific expectations regarding processes that must be implemented in the care of patients. Regulatory authorities usually develop these. In long-term care, the standard created by Medicare and Medicaid requires that all residents have initial assessments completed to a specific format and content within a stated number of days after admission. If doing the admission assessment is part of a particular nurse's job, this standard of care can be used to evaluate the nurse's performance. In an acute care facility, the Joint Commission has a standard of care for effective pain management. Based on this, the nurse could be evaluated for his or her role in achieving that outcome.

Soft Skills Needed in Health Care

The entire world of business is discussing the importance of what are referred to as *soft skills.* Soft skills relate to attitudes, relationships, and communication. These are the skills that cannot be measured as easily as a specific technical skill but that are critical to effective performance. Within health care, some of the soft skills are described in institutional mission and values statements. This is where you find the emphasis on respect and nondiscrimination. Staff members in health care must cooperate in order to carry out some direct care tasks, such as transferring a dependent patient from a bed to a gurney. They also are required to collaborate effectively with people from other departments in order for each person to create an effective schedule for accomplishing patient care. The attitude communicated by staff to patients and visitors creates a strong image of the organization. Although an organization may list these skills or characteristics as essential, there is often no specific behavioral description for each. Therefore, you will discover that spending time reflecting on what behaviors you believe reflect each of these skills will enable you to more clearly communicate expectations to staff.

Critical Thinking Exercise

Consider the clinical area in which you are practicing as a student. Identify one or two staff members on that unit who you believe exemplify excellent soft skills. What behaviors have you seen that are the basis of your determination? Consider the following attributes: What behaviors communicate caring? What behaviors communicate customer service? What behaviors communicate cooperation? What does respectful communication sound like?

■ COLLECTING DATA FOR EVALUATION

When your evaluation of a subordinate is informal, collecting data is relatively simple. You may observe a specific behavior, compare it mentally to the standard, and then provide immediate feedback to the individual about that behavior. Techniques for providing feedback are discussed later.

When your evaluation is formal, that is, you are responsible for a person's performance appraisal, collecting data requires prior thought and attention. There are standards for your data collection as well as for performance. Data used for performance appraisal should be accurate, address the individual's behavior (as opposed to personality characteristics), and be representative of the person's work, with exceptional instances noted as such.

Basing your formal evaluation on specific behavioral information is essential. Without specific behavioral information, you are making assumptions about the behavior of the individual. When you meet for a performance review, the individual may feel that your evaluation has no basis in fact. This is very counterproductive to effective employee relationships. To gather specific behavioral information, you will need to be where you can observe an employee's performance or behavior.

To collect accurate behavioral information, you may need to make special plans to review a person's documentation and observe patient interactions. A good manager learns to hone observation skills so that whenever he or she is in the clinical environment, observations are made. In some instances, you may need information on behavior from others. For example, a unit manager may be writing a performance appraisal when the employee works evenings and the manager works days. In this instance, there may need to be a specific plan for the charge nurse to serve as a data gatherer. The employee should know that this is the plan for the collection of some evaluation data. The unit manager may still be able to personally review documentation, note attendance patterns, review how the report was recorded, and other such behavioral information.

As mentioned previously, you will need to guard against personal bias in your evaluations. Personal bias may occur both positively and negatively. When a person has a good reputation, is well liked and personable, it is easy to overlook behaviors that are marginal, such as being late. Conversely, when an individual does not participate socially with the staff and may not have good soft skills, it becomes easy to accumulate a list of minor problems, such as not straightening up the utility room, and focus on those behaviors.

Bias is particularly problematic when it is related to a person's cultural or ethnic background. Although specific laws prohibit biased actions based on ethnicity, cultural background, gender, or marital status, this would be an unethical practice even if the laws did not exist. Bias may be subtle. For example, if the evaluator is a person who values eye contact and an assertive attitude, the person whose ethnic background teaches that these are disrespectful behaviors may be criticized. If assertive behavior is essential to effective performance in the position, then the manager needs to identify how the individual with a different cultural background can be assisted to meet this standard. Each person deserves respect and to be evaluated fairly.

Another concern is allowing one incident to cloud or overwhelm other data. Again this could be a very positive or very negative event. When an otherwise fine employee makes a serious error, it would be a mistake to focus an entire performance evaluation on the error. The error must be noted and dealt with, but the other fine performance must also be acknowledged. The other extreme is the marginal employee who worked effectively with a very troublesome patient. The tendency is to focus on the work with the troublesome patient and not address the areas in which the individual really needs to improve. Performance appraisals should address the totality of a person's performance. Behaviors chosen for discussion should primarily be representative of the person's work, with exceptional situations noted as such.

Be especially careful not to criticize employees for problems that are outside of their control. This simply creates resentment, because the individual is powerless to change the situation (Langdon & Osborne, 2001). For example, timely initiation of new medical treatment orders may be an institutional goal. This can be monitored on a computerized system that notes when the order was submitted and when it was first carried out. If the order is for a new medication and the medication does not arrive from pharmacy, the nurse cannot be held accountable for late administration.

■ THE COACHING ROLE

You will be functioning in a coaching role when you work with nursing students, when you precept new employees, and when you help current employees to learn new skills or improve practice. Because the role of **coach** is an important role, we offer some suggestions that will assist you when you are working as a coach.

When we talk about the manager functioning in a **coaching role,** we are talking about all those behaviors that result in helping people achieve results. Like an athletic coach, this involves bringing the right team together; providing direction and instruction; and dealing with attitudes, morale, ethics, discipline, and career development (Umiker, 1998). Coaching implies communication that will bring out the best in each person. It results in shaping values, removing obstacles, building on strengths, and strengthening interpersonal relationships. Thinking in terms of **coaching** provides a valuable analogy. A coach for a sport's team is interested in creating a winning team. To do that, every individual must be helped to perform at his or her personal best, and everyone must be helped to work together toward the common goal. A coach accomplishes this by letting people know what they are doing right so that they continue to do it, letting them know where their performance fails to meet the standard so they will attempt to change it, and helping them understand the desired behavior so that they can work toward performing in that way. Even the best player benefits from a good coach who helps that individual work toward his or her personal best. The poor player may be helped to become a solid support for the team even if that individual will never be the star.

The coaching role requires that you possesses strong leadership qualities. You must be competent and emotionally stable, must communicate effectively (see Chapter 5), be willing to take risks, be honest and credible in relationships with others, and must exhibit energy and enthusiasm.

How do you begin to implement the coaching role? First, it is important that this role be a part of your overall management style. That means that it is used in everyday activities, not just when there are problems. It involves letting people know what is going on and what you expect whether you are managing care for a small group of patients or for a whole unit. Coaching involves providing support and encouragement to others on the team. The nurse acting as a coach should set a good example and recognize good work with praise that is provided in public. This role involves listening attentively and providing feedback.

When working in a situation in which a problem exists, it is especially important that you are seen as trying to be helpful. Keep reminding yourself that you are trying to help someone improve. Although there may be some punitive steps to be followed at some point in the future, a caring attitude is important throughout. Show that you care. Be certain that the person understands what you expect in terms of performance. Express your sincere concern about ways the individual must change in order to be successful and to meet those expectations.

Select the right time and place to discuss your concerns with the employee. An old adage states, "Timing is everything," and this is certainly true in these situations also. Although nursing units have little down time these days, typically some of the best times to discuss concerns with staff on a nursing unit are during the late morning hours, right after lunch, or just before the end of the shift. If you believe that your comments are going to disturb and upset the person, planning your meeting just before the person would leave the unit for a break or for the end of the day might be desirable. Such meetings must always be held in a private place, such as an office, where interruptions can be avoided and privacy can be assured.

Avoid using language that is preachy or carries a judgmental impression. It is preferable to discuss the behavior in relation to the standards of practice, avoiding the use of such language as "You should have done. . ." "Should" language often creates the impression that you are rigid. Be sure that you communicate the message that your primary concern is helping the individual improve. Deal with the performance rather than with personalities or personal characteristics.

Give specific suggestions for change. If you are vague, the person may not understand exactly what it is that you expect to change. You also leave yourself open to such comments as, "She wants me to change, but she can't tell me what she really wants." Identify ways in which the person will benefit from making the changes that you are expecting will occur. Your goal should be to motivate the person to improve performance rather than threatening or challenging the individual. It is important to involve the person in setting timelines and goals for change. This is more realistic when working with employees than when working with nursing students who have predetermined timelines for meeting the objectives or outcomes of their particular course. When the changes that you desire take place, it is also critical that you recognize these changes and commend the person for what has been accomplished. This recognition helps build self-reliance and self-esteem and results in the individual feeling more empowered and willing to seek other ways in which performance can be improved. All these result in more positive feelings about work and the work environment.

Critical Thinking Exercise

Reflect on your own life activities. Have you ever had a sports coach or an excellent experienced colleague who helped you become more effective? What behaviors did these individuals exhibit that helped you to grow and develop? What behaviors interfered with your own growth? Analyze your own response to these individuals.

An important part of coaching is helping individuals set stretch goals (Stone, 1999). A stretch goal is one that requires the individual to develop a new skill or ability. In today's environment, this often means that people learn one another's jobs so that when one individual is absent, the job may still get done. Sometimes, to accomplish all the work that is needed, several people must work together on some task even though it is normally the job of one person. As people become multiskilled, the entire organization is enhanced.

You may coach an entire team. This includes helping people to work well together, to consider one another as they make decisions, and to communicate effectively. The coach of a team helps set the direction for the team, facilitates individual functioning, helps organize the work, and teaches skills that people need (Stone, 1999).

Part of effective team coaching is leading meetings of the team. Nursing teams often meet briefly as a part of intershift report. As a facilitator of the team, you will need to assure that everyone understands their assigned roles, expectations for collaborative functioning, and the overall goals for the day. In addition, you should listen to concerns of team members, problems they perceive to be present, and assistance they would like to have in functioning more effectively.

■ MENTORING

Mentoring goes beyond coaching and assists selected individuals to prepare for advancement and greater opportunities. Mentoring is support offered to those with promise and potential. Some people who are interested in career advancement actively seek a **mentor** who can help them grow and develop (see Chapter 10). The person receiving mentoring is referred to as a **mentee.** Becoming a mentor requires that you feel secure in your own role and that you are willing to invest in another person. Mentoring in nursing provides encouragement to the beginner and contributes to the growth of the profession.

According to Stone (1999), mentoring has four purposes. The first is to role model the type of behavior the individual should emulate. You cannot be an effective mentor if your own performance is not excellent. A major part of modeling is to model attitudes and values that are important to advancement. The second is to coach the individual in behaviors that are most productive. The third is to introduce the mentee to those in the organization and in the profession who might contribute to their growth, development, and advancement. This might include introducing the mentee who has an idea for change to the person who could approve a trial of that idea. This provides an opportunity for the mentee to demonstrate abilities and to be recognized. The fourth purpose is to advocate for the mentee when opportunities become available. In a sense, a mentor is a cheerleader for an individual. You might even recommend your mentee for a position elsewhere that offered growth even if you would be losing a valuable member of your team.

■ PROVIDING FEEDBACK

When you are directly responsible for the performance of others, such as unlicensed assistive personnel on your team, an individual you are precepting, or those under your supervision as charge nurse or unit manager, you have an obligation to provide feedback on performance to individuals. They have a right to expect that you will provide them with the information they need to grow in their jobs.

Feedback consists of providing information regarding your evaluation of the person's performance directly to that individual. Feedback can be both informal and formal. Informal feedback occurs most frequently as one aspect of the operation of any unit where it is necessary to give direction, help, instruction, reinforcement, or correction to others. It is provided on an hour-to-hour or day-to-day basis.

Positive Feedback

Positive feedback implies that you are communicating to others what they have done correctly or well. Because constructive comments help an individual develop self-esteem and provide motivation, the wise and mature manager looks for opportunities to let employees know that their efforts are recognized and appreciated. Providing recognition for good performance creates a positive climate. Most persons who are responsible for evaluating the performance of others have little difficulty identifying positive performance. If any problem exists, it is usually that positive feedback is not given frequently enough. Employees may become discouraged if they do not hear positive comments. When the primary nurse says to the licensed practical nurse (LPN) who is assisting with the care of patients, "Mr. Johansen looked so much more relaxed and comfortable after you finished the morning care," the practical nurse knows that her efforts were noticed and valued. Positive feedback also serves to clarify performance expectations and lets employees know they are on the right track. All these factors result in greater job satisfaction and better patient care.

Several guidelines can be followed that make positive feedback most effective. It should occur frequently, for the reasons just mentioned. Positive feedback should also occur in a timely manner. Saving a positive comment until the next formal **interview** delays the gratification that it should provide. Positive comments about a person's work may often be given in public. A manager who finds timely occasions to reinforce the good working behaviors of an individual where others can hear raises the morale in the area as well as increases the self-esteem of the person receiving the compliment. This is only effective if the manager responds to all the employees with positive feedback. If only one or two are ever recognized, others may become resentful that their efforts are not acknowledged. Finally, feedback should always be accurate, sincere, and objective.

Negative Feedback

Identifying unsatisfactory performance constitutes the first step toward correcting performance. The second step is giving **negative feedback,** pointing out to an employee that he or she is doing something wrong. Providing negative feedback is equally important and often more difficult than providing positive feedback. It takes skill and experience to develop methods of providing feedback that will help the employee grow and learn. This is part of the coaching role of a manager and requires that the manager be able to suggest ways to make needed changes. Some managers find it easier to ignore the behavior. Such managers eventually discover that not correcting inappropriate behavior frustrates the whole team and lowers staff morale.

avoidance = bad

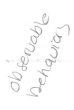

Observable behaviors

When it is necessary to let an employee know that his or her performance must change, certain steps can be followed to make the criticism a helpful experience. Like positive feedback, negative feedback should be timely; it should be given as soon as possible after the incident has occurred. Delaying comment may be construed as approving the unacceptable behavior. Like positive feedback, negative feedback should also be frequent, objective, and accurate. If feedback is provided frequently, it becomes less threatening to those receiving it and easier for those giving it. When we say it should be objective and accurate, we mean it should be based directly on observable behaviors rather than on personality traits or personal likes or dislikes. Negative feedback should also include suggestions for change or alternative behaviors. It should avoid sending put-down or blaming messages. In a similar vein, it should be nonthreatening. Remember, everyone is susceptible to feeling threatened. Highly threatening messages cause individuals to use energy in defense that is better spent on improving care than on reducing the threat. Statements such as, "I don't want to see you doing that again" or "You won't last long if you continue that behavior" are threatening. Finally, unlike positive feedback, which can be given in public, negative comments should always be given in private.

Providing Suggestions for Improvement

Suggestions for improvement can accompany both positive and negative feedback. They should always be present with negative feedback. Suggestions for improvement are most useful when they are specific and descriptive. For a nursing assistant, you might say, "I noticed that you transferred Mrs. Williams to a chair in a way that kept her safe but did not protect your own back. I have a suggestion that might make it easier for you in the future. If the wheelchair is placed at a 45-degree angle instead of perpendicular to the bed, it won't be so far to move her and would be easier for you." Thus, you have clearly communicated your evaluation of her performance, which has both positive and negative aspects, but your suggestion is designed to support improvement.

EXAMPLE *Providing a Suggestion for Improvement*

Mary Wilson noted that the LPN, who was assigned to give medications, was having difficulty getting done on time. She approached her and said, "I noticed that you have been having trouble finishing your medication rounds on time. If you put a small container of juice and one of applesauce on your cart, you would not need to make so many trips to the kitchen and I think it would help you get done on time." She described the problem and gave a concrete suggestion for improvement. She did not dwell on deficiencies or place blame on the individual. She established that she was interested in helping the LPN meet the standard, not simply noting when she does not.

Often is it best to work with the person to develop a plan for improvement.

EXAMPLE *Helping a Subordinate Plan for Improvement*

> Jim Dawson noticed that the nursing assistant was not getting a resident to breakfast on time. He approached the nursing assistant and said, "I see you are having trouble getting Mr. Jones to breakfast on time the last couple of days. Do you have any ideas of how things might be changed to get him there by 8:30?" He noted the problem and then recognized this individual's input was important in solving the problem.

Sometimes general suggestions for improvement can be given to a group with whom you work. You might indicate after report, "We've been having unexpected admissions recently, and they have really thrown our planned schedules off. Let's plan for how we will handle that if it happens again today." By encouraging others to make suggestions for improvement, you are not only solving the problem at hand but are also helping build a cohesive team. Being involved in decision making is also motivating for many people (see Chapter 5).

When a specific error occurs, your feedback should address both the error itself and the reason for the error. One cause of an error is a person's lack of knowledge about the correct procedure or policy. After you have talked with the person and determined that this is the case, your plan for improvement should include providing the needed education or training for that person.

If the cause of an error is a person's carelessness or even deliberate avoidance of known policy or procedure, then you are facing a different kind of remedial task. This kind of concern is addressed in Chapter 12, which discusses the challenge of working with problem employees.

A third cause of an error is a system problem. System problems are often revealed when incident reports are reviewed and a pattern is seen. A system problem might be an ambiguous or unclear documentation method, a poorly designed medication cart on which labels are confusing, or an unrealistic expectation of how many medications one person can pass in a limited amount of time. A system problem might go as far back as a manufacturer's labeling of drugs, the design of intravenous pumps without adequate safety mechanisms, and needle devices that do not protect against injury.

Although we do ask that individuals increase their alertness to cope with system problems, the real answer lies in correcting the system. This often takes time and considerable effort. Acknowledging the system problem and communicating the efforts being made to address this concern provides a positive working climate. Employees become resentful when they know that a system problem exists and that rather than addressing the underlying problem the employer merely demands greater vigilance. When a system problem is identified as presence of drugs with very similar and easily confused labels, the agency might contact the drug manufacturer and the Food and Drug Administration to change the labeling. Meanwhile, a new system for storage that separates the drugs and places special alert notices may help alleviate the potential for error. Nurses have been instrumental in initiating the process of change. (See Chapter 4 on evaluating care.)

A fourth type of error occurs when an otherwise good employee makes a human error. Although some would argue that health care must be 100% error free, most of us would acknowledge that when working with people and the ever-changing environment of health care, this would probably only be an elusive goal. Processes and procedures must be reviewed, but then we must forgive the error and move forward. Punitive actions taken in such instances seldom lessen the chance of error, but rather may increase it by raising the level of anxiety. Punitive actions also signal that the employer believes that this was a willful error. Thus, the sound employee feels unfairly libeled. When a punitive approach is the pattern, good employees may try to cover up errors rather than acknowledge them. This then blocks any effective plan to work on the system problems.

■ FORMAL PERFORMANCE APPRAISAL

Formal feedback in the form of **employee performance evaluation** may also be referred to as **performance appraisal.** The nursing unit manager usually conducts the evaluation, which typically occurs at designated time intervals. Such intervals may be every 3 months for the first 6 months after hire and then on the employment anniversary and annually thereafter. Some workplaces are increasing the use of self and peer evaluations as well as supervisor evaluation as part of this process. Patient or consumer evaluations may be added to the overall evaluation if they are available. This has been termed *360-degree evaluation* (Arney, 2001). This reflects that evaluation from all these sources provides the most comprehensive view of an individual's performance.

Self-evaluation requires that you try to look objectively at your own performance and identify areas in which you are doing well and those areas in which you hope to grow and develop. Self-evaluation is critical to professional growth regardless of whether the workplace requires it to be done in a formal way.

In **peer evaluation,** nurses are asked to evaluate other nurses as a contribution to their growth and development in nursing. We often informally evaluate coworkers and make a judgment about their performance, but we may not ever share our evaluation because that may seem inappropriate or uncomfortable. Our informal evaluation may lack clear standards of measurement, may be based on one or two isolated instances, and may be greatly affected by our personal biases. If you are asked to participate in peer evaluation, you have an obligation to those peers.

Purposes of a Formal Appraisal

An effective performance appraisal system has at least two major purposes. The first is to improve the functioning of the organization; the second is to foster the personal development of the employee within the organization. Some would also give a third reason for evaluation: to provide a basis for termination of an employee from a position, should that be necessary.

For the organization, performance appraisals can provide information on which to base management decisions regarding such matters as salary increases, merit wage increases, promotion, transfer, demotion, and termination. The performance appraisal helps assess the effectiveness of an organization's hiring and recruiting practices. It can also help identify training and development needs of the employees so that staff development programs can be structured appropriately. Inherent in this process is the establishment of standards of job performance that benefit any organization.

Any effective performance appraisal must be legally defensible. That means that it is set up to be objective and to avoid bias, as discussed under data collection. Also important are the records and documentation used to support any actions taken. If an individual grieves a performance appraisal or any disciplinary action taken, the process is very like a judicial process in its demands for timely documentation and appropriate processes. If a former employee sues the agency in regard to discipline or termination, these same records must be of a quality that they meet standards of evidence.

Employees are assisted in effective professional development through well-done performance appraisals. The employee and the supervisor can develop plans that will result in personal growth, including increased skill performance, technical training, or a formal advance in education that will help improve future performance. In addition to providing information about the employee's performance, the performance appraisal can make known to management the employee's goals and aspirations. A performance interview, properly conducted, results in improved communication between the supervisor and the employee. It provides an established opportunity for the supervisor to recognize the accomplishments of the employee. Receiving recognition for a job well done motivates employees to continue doing their best (see Chapter 5).

Characteristics of an Effective Performance Appraisal System

You can probably recall some instance in your life when you were unhappy about the way you were evaluated. It might have been an experience in which the way an instructor conducted a clinical evaluation or the criteria that were used seemed unfair. It might have been an actual employment situation. You may also remember an instance in which the review of your performance was conducted so positively that it helped you move forward professionally and increased your respect and admiration for the person who assisted you in that process. What factors must come together to ensure that the evaluation process has a positive outcome? What must occur for all parties involved to believe it is a meaningful investment of time and energy? Display 7-1 lists the characteristics of an effective performance appraisal system.

First, a well-developed evaluation process is one that has the support of top administration within the organization and that is viewed as fair and productive by all

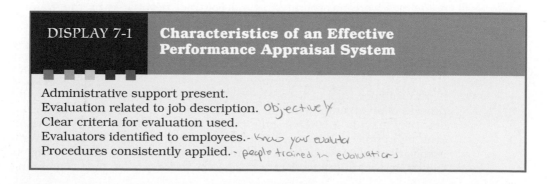

| DISPLAY 7-1 | **Characteristics of an Effective Performance Appraisal System** |

Administrative support present.
Evaluation related to job description. *Objectively*
Clear criteria for evaluation used.
Evaluators identified to employees. - *Know your evaluator*
Procedures consistently applied. - *people trained in evaluations*

who participate in it. Administrative support creates the staff time and budget that must be invested to develop an effective system.

Similarly, the purposes of evaluation need to be identified, communicated, and understood by both managers and employees. For what purpose will the evaluation results be used? In decisions regarding salary? In decisions regarding ability to transfer to another nursing department?

Procedures that will be used, such as the frequency of formal evaluation interviews, also must be defined. In many instances, if nurses operate within the guidelines of a negotiated contract with the hospital administration, the processes of evaluation will be described in the contract itself.

Another important factor in an effective performance appraisal is reliance on job descriptions. The importance of job descriptions was discussed earlier in this chapter. All individuals have a right to know the criteria by which they will be evaluated. These criteria, which evolve from the job description, should be shared with the employee at the time of orientation to the job.

All individuals employed in an organization must know who in that system is responsible for evaluating their performance. For example, you might be very distressed to learn that your evaluation was written by the day supervisor on your unit if you believed you would be evaluated by the charge nurse with whom you worked on the evening shift. In most organizations, the employee will be evaluated by the immediate supervisor, because that person is most familiar with the employee's performance and the expectations of the position. Evaluations should be based on many different observations of performance, and the immediate supervisor usually works most closely with the subordinate. However, the evaluation process may vary in certain institutions. If the immediate supervisor is not conducting the evaluation process, the person formally responsible for the process should make every effort to solicit accurate information about an employee's performance.

It is also critical that the person doing the evaluating be trained in the use of the evaluation tool and be skilled in conducting the appraisal interview. Besides giving the employee verbal feedback in an interview, the evaluator should prepare a written evaluation, and the employee should be given the opportunity to respond in writing. If the employee disagrees with statements in the evaluation, there should be a process for appeal. The employee should know what is to be done with the written evaluation. Is it shared with the employee only? Is it also placed in the employee's personnel file? Is it transmitted to a person of higher authority in the organization? Well-developed and well-implemented plans for monitoring the evaluation process and the tools used for appraising performance must also be in place. For an example of guidelines for performance evaluation, see Display 7-2. These guidelines were incorporated into a contract negotiated by the Washington State Nurses Association.

Common Problems Encountered in Appraisal Programs

A performance appraisal can be one of the weakest elements in the management process of an organization. When individuals feel uncomfortable with evaluating others, they may do it poorly. Some people, both employees and supervisors, view the evaluation process negatively. For the employee, this may be a carryover from earlier associations with evaluations that resulted in grades and admonitions such as "You can do better." Supervisors may believe the process is too time consuming, requiring

DISPLAY 7-2 **Guidelines for Performance Evaluation**

PHILOSOPHY

An evaluation program should be considered as a step in bringing about, as well as determining progress in achieving, personal and professional growth and development resulting in better patient care.

PRINCIPLES AND GUIDELINES

To meet evaluation criteria, a performance appraisal must be:

a. Developed within the framework of the institution's written policies.

b. Based on expectations as stated in the job description for the position.

c. Written and presented by an evaluator who has:
   1. Been oriented to these guidelines for performance evaluation and to the method of evaluation used in the particular institution.
   2. Made actual and frequent observations of the performance of the evaluatee.
   3. Been involved in the evaluatee's growth and development.

d. Prepared prior to and presented in an evaluation conference, which must be conducted by the person writing the evaluation. This conference must be conducted on a planned basis with foreknowledge of the evaluatee as to time and place.

e. Prepared and presented prior to completion of the first ninety (90) days, no less than annually thereafter, and, if possible, at termination of employment.

f. Presented with the understanding that:
   1. The evaluatee has been oriented to these guidelines for performance evaluation and to the method of evaluation used in the particular institution.
   2. The evaluatee has the responsibility to participate in the evaluation conference by mutually planning with the evaluator personal and professional goals for further development.
   3. The evaluatee may comment in writing on the evaluation form.

g. Signed and dated by both the evaluator and the evaluatee to signify that the evaluation has been reviewed in conference.

h. Reviewed, dated, and signed by a member of management in line authority above the evaluator.

i. The nurse shall be given a copy of the reviewed, dated, and signed evaluation on request.

j. If a permanent nurse shall receive an evaluation that indicates unsatisfactory performance in some areas of practice, the nurse shall have a reasonable opportunity to improve, and then another evaluation shall be prepared and presented as above to indicate any change in performance, unless there is a clear and present danger to patients if the nurse remains in the nurse's regular assignment.

Collective Bargaining Agreement by and Between the Washington State Nurses Association Northwest Local Unit and Northwest Hospital, July 1, 1985 to June 30, 1987.

judgments that they believe they lack the knowledge or skills to make. Both these opinions can be valid if the process is not clearly defined and soundly implemented. Employees need assistance in seeing evaluation as an opportunity for growth, and supervisors must learn to view it as an opportunity to do a better coaching and counseling job. Both coaching and counseling of subordinates are important aspects of the supervisory role. An understanding of the process will help you be an effective evaluator.

Oberg (1972) identified some common problems that interfere with the success of formal appraisal programs. These are identified in Display 7-3. They include an unwillingness to devote the time needed, difficulties with consistency across employees by one supervisor and across supervisors, lack of clarity in expectations, poor selection, placement, and training programs, lack of skill on the part of supervisors, and a concern about the effect of performance appraisal on relationships in the workplace.

When all persons involved in the evaluation system are aware of these common concerns, steps can be taken to diminish or eliminate them. All employees need and want to know how they are doing, and a properly conducted evaluation session can effectively provide that information.

DISPLAY 7-3   Common Problems That Interfere With the Success of Formal Appraisal

1. Performance appraisal programs may be viewed as demanding too much from supervisors, in that it is difficult for a first-line supervisor to know what each of 20, 30, or more subordinates is doing.
2. Standards and ratings tend to vary widely, with some raters being tough and others more lenient.
3. An appraiser may replace organizational standards with personal values and bias.
4. Because of lack of communication, standards by which employees think they are being judged are sometimes different from those their superiors actually use.
5. Appraisal techniques tend to be used as performance panaceas and cannot replace sound selection, placement, and training programs.
6. The validity of ratings may be reduced by supervisors' resistance to making the ratings, due to the discomfort they feel when having to confront the employee with negative ratings and negative feedback.
7. Ratings can boomerang when communicated to employees, because negative feedback fails to motivate the typical employee and may cause the employee to perform more poorly.
8. Performance appraisals may interfere with a more constructive coaching relationship between the supervisor and the employee. Supervisors may see the evaluation process as placing them in the role of judge.

From Oberg, W. (1972). Make performance appraisal relevant. *Harvard Business Review*, 44(1), 62.

Types of Performance Evaluation Tools

Grote (1997) suggests that there are three parts to an effective performance appraisal. The first two, collecting the data and evaluating the performance, we have already discussed. The third is writing an effective review. A number of different kinds of evaluation tools exist to facilitate this process. We will not attempt to discuss all the forms in current use, but we will share with you some of the more commonly used ones. The most common evaluation tools are the **narrative or essay technique** and the various forms of **rating scales. Checklists** are also common. Less common is the use goals and objectives as a basis for evaluation. Several evaluation methods have been designed to avoid evaluator bias. Three such methods are the **field review** method, the forced-choice rating method, and the **critical-incident technique.** Although many of these forms focus on scales, providing behavioral examples remains the foundation for any effective written report (Grote, 1997).

THE NARRATIVE OR ESSAY TECHNIQUE

In the narrative or essay technique, the evaluator writes a paragraph or more (usually more) outlining an employee's strengths, weaknesses (or areas for improvement), and potential. It often begins with a brief description of the position the employee occupies within the organization and should always be reflective of the employee's performance in relation to the job description. It may also include some comment on personal attributes if pertinent to the job (e.g., "ability to function well under stress").

This format for evaluation has the advantage of providing an in-depth review of an employee's performance and may be especially suitable for identifying problem areas and areas on which to focus further development. However, its preparation can be quite time consuming, can vary tremendously in length and content, and depends on the evaluator's ability to write. Narrative evaluations are difficult to compare, because each may touch on different aspects of performance. This form of evaluation is widely used in letters of recommendation.

RATING SCALES

The rating scale is probably the most widely used tool for evaluating nursing performance. The tool consists of a set of behaviors or characteristics to be rated (again based on the job description) and some type of scale that will indicate the degree to which the person being evaluated demonstrates each behavior. The rating scale may take several forms as outlined in Table 7-1. The development of a valid and reliable rating scale is very time consuming and requires special skills.

Rating scales have the advantage of usually being very acceptable to the rater and providing information that is generally more consistent than that obtained in a narrative approach. However, it does not provide the depth of information that the narrative can make available, and its validity and reliability when used by different raters might be challenged. For example, what one head nurse may see as *A* performance may be rated as *B* performance by another.

TABLE 7-1	TYPES OF RATING SCALES
Type of Scale	**Description**
Numerical rating scales	On numerical rating scales, the degree to which the employee performs a desired behavior is rated by circling the appropriate number. Instructions on the evaluation instrument explain the ratings. For example, if the numbers 1–5 are used, the instructions may indicate that 5 is outstanding, 4 is above average, 3 is average, 2 is below average, and 1 is unsatisfactory.
Lettered rating scales	Lettered rating scales function in the same way as numerical scales, except that letters are used instead of numbers. For example, the letter A may represent outstanding performance, B above average, and so forth. One can quickly see how this system could easily be equated with the giving of grades in our educational system.
Graphic rating scales	Graphic rating scales rate performance by placing a mark somewhere along a horizontal line that is divided into sections with labels such as "always," "frequently," "usually," "seldom," and "never." Each standard of performance is listed on the evaluation tool and rated by this scale.
Descriptive graphic scales	Descriptive rating scales describe in varying terms the performance in relationship to each standard. Descriptions are placed along a continuum. For example, if the standard of performance relates to documentation, the description at one end of the continuum might state, "Documentation is accurate and complete on all patients assigned, includes meaningful examples and observations." The statement at the opposite end of the continuum might state, "Documentation omits essential aspects and does not accurately reflect patient condition. Contains many misused and misspelled words." These descriptions represent the best and worst behaviors, and two or three additional statements describing other degrees of performance would be included between them.

THE CHECKLIST

Another type of evaluation form is the checklist. It describes the standard of performance, and the rater indicates by placing a check mark in a column whether the employee demonstrates that behavior. The columns are usually titled "yes," "no," or "not applicable," although other words carrying the same meaning can be used. These evaluation forms are efficient when evaluating a large number of employees but do not provide a way to indicate the degree to which or frequency with which a behavior occurs. Behavior is seldom either totally "yes" or totally "no."

GOALS AND OBJECTIVES

During the 1960s, **management by objectives** gained a great deal of attention. As a result, evaluation tools were developed that incorporated this philosophy of management. They focus on the evaluator's observations of the employee's performance as measured against very specific, predetermined objectives or goals that have been jointly agreed on by the employee and the evaluator. During the feedback interview, the results are discussed and new goals for the next period of evaluation are established. This form of management and evaluation encourages employees' participation in setting their own goals and objectives and probably discourages complaints that they are being judged unfairly. You can quickly imagine how this system would break down if an employee's goals differed from those of the organization or if the employee was not interested in establishing personal goals on which to base evaluation. Management by objectives may not work in hospitals, where the tasks (and therefore the job description) of the nurse are based on patient needs that may vary and are thus difficult to quantify and describe clearly.

METHODS TO DECREASE RATER BIAS

Because **rater bias** in evaluation is an ongoing concern, decreasing rater bias is the goal of other techniques. The ones most commonly used, the field review method, the forced choice rating scale, and the critical-incident technique, are designed specifically to decrease rater bias. Because of their complexity and time demands, they are used less frequently than other methods (Table 7-2).

TABLE 7-2	TECHNIQUES TO DECREASE RATER BIAS
Method	**Description**
Field review method	Allows the ratings of several supervisors to be compared for the same employee.
	A small group of raters is identified for each supervisory unit, and each rates an employee's performance.
	A member of the administrative staff then meets with the members of the rating group and identifies areas of agreement.
	The administrative staff member helps the group arrive at consensus and helps each rater perceive the standards similarly.
	The process can be very time consuming.
Forced-choice rating method	Requires that the evaluator choose from among a group of statements those that "best describe" the individual being evaluated and those that "least describe" this person.
	Statements are then weighted or scored by another individual in the organization; high scores represent better employees.
	The evaluator does not know the scoring value of each statement while scoring, thus, bias is reduced.
	This method has the disadvantage of being costly to develop.
Critical-incident technique	Used to collect data for use in other evaluation methods (e.g., the narrative technique) or used as an evaluation method itself.
	Requires that the supervisor observe, collect, and record specific instances of the employee carrying out responsibilities critical to the job.
	These observations are used to prepare the evaluation, or they serve as the evaluation itself, to be reviewed with the employee during the feedback interview.
	To be free of bias, it is important that incidents be recorded regularly and that they relate to job performance and job descriptions rather than focus on personality traits.
	Such written accounts of behavior may assist supervisors in their role as coach and communicator. Having to record incidents helps the supervisor remember more accurately and completely the aspects of an employee's performance that will be reviewed during the feedback interview.
	One disadvantage of this method is that it is time consuming, because the supervisor must write down incidents on a regular basis.
	A second disadvantage is a tendency to record behaviors that are not desirable and to fail to write down those that represent expected performance.

■ THE EVALUATION INTERVIEW

Once the supervisor completes an employee's evaluation, time needs to be set aside to discuss the evaluation with the employee. Remember, this should not be the only time the supervisor communicates with the employee, but it can be one of the most meaningful times. Certain characteristics can result in a more successful interview.

Planning for the Interview

The review of an individual's performance should never be conducted haphazardly. The feedback interview may be more important to the performance evaluation system than the evaluation tools used to rate an employee's performance. A good interview requires thought and planning, just as other management activities do. Because providing a performance appraisal is uncomfortable for managers, some are tempted to provide the written document for an employee to read and sign and omit the face-to-face discussion. This robs the employee of the opportunity to discuss concerns or ways to improve.

A specific, mutually convenient time should be planned for the interview session. It should be a time that will allow for exchange of ideas and perceptions. An interview conducted when the employee is concerned about completing the morning care of patients will not be as effective as one conducted when the employee can focus on the content of the interview. Similarly, an interview scheduled during a time when the supervisor is distracted by many other urgent items will be rushed through. The interview should not last longer than is necessary to accomplish specified activities; that is, it should not become the occasion for social chit-chat. Most interviews can be conducted in an hour or less. A specific time frame, such as 2:00–2:30 p.m., tends to focus both individuals on the needed topics and avoid time wasting (Langdon & Osborne, 2001).

You will also need to plan carefully for the location of the interview. The interview should be conducted at a convenient, private location. A busy workroom or a corner of the nurses' station is not conducive to achieving performance review goals.

Planning for specific content includes having appropriate copies of any evaluation tool so that they can be reviewed. Making a list of the items you want to be sure to discuss will facilitate your organization and prevent you from forgetting either positive or negative comments that you had intended to make. If you have specific behaviors to discuss, have available your notes regarding those behaviors, attendance records if that is an issue, or copies of documentation that illustrate a particular concern. Preparing thoroughly helps an evaluation interview to proceed much more smoothly.

Conducting the Interview

A good feedback interview allows both persons an opportunity to become comfortable in the session. Beginning with socializing will help the employee feel more at ease. Socializing is an informal conversation about ordinary matters. Socializing about work-related situations tends to be more desirable than about personal matters (Arthur, 1996).

Begin the main focus of the discussion by asking the employee to identify either previously agreed on objectives or the major aspects of the job on which he or she will be evaluated. Plan to use your active listening skills to understand the employee's viewpoint. Whereas Arthur (1996) suggests that using 50% of the time to listen is appropriate, Langdon and Osborne (2001) suggest that the manager spend 80% of the time listening. Watch the employee's body language, and rephrase and summarize as needed to assure that you accurately understand the message of the employee and that he or she accurately understand your message.

All information about performance provided to the employee should be job related and based on observed behavior. The ratings should be based on clearly defined expectations. There should be no surprises for the employee.

The manager should also anticipate that the employee might disagree with some of the comments made. The employee may have perceived his or her performance to be better than the supervisor did. Generally, open and candid responses are desirable in these situations, as is the ability to be a good listener.

The nurse manager must maintain control of the interview and ensure that productive communication patterns are used throughout. To accomplish these goals, the nurse manager can point out when a pattern or topic is not productive and redirect the conversation. Calling the employee's attention to particular response patterns, such as excuses, that are nonproductive may also prove useful. Refocusing an interview is another technique that allows the manager to maintain a positive discussion. Focusing evaluative statements on performance rather than on personality characteristics helps avoid areas that can disrupt the communication process (Haar, 1978).

Any performance review should be future oriented as well as reviewing the past. Suggestions for improvement or growth should always be present. Part of the role of the manager is helping people grow in their jobs. These ideas for improvement or growth also may originate with the employee. The manager can then identify a way to support those goals.

If you have identified areas of deficient performance, it is often productive to ask the employee to problem solve possible avenues for improvement. A useful strategy is to say "What strategies can you identify that would alter this?" When strategies have been identified either by the employee or the manager, asking for commitment is important. Use a phrase such as "Can I have your agreement to work on this improvement?" This requires that the person actively enter into the plan. If asked to make a commitment to a behavior change, an individual is less likely to ignore the concern. However, you want to move beyond a glib "yes" to a discussion of behaviors that will be implemented (Langdon and Osborne, 2001).

When it is necessary to make a number of recommendations for change during the evaluation conference, a follow-up session should be planned. Arranging for a second meeting provides an opportunity for the employee to change his or her performance and receive immediate feedback. If the supervisor expresses confidence in the employee, the employee is more likely to understand that the manager believes the improvement will occur.

EXAMPLE *Conducting an Evaluation Interview*

Alma Jeffers was scheduling her first set of evaluation conferences since she had become unit manager. She was nervous about the process and especially concerned about talking with Bob Monroe, one of the RNs, on the unit. Bob's charting had frequently been identified as deficient when audits were done. She carefully planned to talk about the good quality of care that Bob provided but knew she must discuss the need for improvement in documentation. After discussing his good work and asking him to identify goals, she stated, "There is an additional concern that I have. When audits of charting from our unit are done, there have been four occasions when your lack of documentation regarding teaching made it appear that appropriate patient care was not being done. Do you remember when you received those individual notices?" He replied "Oh that—I have always felt that charting was the last priority. Patient care comes first." Alma responded "It really isn't a situation of either–or. It is a situation of both being important. This is not only important for legal reasons, but also assures that there is continuity of patient care. Can I have your agreement to work at changing this situation?" He replied "Well, I guess so." She concluded with "I will be checking with you periodically to see how things are going. I would like you to let me know if you need any assistance."

Potential Errors in Performance Evaluations

There are a variety of errors that an individual may make in conducting performance evaluations. These are primarily based on failing to use effective communication strategies.

Failing to investigate facts before expressing opinions means that your evaluation is not based on specific behaviors. If you do this, you lose credibility with staff. They will feel that you are not fair and unbiased in your comments. When this occurs, even appropriate feedback may be discounted.

Conducting a one-way conversation blocks input and response by the person being interviewed. By not listening as well as speaking, you lose an opportunity to connect with an employee whom you supervise. Asking for input does not imply that you will be changing the evaluation but establishes that you are willing to communicate.

Interrupting the employee's thoughts, explanations, or questions implies that these are not worth your time and attention. This makes the employee feel disrespected. Whatever the value of the information you provide, the climate in which it is given contributes to the perception of the employee.

Criticizing the employee rather than the performance is a common pitfall. When an individual has not performed well, remember that you should be focusing on behaviors in relationship to standards. Avoid vague generalizations and personal comments.

Smoothing over real deficiencies and problems too fast happens when the supervisor is uncomfortable with providing negative feedback. For most people, providing negative feedback creates personal discomfort. There is concern about the reaction and sometimes a concern that the negative comments will interfere with previously good relationships. Your language should be clear and direct so that the person understands the problems. Accompanying the negative feedback with suggestions for improvement is a positive step to help with this.

Blaming your own supervisor by claiming that your corrective measures originate "higher up" is usually done to avoid the discomfort of confronting someone

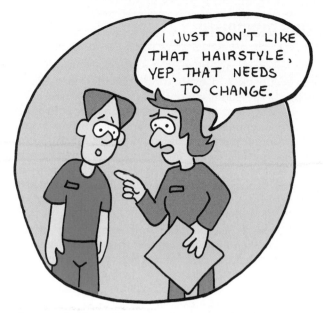

Effective employee evaluation addresses performance rather than personal attributes.

with a poor evaluation. This undermines your own authority in the eyes of those you supervise and does not really make the person feel better about the negative feedback. As a supervisor, you must take responsibility for your own decisions and behavior.

Allowing the interview to deteriorate into a social visit can occur when there are good interpersonal relationships between people in the work environment or when the supervisor is very uncomfortable with the evaluative role. This is really unfair to the employee. Employees deserve to hear clear feedback about their performance. If they are doing well, it will be motivating for them. If there are areas in which they can grow, these need to be explored.

Critical Thinking Exercise

Jane Adams is an older LPN (LVN) on your unit. She has indicated that she plans to retire in 2 or 3 years. She provides good care to her patients and is a loyal employee, but she is very sensitive to criticism. The hospital in which you are employed includes attendance at staff development programs as a significant part of the annual evaluation of employees. You know that Jane has not attended any programs or workshops in the past year because, as she states, "I'll be retiring soon." As the person responsible for evaluating her performance and conducting the performance interview, how would you deal with this item? How would you conduct the interview? How would you present your evaluation of Jane to your superior?

■ PROGRESSIVE DISCIPLINE

In the previous discussion, the focus has been on the satisfactory employee who needs feedback and evaluation that identifies both positive actions and areas for growth. At the point where the quality of patient care becomes jeopardized, an organization may need to terminate an employee. **Progressive discipline** is the process by which an employee's performance is evaluated with feedback and increasing sanctions on unacceptable behavior. The goal of this process is to correct employee performance but also to set the stage for termination if that is needed. Actions taken in this situation are often termed **disciplinary procedures.** The need for progressive discipline occurs when, despite coaching and assistance, the employee's behavior continues to fall below the expected and allowable standard. This situation is taxing to the most experienced manager.

Progressive discipline is the responsibility of a person with administrative authority, such as the unit manager, and is not the responsibility of the team leader or other nurses on the unit. Managers typically dread these situations. However, there will be times when patient safety or quality of care will demand that action be taken.

An employee faced with possible sanctions and termination is entitled to **due process** in most instances. Due process includes being notified of the problem, being told what must be done to correct the problem, receiving help (coaching and/or teaching) in remedying the problem, and time for this to occur. When the manager first realizes that a serious problem requiring significant change may exist, it is wise to contact the human relations department and the manager's immediate supervisor. Most contracts or policy manuals have sections that spell out specific steps for dealing with disciplinary problems and provide directions on the timelines to be followed. By knowing and following the established protocols, the manager would be using correct evaluation procedures and providing due process for the employee.

The person to whom the manager reports will want to be aware of any problem that may involve disciplinary procedures. The situation should be discussed with him or her and approval obtained before moving ahead. The administration will want to be certain that the disciplinary steps are carried out fairly and are legally defensible.

Steps in Progressive Discipline

If progressive discipline becomes necessary, a series of steps should be followed. These start with the least severe and move to the more critical. We identify five major steps. A specific protocol used by a particular organization may specify more.

PROGRESSIVE DISCIPLINE STEP ONE: COUNSELING

First, the employee must be counseled in regard to the performance and the expectations for improvement along with a time frame for improvement. When this takes place, the counseling should embrace all the guidelines consistent with effective performance evaluation described previously. Managers must have a good understanding of the strengths and limitations of their counseling skills. In most situations, matters discussed should be confined to those related to job expectations. Managers must avoid labeling causes of behavior (such as mental health problems or attitudes) and focus on behavioral descriptions. Additional counseling of a personal nature should be referred to a competent professional counselor and not be intermingled with the disciplinary process. The manager has an obligation to inform the employee of the consequences of a failure to change behavior. These consequences are discussed next.

PROGRESSIVE DISCIPLINE STEP TWO: OFFICIAL REPRIMAND

If the employee does not correct the problem behavior within the designated time frame, the process moves to the second step. The second step involves again informing the employee about the problem behavior, identifying acceptable behavior, and officially reprimanding the employee for the poor performance. Some authorities suggest that this **first reprimand** be a verbal reprimand. The verbal reprimand is given to the employee verbally, and then the manager records in the file that a verbal reprimand was given. Some policies require that the first reprimand be in writing. Some organizations continue to call the first reprimand a verbal reprimand but still require it to be in writing. (Although this terminology may seem strange to all involved, the terminology officially designated by the organization must be used.) The employee is given a copy and another copy is placed in the employee's file. Because of the legal implications, most authorities now recommend that all reprimands be in writing.

PROGRESSIVE DISCIPLINE STEP THREE: SECOND REPRIMAND

If correction does not occur, the next step is a **second reprimand.** This reprimand must be a **written reprimand.** The employee must see and sign documentation that will verify that they are aware the problem has been discussed. This does not mean that the employee agrees with the reprimand but simply that the employee is aware of it. Such documentation is usually placed in the employee's personnel file and the employee is also provided a copy.

PROGRESSIVE DISCIPLINE STEP FOUR: SUSPENSION

If the unacceptable behavior continues, the next progressive step is **suspension.** The employee will be told that he or she is not to return to work for a period of time, for instance, 2 weeks. It is hoped that this suspension will help the employee see that the behaviors being exhibited are considered serious. Sometimes, a suspension gives the employee the needed time to make some corrections.

PROGRESSIVE DISCIPLINE STEP FIVE: TERMINATION

The employee is then allowed to return to work. If the unacceptable behavior has not changed after the suspension, the final step is **termination.** Many people will terminate their employment voluntarily before reaching this stage in the process, but one cannot expect that this will always occur. (See Display 7-4 for a summary of the steps in progressive discipline.)

Critical Elements in Disciplinary Actions

Fortunately, most behavioral problems can be handled informally. However, if the process becomes more formal, there are certain assurances that the manager must be able to make. Most institutions have appeal boards or other processes for review-

DISPLAY 7-4	**Steps in Progressive Discipline**

1. Counsel the employee regarding the performance problem and expectations for improvement. Timelines for improvement are given.
2. Reprimand the employee for the first time if the unacceptable behavior continues. This may be oral or written, depending on policies or contracts.
3. Reprimand the employee for the second time if the unacceptable behavior continues. This must be written.
4. Suspend the employee for a given period of time if the unacceptable behavior continues.
5. Terminate the employee if the unacceptable behavior continues after return from suspension.

ing disciplinary cases. If these do not exist, individuals who believe they have been improperly treated may always seek retribution in civil courts. To present a sound appearance if the evaluation process is challenged, certain elements are critical.

It is up to the employer to prove that the alleged acts did, in fact, occur and they were sufficiently serious to warrant disciplinary action. The burden of proof is placed on the institution. When cases go to higher hearing boards, or perhaps into a court of law, the tendency is for judges and juries to see the individual employee as being at a disadvantage compared to a large institution. It may appear as though a large, profitable institution is against one little person who is trying to do his or her best. At times like these, the critical incidents or anecdotal notes the manager has collected for discussion with the employee during evaluation interviews are especially significant.

Proper and adequate documentation must be collected regarding the problems. This documentation must include a history of the incident or incidents. It is important that the situation not appear to be one person's word against another's. Quick notes scrawled on a calendar or in a diary are useful data for documentation. Most of us live busy lives, and it becomes difficult to recall exact times and dates if time has passed. This emphasizes the importance of making some type of note at the time that the incident occurs. The quick note should include a short statement reminding you of the nature of the meeting, telephone call, message, or conference.

Information should be gathered that indicates that the misconduct was not of a temporary nature. We all have had bad days and sometimes bad weeks. A consistent and recurrent pattern that is unlikely to change in the future must be demonstrated.

Records of all evaluations and evaluative sessions are essential. A written record of all conferences with the employee must be kept. These records must be shared with the employee, and, in most situations, opportunity must be provided for the employee to respond to them. A copy of the record of the conference should be given to the employee in person. Leaving it in a mailbox or in some other place to be picked up provides no assurance that the employee will actually receive it.

If the manager anticipates that the conference with the employee will not go smoothly, having a third person present provides another individual to validate what has occurred. The employee should know prior to the conference that the third person will be present and may want to bring someone to represent his or her interests. If a contract is in effect in the organization, the employee's advocate may be a representative from the bargaining unit.

The conduct that is being criticized must not have been condoned earlier. This means that it should not have been ignored or forgiven. Instead, the employee must have been specifically warned of the consequences of continuing the unacceptable behavior. It is important that employee problems be dealt with directly as soon as it is established that a problem exists. When unacceptable behavior is not dealt with openly, it is in reality being condoned. Think, for example, of the employee who frequently calls in ill when scheduled to work weekends. If the manager overlooks this behavior, the employee is given the message, "It's okay" or "You're forgiven."

The information provided must show that the employee has not been singled out for disparate treatment. In other words, other people who performed the same acts must not have been excused. This may be one of the most difficult standards for a manager to maintain. For example, an employee who in other ways is an outstanding nurse cannot be allowed to be consistently late without a reprimand if another individual is reprimanded for being late. Further, if a reprimand is given, it can only be for those behaviors that have occurred since the counseling session held earlier. For example, let us assume an employee is consistently late for work, is counseled, and improves. Then the employee starts making serious medication errors. The reprimand can deal only with the behavior related to failing to give medications correctly, because the previous problem has been corrected. Of course, if the earlier problem still exists, conferencing about it is appropriate and necessary.

Common Pitfalls in Progressive Discipline

Like other areas of working with employees, progressive discipline has some common pitfalls. These include lack of adequate documentation, starting too late with intervention, poorly described standards and expectations, lack of clarity about who is responsible for evaluation, and a manager's attempt to be "nice" at the expense of being direct about poor performance. Two pitfalls of the progressive discipline system need to be discussed in more detail than a list allows. The first of these is the tendency of a manager to wait until he or she can no longer tolerate the person's behavior. Because managers are busy people, behavior that can be a serious problem is sometimes not addressed even when it is identified. Then as the behavior continues without change, the manager may overreact and respond out of anger. An angry person may say things inappropriately, fail to communicate effectively, and create angry or resentful feelings in return rather than create an intent to change.

Another pitfall is the tendency to write a positive terminal evaluation for the employee who has performed unsatisfactorily if that person agrees to resign rather than continue in a disciplinary process. Such an evaluation could be used to discredit your previous statements if the matter were to go to a court of law. Further, if that person performs in an unsatisfactory manner for another employer you have undermined your own credibility as a professional. In summary, it is not easy to work with problem employees. Sometimes, little progress can be made. Other times, you will be limited in what you may do because of rules or regulations. You may experience frustration. It is helpful to remember that the skills you will learn to use as a manager have some commonalities with the skills you learned to become a competent clinical nurse. For example, you will remember that the more that you used the skills, the easier it became to perform the expected behaviors. Your self-evaluation of the manner in which you functioned was critical to improving your performance the next time. When you were in doubt about a particular approach to a task, you asked a more experienced person or researched the topic in a textbook. You gave yourself credit for things that went well and made a mental note to continue to use that approach in the future. These same approaches will serve you well in the interpersonal aspects of the management role just as they have as you worked to improve your clinical performance.

■ PROBLEMATIC RESPONSES TO EVALUATION

Some individuals when given a negative evaluation respond emotionally in crying or anger and hostility or by trying to excuse poor performance. For most people providing evaluation this creates distress and sometimes a feeling of helplessness to respond effectively.

Crying in Response to Evaluation

An individual who is presented with negative feedback may respond by crying. The person who cries when criticized may be simply an individual who cries easily and is unable to control expressions of emotion. A matter-of-fact response, offering a tissue and acknowledging that this situation must be difficult, allows the person to regain control and continue with the interview. Crying may recur throughout the interview. If you respond in the same calm way each time, you encourage the person to manage his or her own emotions. A common mistake is for the inexperienced evaluator to apologize for causing distress and to become very solicitous. This diverts attention from the performance problem that needs to be discussed.

Another concern when a person cries is whether the person may be attempting to manipulate the evaluator and divert attention from the behavior in question. In general, it will not be possible for you to determine this. However, you do not need to know the origin of the behavior in order to respond appropriately. Whatever the response, be calm and matter-of-fact and continue to focus on the behavioral concern and the changes needed.

Anger and Hostility

Some individuals who are evaluated negatively respond with anger and hostility. This individual may provide countercharges to the behaviors, that is say that others behave the same way, your evaluation is biased, or you are not there enough to really know. Individuals who do this often "hook" the supervisor into aggressive behavior in return. Once the supervisor succumbs to this exchange, it creates a no-win situation for the supervisor. When the response is aggressive, the supervisor must carefully maintain an assertive response, focus on the facts and behavior, and clearly state the corrective action in an assertive manner. The supervisor may have to keep returning to and repeating the basic facts. If the person becomes angry, it is sometimes necessary to acknowledge the person's feelings and suggest that the interview be terminated for that time and continued when the employee has had a chance to think about the evaluation. You will need to guard against meeting anger with anger and creating a hostile environment.

Providing Excuses in Response to Evaluation

Some individuals respond to negative evaluation by offering multiple excuses for their behavior. Although you do need to listen to the person and hear his or her side of the situation, you need to consider your response carefully. There may be a system problem of which you were unaware. However, this may simply be an attempt to deflect criticism. Participating in a charge–excuse cycle allows the employee to believe that the poor performance could be acceptable. Failure to listen may mean that you are making decisions based on poor data. One way to stop the excuse cycle is to use the same assertive response used for the aggressive person, in which the behavior and standards are carefully repeated and the expected changes in behavior are outlined.

Critical Thinking Exercise

Elizabeth Marshall, LVN (LPN), has worked on your unit for 5 ½ months. In that time, she has been late on at least six occasions. She tends to take 45 minutes for her lunch breaks instead of the expected 30 minutes. On occasion, her uniform has been wrinkled and stained, and her shoes usually need polishing. Her patients make positive comments about the care they receive, and she is willing to make adjustments in her own schedule to work around the needs of others on the staff. In preparing for her 6-month performance appraisal, what factors should you consider? How will you present that information? What are the positives and what are the negatives? How do you plan to proceed?

■ SELF-EVALUATION STRATEGIES

Self-evaluation is a critical component of professional practice. Self-evaluation guides your growth and development as a nurse, directing you to education sources and focusing your career directions. In addition, in many institutions employees are asked to come to their formal performance appraisal meeting having completed their own self-evaluation. The employee is asked to use the same criteria and even the same form that will be used by the supervisor. At the performance appraisal interview, the two documents are compared. Areas of agreement are noted and areas of discrepancy are then discussed.

There are differences in how the two evaluation forms (supervisor and employee) may be used. In some agencies, both forms go into the file. In others, the two documents are synthesized and one document goes into the file. This format often relieves the meeting of some stress. The employee may know the final document to be placed in the employee personnel file will be a synthesis of the two documents. This leads to a collaborative approach to evaluation.

Formal self-evaluation is more often a successful strategy when it focuses on either personal goals and objectives or areas for growth rather than areas of deficiency. Most people are reluctant to introduce the idea that they might not be meeting minimum standards of performance. Some individuals are concerned that they not sound immodest so they will not rate themselves highly. If you are doing a self-evaluation, try to be as objective about yourself as possible. Use the criteria and provide behavioral examples to support your self-evaluation. Do not hesitate to recognize areas in which you are demonstrating very good or even excellent performance. On the other hand, be sure to identify areas in which you seek to grow and improve.

Critical Thinking Exercise

You are due to receive your first performance appraisal after 6 months working the 3 p.m. to 11 p.m. shift on a general medical unit. You feel that you have done very well at making the transition to the registered nurse's role. You know that you may be approved to train for the relief charge nurse role if the unit manager believes you have the skills. You think you do have the skills, but are concerned that she may not think so. After all, the unit manager has had minimal opportunity to directly observe your performance. You spent some time in initial orientation on days and then moved to evenings where the charge nurse has provided your supervision. How will you prepare for this performance evaluation? What can you present that will help the unit manager to positively evaluate your skills and abilities? What communication skills will be important in this interview?

■ PEER EVALUATION STRATEGIES

Some facilities are using peer evaluations as one component of the formal evaluation system. When peer evaluation is used, the individual often is allowed to choose the peers who will be involved in the evaluation process. Peers are given a specific evaluation form and asked to complete it regarding the individual. These may be used along with a self-evaluation to try to build a more comprehensive picture of the person's performance. Peer evaluations may be especially important when a supervisor has a very broad span of control and has limited contact with individuals to be evaluated, and, therefore, limited behavioral observations to support evaluation.

If you are participating in peer evaluation, you need to be clear about how your evaluation will be used by the supervisor. For peer evaluation to be effective, everyone must take the responsibility seriously and approach it the same way they would if they were the supervisor. Education of staff in the process of peer evaluation makes a significant difference in the value of this approach. Dancer et al. (1997) found that initially peer evaluations were sketchy, did not contain specific behavioral examples, and were sometimes not completed. Providing written guidelines facilitated this process. They also found that some individuals continued to be very uncomfortable with peer evaluations. Building trust between employees and focusing on potential growth helped develop a foundation for effective peer evaluation.

■ RESPONDING TO PERSONAL EVALUATION

Much of this chapter has been written from the perspective of the nurse who is evaluating others. However, throughout your career you will be receiving employee evaluations regardless of your position in the organization. You will be receiving feedback and participating in evaluation conferences as the follower rather than the leader. There are steps you can take in the follower role to ensure that this process runs smoothly.

There may be occasions when you actually seek feedback. Comments such as "Were my assessments of Mrs. James accurate?" or "Please check to see that I have programmed this monitor correctly" are asking for feedback. The reasons for seeking feedback are the same as the reasons for providing it. Not surprisingly, then, the skills in receiving feedback are similar to those for providing it.

Responding to Positive Feedback

Some people are uncomfortable when receiving any type of feedback, especially positive comments. In trying not to appear overconfident or self-important, many individuals verbally discount any praise they receive. They may make comments such as "Oh, I really didn't do so much" or "It wasn't as good as I'd have liked." Compliments about your performance, behavior, or professional demeanor should be accepted with dignity. It is appropriate to express your appreciation by a simple and sincere "Thank you." A statement such as "Thank you for noticing" or "Thank you. I've been trying to improve that skill" graciously accepts the compliment given. A response such as this also reinforces the action of the person providing you with feedback.

Responding to a Negative Performance Appraisal

If you are a conscientious employee, you will give some serious thought to the type of feedback you are receiving. If the feedback you are receiving is negative, it may be very difficult for you to discuss it further. You may feel defensive about the comments that have been made. In such situations, it is important that the communications be clarified. Such questions as "How might I improve my skills?" or "How can I be of greater assistance?" may be good openers. Restating a message is valuable in determining that you understood what was being said. Statements such as "What I heard you say was that I need to look for opportunities to help others" or "Am I too slow in completing my care?" provide opportunity for verification, clarification, or expansion. Notice that all messages are in the form of "I" statements.

Most formal performance interviews are positive. The performance of an employee over the past 6 months or 1 year is reviewed against standards, goals may be set for the next period of time, and future plans may be discussed. If, however, the content of the interview is negative, you may find yourself feeling very defensive and perhaps emotionally upset. Continuing with the interview under these circumstances may not be desirable. It would be appropriate to request that the interview be continued at a later time, after you have had an opportunity to think about the comments that have been made. A second interview session could be scheduled for about

2 weeks later. You could accomplish this purpose with a statement such as, "I'm a little overwhelmed by the comments you have made. Could I have a little time to think about them before I respond—say, about 2 weeks?" You may be asked to respond in writing to a written evaluation that you will have discussed. You may also be asked to sign the evaluation indicating that you have read it. Signing the document does not necessarily indicate agreement. If you truly disagree with comments that have been recorded, it is acceptable to make a written comment to that effect when signing the written document.

If you are granted time to reflect on a poor evaluation and return to talk about it later, use the time well. Try to avoid being defensive. Look at the behavioral descriptions. Be clear in your mind about the concerns. You should construct a self-improvement plan to present to your supervisor. This plan should include specific steps you will take to change your behavior. Include a plan for future conferences with your supervisor. Put this plan in writing. When you meet with your supervisor, take a proactive role rather than a passive role. State that you are interested in becoming the best nurse you can be. Share your plan with your supervisor. Ask the supervisor for suggestions to augment the plan and make it more effective. Set up a plan for ongoing feedback as you work on your performance. This approach will demonstrate your professional commitment and be looked on very favorably by a supervisor.

Critical Thinking Exercise

Mary Peters, a nursing student, is completing her final semester. She has just received a very critical midsemester clinical evaluation from her instructor. Mary believes that her performance is better than the evaluation presented. How should she proceed? What guidelines should be considered? What suggestions would you make for others who might encounter a similar situation?

If after reviewing the evaluation you believe that your behaviors did not reflect poor performance and are concerned that the evaluation might be marred by bias, lack of information, or system problems, you are faced with a different problem. Above all, resist the temptation to take the offensive and attack the supervisor either directly or indirectly by talking with other staff. You can rarely improve the situation by such action. Approach this as a problem-solving process and seek to avoid an adversarial relationship with your supervisor.

If you work in an agency with a collective bargaining contract, you might want to consult with a representative of your bargaining group. If there is no bargaining group, you might check relevant personnel policies to determine what might be your next action. You might consult with an experienced nurse before proceeding. You could also take the evaluation and provide behavioral examples to show your work more positively. Consider whether some of the comments have merit and acknowledge them. You might ask the supervisor to include your immediate charge nurse in the next conversation if that person was not a part of this evaluation. Sometimes you may need to provide data about the staffing pattern during the times in question if this was a complicating factor. You are trying to be specific and factual when you meet again with your supervisor.

In most instances, your career is best served by your seeking to make your performance meet the expectations and standards of your supervisor. Even if you decide that you do not want to continue working in that environment, if you can create a positive view of yourself and your abilities before leaving, you will have a stronger reference and be in a better position to seek a different position. There may be an instance in which you feel that you cannot ethically conform to expectations. If that is the case, then you may want to resign. However, even in this instance, attempt to do so without attacking individuals or creating a hostile relationship.

■ KEY CONCEPTS

- Supervision involves oversight of performance in order to determine whether outcomes are being met.
- Ongoing performance evaluation, which is essential to effective management, may occur both formally and informally, and it should be based on clear standards of performance, such as job descriptions, policies and procedures, standards of nursing practice and standards of care. Soft skills related to attitudes and interpersonal behaviors are also an important component of evaluation.
- Data collected for the purpose of evaluation need to be behavioral in nature, free of bias, and representative of the person's overall performance.
- Providing feedback is a skill demanded of all managers. It requires that the individual be knowledgeable about both verbal and nonverbal communication skills and be able to use each effectively.
- Informal feedback involves giving the employee day-to-day or hour-to-hour information about his or her performance. It lets the employee know whether he or she is meeting the standards of the organization, reinforces good care, motivates the employee, helps correct inappropriate or incorrect behaviors, and supports the development of more effective performance.
- Coaching involves using feedback to assist others to achieve their own personal best and to support the entire team in achieving desired outcomes.
- Formal feedback is known as performance evaluation. The most effective performance appraisal systems are supported by administration, use evaluation tools with clear criteria that are built on the employee's job description, have clear procedural guidelines, and are conducted by supervisors trained in the process.
- The tools used in the performance evaluation process may take any one of several forms, but should be based on specific behavioral feedback and be as free of bias as possible.
- Evaluations lead to a performance interview that should be well planned and conducted to allow for exchange of communication and feedback.
- Evaluators may encounter problematic behaviors such as crying, anger, hostility, and excuses in response to negative evaluation. Continuing to be specific and factual in describing behavior as it relates to standards will assist in focusing the interview on behavior change.
- When problems cannot be corrected through other measures, progressive discipline may have to be used. Progressive discipline involves a series of steps of which the manager should be knowledgeable. Managers must assure that critical elements in disciplinary action can be met.
- A number of pitfalls can be encountered during progressive discipline. Being aware of common pitfalls can help guide the manager toward positive action.

- Self-evaluation is an essential professional responsibility and can lead to growth and professional development.
- Peer evaluation requires the same careful attention to standards and behavioral descriptions that are a part of a manager's evaluation. Peer evaluation can strengthen the workplace when done carefully.
- When receiving positive feedback, you should strive to accept it and acknowledge it with a simple statement of thanks.
- When receiving negative feedback, you should consider it carefully and then formulate a response that is based on a well-thought-out plan for improvement.
- If you receive a negative performance evaluation that you do not believe is accurate, think and plan before you respond. Avoid actions that will establish an adversarial relationship, if at all possible.

REFERENCES

Arney, S. (2001). Examining employees from all angles: the 360-degree evaluation. *Behavioral Health Management, 21*(4), 60–62.

Arthur, D. (1996). Performance appraisals: face-to-face with the employee. *HR Focus 73*(3), 17–19.

Dancer, S., Johnson, T., Zauner, J. et al. (1997). Peer evaluation: a visual picture. *Nursing Management, 28*(11), 57–60.

Drogosz, L. M., & Levy, P. E. (1996). Another look at the effects of appearance, gender, and job type on performance-based decisions. *Psychology of Women Quarterly, 20*(3), 437–446.

Grote, D. (1997). Getting the most out of the review process. *HR Focus, 74*(1), 15.

Haar, L. P. (1978). Performance appraisal. In A. G. Rezler and B. J. Stevens (Eds.), *The Nurse Evaluator in Education and Service.* New York: McGraw-Hill.

Langdon, K., & Osborne, C. (2001). *Performance Reviews.* New York: Dorling-Kindersley.

Oberg, W. (1972). Make performance appraisal relevant. *Harvard Business Review, 44*(1), 62.

Stone, F. M. (1999). *Coaching, Counseling, & Mentoring.* New York: American Management Association.

Umiker, W. (1998). *Management Skills for the New Health Care Supervisor* (3rd ed.) Gaithersburg, MD: Aspen Publishers.

8

The Nurse as Change Agent and Advocate

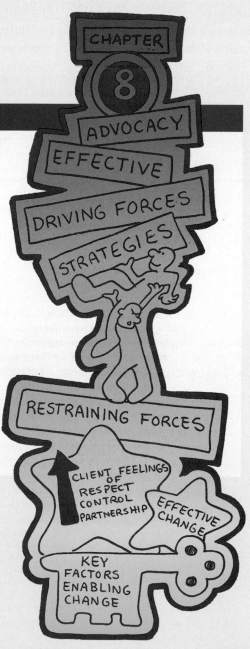

Learning Outcomes ■ ■ ■ ■ ■

After completing this chapter, you should be able to:

1. Explain how external forces cause change.
2. Apply Lewin's force-field analysis to assessing the need for change in your clinical practice.
3. Identify key factors in enabling change and overcoming resistance to change.
4. Apply an understanding of change to initiating and participating in change.
5. Compare the effect on nursing practice of adopting each of the several definitions of advocacy.
6. Identify prerequisites and general goals for effective advocacy.
7. Outline the general goals and objectives of client advocacy.
8. Apply knowledge of advocacy in advocating effectively for clients.
9. Apply knowledge of client advocacy to advocating for other health care workers.
10. Discuss constraints on and supports for the advocacy role.

Key Terms ■ ■ ■ ■ ■

advocacy
advocate
champion
change
change agent
coercion
constraints on advocacy
consultant
co-optation
driving forces
empirical-rational strategy
empowered

external forces
force-field analysis
internal forces
mediates
mediation
movement
negotiating
negotiation
normative-reeducative
   strategy
ombudsman

paternalism
power
power-coercive strategy
reactive change
refreezing
resistance
responsible model
restraining forces
stakeholders
story board
unfreezing

A dramatic, sweeping change of the entire health care system in the United States began in the 1990s and has not abated as we move into the twenty-first century. There are many drivers of this change; high in importance is the concern about the continuing increase in health care costs (see Chapter 3). Many health care organizations are changing their mix and types of workers. Employees are expected to cross-train and become multiskilled. Organizations are increasingly adopting continuous quality improvement (CQI), whereby all employees are **empowered** to fully participate in bringing about changes that improve care (see Chapter 4). Health care consumers are faced with changes in policies and procedures, new ways of caregiving, and new expectations for their own participation. Thus, change presents challenges for both providers and consumers of health care.

The government, providers of care, and recipients of care agree that changes must occur. However, there is great debate about what changes are necessary and how those changes should be accomplished. For professional nurses to participate in and influence the outcome of health care reform and assist clients in the midst of this system, nurses must not only understand the issues but also know how to be effective participants in the process of change itself. By understanding change theory and its application and the basic principles of **advocacy,** nurses can become valuable leaders in meeting the health care challenges for nursing units, healthcare organizations, and clients. Nursing leaders use the change theory to ensure that the contributions of nursing are included in our national plans for ever-changing health care. This chapter provides you with the basic principles for achieving successful change and advocating for clients.

■ DEFINING CHANGE

To **change** simply means to alter, to become different, or to transform. Changes occur as a result of **internal forces** or **external forces** impinging on an individual or organization. External forces for change are those that originate outside the person or organization. Insurance companies, state and federal government, consumers, new technologies, physicians, and competitors are some of the external forces to which health care institutions must respond. The federal Health Insurance Portability and Accountability Act (HIPAA) legislation that mandated privacy protections for health care clients became effective in 2003 and demanded massive changes in training and operating procedures for all affected organizations and their employees. As a professional nurse, you will participate in many changes due to external forces such as technological advances, practice models, economics, consumer demands, and regulatory requirements.

Internal forces come from within the organization (for organizational change) or from within the person (for individual change). These forces may include a strategy for success formulated by top management, the decision to purchase new technologies, or a need for change in employee behavior. For example, a decision to adopt a computerized nursing documentation system means that all staff will need to change their method of documentation. When you entered the nursing program that you are currently attending, you were motivated by an internal desire for change, the desire to prepare yourself to become a nurse.

Nursing advances, such as collaborative governance and career ladders, have come from the visions of nursing leaders who felt that these internal changes would lead to an empowered work force that would add quality to the organization. Often, these internal forces for change are a result of the organizational vision and strategies to position the institution to better meet the challenges of external forces.

Change may be unplanned. Unplanned or **reactive change** occurs in response or reaction to some event or problem as it arises. We make adjustments to unplanned change daily. Examples for nurses might include making a change in priorities because of an unexpected admission; an employee who calls in sick, resulting in short staffing on a unit; or a sudden need to transfer a patient to the intensive care unit (ICU). Not all unplanned change is unpleasant. A patient may take a turn for the better and require less time than planned. You might be asked to assume the charge nurse role because of your problem-solving skills. You might not have planned to make this change, but when the opportunity is offered you welcome the challenge.

Planned change is defined as "the deliberate design and implementation of a structural innovation, a new policy or goal, or an overt change in operating philosophy, climate, and style" (Thomas & Bennis, 1972, p. 289). Planned change involves a deliberate and conscious set of carefully orchestrated actions whose purpose is to create a better product, work environment, service, or other factor affecting an organization. Your decision to enter nursing was a planned change. Planned change is used for projects that are complex or large in scope and require greater time, resources, or skills for successful implementation. Planned change is essential for nurses to achieve full participation in the process of reform that is occurring in the U.S. health care system.

A **change agent** is the person who seeks to cause or create change. This person may originate the ideas for change or may be an individual who recognizes the value of new ideas originated by others. Nurses may need to be change agents in regard to themselves, clients, and the institutions in which they practice. Individuals who understand the process of change and how they can best adapt to the uncertainties it brings more often become the agents of change rather than the targets of change. It is this involvement and participation that will give you a sense of control and allow you to be successful in this ever-changing world. The nurse who is able to embrace rather than resist change will be positioned for a career of unprecedented opportunity and reward.

■ UNDERSTANDING THEORIES OF CHANGE

Theories of change help us study and understand what is happening in the process. One individual who contributed significantly to our understanding of change and the change process was Kurt Lewin (1951), who is noted for a identifying a planned change process called **force-field analysis.** He identified three phases through which a change agent must proceed before a planned change can be realized. He designated these phases or stages **unfreezing, movement,** and **refreezing.**

In the unfreezing stage, the change agent loosens or unfreezes the factors or forces that are maintaining the status quo or keeping the situation as it is. This involves increasing the perceived need for change and creating discontent with the situation as it is.

The second stage identified by Lewin involves movement. During this stage, the change agent identifies, plans, and implements appropriate strategies to bring about the change. Changes should occur gradually whenever possible. Bridges (2003) in his description of change calls this a neutral period. The changes are not yet solidified, people have not gotten comfortable with the new way things are, and they are often ambivalent about going forward or retreating into old ways.

The final phase is referred to by Lewin as refreezing. During this period, the changes are integrated and stabilized. It is a time when positive feedback and encouragement help solidify the changes. Bridges refers to this phase as acceptance and adaptation. These terms help us see the underlying feelings that are occurring in those participating in the change. When people have accepted the change as the new reality and adapted their worklife to the change, then the change process is complete.

Lewin's theory is based on the concept that individuals will strive for equilibrium. Thus, in the change situation, there must be a balance between the forces that call for the change, which Lewin referred to as **driving forces,** and those that oppose the change, called **restraining forces.** People prefer things with which they are familiar and have a natural tendency to resist change, especially if it requires a change in values or beliefs or if it appears it will require something extra. The results of change may be unknown and thus represent a threat to some. Therefore, the need for change must be clear and powerful enough to motivate the individual, group, or organization to see and accept it. The driving forces must be increased and/or the restraining forces must be decreased so that the need for change is greater than the desire to retain the current pattern. In reality, the process of change may flow back and forth between the two.

■ STRATEGIES FOR CHANGE

Although a number of strategies to create change may be used, in general they fall into three categories: empirical-rational strategies, power-coercive strategies, and normative-educative strategies.

Power-Coercive Strategy

power & fear (handwritten)

The **power-coercive strategy** is employed when a leader orders change and those with less **power** comply (Benne et al., 1976). By using this strategy, the nurse who wishes to be a change agent would need official authority in order to mandate a change. Compliance originates in the desire to please a supervisor, fear of losing employment, fear of sanctions for noncompliance, and rewards for compliance. Regulations and laws originate from the strategy of power-coercive change. For example, failure to comply with state registered nurse (RN) licensing requirements can lead to loss of license to practice.

Laws regulations (handwritten)

A power-coercive strategy may be used to force a change for the common good when it is assumed that experience with the change will lead to a change in values. Desegregation laws are an example of this strategy. Change in behavior was forced despite great conflict in an effort to provide equality of opportunity and experience. It was then hoped that the experience of living with desegregation would lead to changes in attitudes, beliefs, and values regarding those of other ethnic and cultural backgrounds.

There are times when a power-coercive change is so incongruent with the beliefs and values of an individual or group that it does not succeed. The amendment to the U.S. Constitution prohibiting the sale of all alcoholic beverages provides one such example. Despite the consequences of using or selling alcohol, people violated the law in large enough numbers that the law created extreme enforcement problems. Because the law did not reflect the values of the majority, the amendment was subsequently repealed.

In organizations, power-coercive strategies may become very costly and fail due to the **resistance** this strategy invokes. Many professional staff are deeply offended by a power-coercive strategy that does not acknowledge their own expertise and concern for the outcomes of their actions.

Empirical-Rational Strategy

The **empirical-rational strategy** maintains that people will follow their rational self-interest once it is revealed to them (Benne et al., 1976). In other words, a change will be accepted by a person, group, or organization when it is seen as desirable and is aligned with the interest of those affected. This strategy emphasizes reason and knowledge. It is primarily used for technological changes. The recipients of change do not actively participate in planning the change. The "right" person for the job educates the targets of change so that they understand the benefits of altering the status quo. By using this strategy, the nurse who identifies the need for change can become a change agent by identifying a better approach and then educating others about the value of this approach.

An example of this strategy might be the introduction of an automated medication-dispensing machine on the nursing unit. If the manager explained to you that you would no longer have to count narcotics each shift, that patient charges would now be automatic, and that you could learn to use the machine in 30 minutes, you might see the change as desirable because it would save you time. It would be in line with your self-interest; you could get finished with your shift on time. In this example, the change would probably proceed easily and quickly.

EXAMPLE   *Using the Empirical-Rational Approach to Change*

Staffing on a nursing unit at Community Hospital needed to be changed from total patient care (in which an RN performs all nursing duties and tasks for a group of patients) to partners in practice (in which one RN and one nursing assistant care for a group of patients). This change was necessitated by the shortage of RNs in the area. RN positions could not be filled, and the unit was working with short staffing, overtime, and missed days off. By using an approach developed around the empirical-rational strategy, the manager educated the staff on the desirability of the change and how it would affect working conditions for the nurse. There would be the immediate alleviation of some things contributing to poor work satisfaction. With fewer RNs needed for each day, the current staff could fill the staffing needs. In addition, there might be increased efficiency, more time for the nurse to spend on professional patient activities such as teaching, and more staff at an equal or lower cost. The nurse's beliefs or feelings about the abilities of the nursing assistant or supervising others were not discussed.

The RNs on the unit were very upset when presented with the completed plan and a date for implementation. They insisted that nursing assistants could never provide the quality of care expected on their unit. They vowed that they would quit before they would compromise their priniciples about nursing care.

This situation demonstrates the pitfall of using a completely empirical-rational approach to change. Failure occurred because feelings, beliefs, and values were ignored in the change process. Bridges (2003) points out that omitting feelings, beliefs, and values contributes to the failure of planned changes in many businesses. He provides several examples of major changes by national corporations that appeared to be appropriate from an empirical-rational point of view. These changes failed because those initiating the change had failed to consider feelings, values, and the shared culture of the businesses involved as they planned and implemented the change process.

Normative-Reeducative Strategy

Lewin

People
attitudes
norm
values
skills
relationship

The third strategy of change is the **normative-reeducative** approach. The normative-reeducative strategy states that change will take place only after changes in attitudes, values, skills, and significant relationships have occurred (Benne et al., 1976).

This model emphasizes that involvement of those affected by the change is essential in achieving changes in attitudes, beliefs, and norms. This view of change differs from the empirical-rational strategy in the assertion that self-interest and knowledge are not sufficient to bring about change.

In using this strategy, the change agent must involve those most affected in working out the plans for achieving the change. Mutual trust and collaboration facilitate this process of change. The assumption that successful change requires alteration of attitudes, values, norms, or external relationships means that "people" factors are as important to progress as are technology, knowledge, and information. Therefore, when the change agent and those participating in the proposed change experience conflict, the progress must be halted until the conflict has been resolved. In this strategy for change, the input of ideas, information, and technology must be aligned with norms and values for the change to successfully occur. This theory was developed by Kurt Lewin, Warren Bennis, and others and is the foundation for most major organizational change today (Benne et al., 1976).

EXAMPLE *Using the Normative-Reeducative Strategy for Change*

At General Hospital, the nurse manager was confronted with the same shortage of nurses experienced at Community Hospital. She also decided that changing the pattern of care delivery could solve this problem. This nurse manager, following the principles of the normative-reeducative strategy, introduced the potential change to the staff for its reactions. As in the empirical-rational method, information and rationale for the change were given, but then the group was invited to discuss its concerns and feelings about the potential change. The nurse manager listened carefully to cues about attitudes, beliefs, and values that could affect the success of the change. After listening to the staff discuss its concerns about the qualifications, abilities, and commitment of the proposed nursing assistants, the manager asked for suggestions for making the plan more acceptable to the RNs. One of the RNs suggested that the plan be modified to include having the RNs from the unit assist with screening, hiring, and training the new nursing assistants they would be working with. This modification was discussed and most agreed that it would assure that the care met their standard. The RNs began to discuss how changing might help with some of the concerns they had about the old staffing pattern. At the end of the discussion, the staff agreed to use a trial unit and participate in this change of staffing.

Most modern experts would assert that large-scale organizational change will not be successful until normative-reeducative principles are addressed. It is from this point of view that we proceed with describing the implementation of change.

■ THE ROLE OF THE CHANGE AGENT

When the need for change has been identified, some person or group must be responsible for leading the change. This individual, as we mentioned earlier, is called the change agent. The recipients or targets of the change can be an individual, a group, or an entire organization. In organizations that have adopted CQI, the change agent is called the **champion** and the others affected by the change are referred to as **stakeholders,** a term we hear frequently today. Under this model, anyone in the organization can have an idea for improving the system (become a champion) and present that idea to those who would be affected by the improvement (the stakeholders).

EXAMPLE   *Changing the System for Handling Supplies*

Ed Wilson, a staff nurse in a local hospital, had an idea for a better system for handling supplies on the new labor and delivery unit that was under construction. He proposed that there be case carts in each room instead of a centrally located supply cart. Ed became the champion of the project and enlisted the support and input of management and his peers. The result was a system whereby supplies were at the fingertips of the nurse when needed and patient care was improved. Most importantly, this nurse earned the respect and gratitude of colleagues for creating an improvement in their work environment.

The change agent may be an employee of the organization or an outside **consultant.** Consultants are often used when the change requires specialized expertise and skills, freedom from day-to-day organizational responsibilities, or the objectivity of an outsider.

■ DRIVING OR RESTRAINING FORCES

The theory of force-field analysis by Lewin (1951) describes the forces that push toward change balanced against the forces that restrain change. The external and internal forces that push toward change are called the **driving forces.** Forces that push against change are called **restraining forces.**

When these forces are in equilibrium, the current status is maintained. For change to occur, driving forces must be increased or the restraining forces must be decreased so that the balance becomes upset. The tendency for those who want a change is to push. However, the tendency of the target of change is to push back and thereby maintain balance. The change agent must identify the driving and restraining forces in order to determine the best plan for implementing change.

In an example of a nursing unit changing from total patient care to partners in practice, let us list the driving and restraining forces. The driving forces (forces for change) might include decreased cost, increased care hours for the patient, and elimination of nonprofessional duties for the RN. Restraining forces might include the RN's loss of control of all aspects of patient care, loss of personal contact with patients, and concern about quality of care. Until the balance of the forces is disturbed, change will not occur.

In the example of General Hospital, having the RNs participate in the hiring and training helped decrease the restraining forces. The workload was a strong driving force for change. Thus, the balance was changed so that the system con-

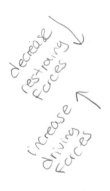
decrease restraining forces ↓

increase driving forces ↑

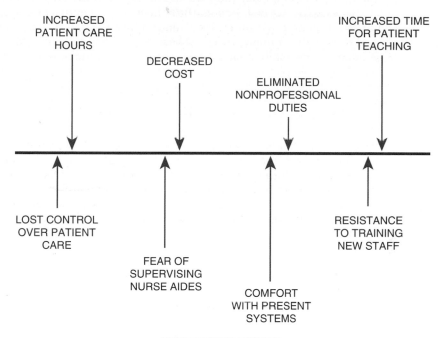

DRIVING FORCES

INCREASED
PATIENT CARE
HOURS

DECREASED
COST

ELIMINATED
NONPROFESSIONAL
DUTIES

INCREASED TIME
FOR PATIENT
TEACHING

LOST CONTROL
OVER PATIENT
CARE

FEAR OF
SUPERVISING
NURSE AIDES

COMFORT
WITH PRESENT
SYSTEMS

RESISTANCE
TO TRAINING
NEW STAFF

RESTRAINING FORCES

FIGURE 8-1
Force-field diagram.

tained more driving forces than restraining forces. Successful change was more likely to occur.

Reduction of restraining forces is generally a more effective way to encourage change than is increasing driving forces. Increasing driving forces may lead to hostility and the emergence of additional restraining forces.

Lewin's force-field model illustrates the need to look at multiple factors that can affect the tendency to change. As we learned from the normative-reeducative strategy, factors affecting change include attitudes, beliefs, and norms, as well as knowledge and technology. A chart of the force-field analysis for our partners in practice example illustrates the application of these many factors (Figure 8-1).

■ OVERCOMING OBSTACLES TO CHANGE

Lewin (1951) also identified underlying obstacles to change and constructed a model of the process to overcome those obstacles. This three-stage sequential model begins with unfreezing the status quo. People prefer familiarity and have a natural tendency to resist change, especially if it requires a change in values or beliefs. Therefore, the need for change must be clear and powerful enough to motivate the individual, group, or organization to see and accept it. It is during this unfreezing stage that the driving forces are increased and/or the restraining forces are decreased so that the need for change is greater than the desire to retain the current pattern.

The feelings and emotions of those involved in change are critical components of what is happening. Perlman and Takacs (1990) listed 10 emotional phases experienced during the change process. These phases (equilibrium, denial, anger, bargaining, chaos, depression, resignation, openness, readiness, and reemergence) may help the individual implementing the change to understand the reactions and feelings of those involved and take appropriate actions. This long list recognizes that many emotions occur and that emotions may differ from person to person.

The next sequential step is to formulate and try out a plan. This step requires the change agent to work with stakeholders in fostering new values, attitudes, and behaviors. If the change is sweeping, a pilot, or trial, is a desirable and often effective way to introduce a change before the program is implemented over a large area of the organization. A pilot program involves implementing the change (or trying it out) in a selected area or with a small group before making a major change. In the case of change from primary nursing to partners in practice, one nursing unit might be selected to do the trial, evaluate it, and "work out the bugs" before the change is implemented on all nursing units.

The last step in Lewin's sequence is called refreezing. At this stage, the new pattern of behavior becomes the norm. Without this step, there is a tendency to revert to the old "tried and true" patterns. Refreezing occurs when new patterns become frequent enough to be comfortable and are rewarded. In our example of conversion to the use of nursing assistants at General Hospital, rewards might include lower patient-to-staff ratio, recognition from administration for a job well done, or even bonus pay at the completion of a successful trial.

■ ENABLING CHANGE

Because change is a reality that we must all learn to accept, attention has increasingly turned to enabling change or helping it occur. As we discuss the various steps in enabling change, you will recognize many of the steps that you have learned previously as the nursing process.

Assessing the Situation

It is important that you assess the situation in which change is to take place. What are the difficulties or problems that this change is designed to alter? Is the change designed to improve a system that is currently working satisfactorily? Is the change being driven externally or internally? Who supports the potential for change? Who is critical of any change? Who will gain from the change and who will lose?

Bridges (2003) suggests that there are many losses in any change and failure to acknowledge that loss is present is one reason for the failure of change. A new computerized documentation system may be efficient, but nurses who have felt expert at using the current system lose their feelings of being expert and must face being novices again. A change in care delivery systems may remove responsibilities that gave meaning and feelings of accomplishment to an individual. For example, the nurse who feels deep satisfaction from providing total care for all a patient's physical

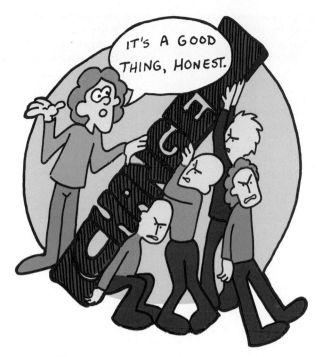

Many factors result in resistance to change.

needs faces loss of that special relationship when personal care is assigned to an assistant and the nurse spends less time with the patient.

Do you expect the change to be resisted? It is critical that you understand why the change might be resisted. Resistance may have its roots in the presentation, timing, or pace of the change. However, resistance may relate to weaknesses of the proposal. Those planning for change may not have explored the potential effects or considered problems that might be confronted. Some resistance to change is a result of the group's fears or unwillingness to give up benefits that exist in the current system.

Inertia, habit, and comfort with the known are characteristics traditionally grouped under resistance to change. For most people, change isn't actively sought; the established routine is preferred. However, routine may be preferred because it provides some control. Because change, at its onset at least, involves some ambiguity if not outright confusion, control is threatened. That is, resistance is frequently a reaction to a loss of control, not necessarily to the change itself (Jick, 1993).

In addition to the fear of loss of control, excess uncertainty can lead to resistance. Employees want to know why, when, and how changes will occur. They also are concerned about how an anticipated change will affect them. It takes extra effort to accomplish change, and the reasons for putting forth that extra effort are need to be adequately explained. Lack of trust is another key factor in resistance to change. For a group to follow a change agent through the uncertainty, loss of control, and expenditure of extra effort, it needs to feel that the leader is sensitive to its needs. When trust is absent, resistance to change increases (Display 8-1).

Out come #3

4

DISPLAY 8-1	Factors That Result in Resistance to Change

Poor timing of the change
Poor presentation of the proposal for change and its effects
Weaknesses in the proposal for change
Improper pacing of the change   *too fast too slow*
Comfort with the present way of doing things
Fear of loss of control
Excess uncertainty of the effects of change
Lack of trust
The expenditure of personal energy required for change to occur

A variety of resistive responses may be seen. Asprec (1975) described four ways in which resistance to change may be revealed. Active resistance is seen in voiced frustration and aggression toward those proposing change. Organized passive resistance or resisting change collectively involves people coming together and simply ignoring the change and continuing with the old and familiar. Indifference seen as stakeholders attempting to divert attention elsewhere is another way change is resisted. Some resist by acceptance on the surface or by not openly opposing a change but not getting the change quite right. Management is then challenged to identify and manage those reactions so that change can occur.

Planning for Change

Change can be an exhilarating, exciting process. Groups that experience one success are ready, willing, and able to approach the next opportunity; one success leads to future successes. These successes result in teams that see themselves as powerful and competent. Thus, empowered teams develop in an environment that manages resistance effectively and supports stakeholders. However, becoming a successful change agent, developing positive attitudes, and enabling change require skills in planning for the change.

Several factors need to be addressed when planning any change. The first factor to be considered is the timing of the change. At times, extraneous factors may affect the success of the change. In our example of conversion from primary nursing to partners in practice, we would be ill advised to begin the pilot program on a nursing unit during a time the nurse manager was on vacation.

A second important factor is planning how fast the change will proceed. Here, the benefits of rapid results must be weighed against the potential for success. Is there enough time for trial-and-error adjustments to the plan? Would adjustments lead to a more efficient result? Is time of the essence for financial reasons? The best guidelines for determining the right pace are judgment and experience.

The scope of planned change is also a factor to be considered in permanent success of a change. In our example of partners in practice, a pilot study on one nursing unit to try out and perfect the change would be advisable before implementing the change in an entire hospital. Modifications and adjustments are to be expected and can be handled more easily in a smaller area.

The most fundamental step is to develop a trusting relationship with those involved in the change through open communication and full participation. Lack of trust is a key factor in resistance to change, because resistance increases when trust is absent. For a group to follow a change agent through the uncertainty, loss of control, and expenditure of extra effort, it needs to feel that the leader is sensitive to its needs. You should explain in advance the need for change and how it will benefit the group. Allow for questions and suggestions. If your group believes that you value its ideas and that it can be free to voice its concerns to you, then you are off to a positive beginning. Give and receive feedback; be sure you are understood. Accept feedback as constructive, and refrain from value judgments or criticism. Attempt to gain consensus and establish a receptive frame of mind for the change plan before proceeding with implementation.

Bridges (2003) suggests that listening is critical at this stage. People need an opportunity to describe their fears, the losses they perceive will occur, and their feelings about the situation. As you listen, acknowledge their feelings. Don't argue with their expressions of feelings. Remember what you learned in your clinical courses. Feelings are real and the losses that may occur are real also. People need to grieve these losses. However, you cannot stop with that. If you are to plan a successful change, you need to consider what you might offer individuals to help with resolution of their losses. For example, will there be training and support to help restore feelings of expertise in a new system? Listening actively to all objections to the new proposal will help you identify those that must be addressed in the process. Alterations in the process or plan may be needed.

Participation and involvement are crucial in achieving permanent changes, because they address the issue of loss of control described by Jick (1993). The degree of involvement must be balanced with the time available; full participation can be very time consuming if the group is a large one. Often, a smaller task force of individuals with information to contribute, as well as recognized credibility within the workgroup, is assigned to formulate a plan based on input from the larger group. This strategy allows the plan and its implementation to proceed more efficiently.

To become a successful change agent, you must be able to demonstrate to others your commitment to the change. Foley (1993) states, "The leader's commitment must shine through her or his every behavior, every decision and every statement. . . . When others see and feel our commitment, they more readily join in and want to become a part of the program." Thus, your personal enthusiasm for a task will greatly affect the outcome. The change agent needs to believe in the necessity for planned change. It is very difficult to enlist support and trust when you lack a personal desire to succeed. As a committed champion of the change plan, you can communicate your enthusiasm and help others get on the "bandwagon." Humor should not be overlooked as a method of reducing tensions and creating an atmosphere of camaraderie. A leader's enthusiasm is contagious. People want to be a part of events that are exciting, important, and fun.

Provision of resources and support also facilitates the process of change. A manager may be able to offer extra paid time or a stipend for the work of the group or be able to enlist other members of the organization with special skills to manage parts of the change. This provision could include assigning some of the tasks of the workgroup to others to free the workgroup to devote time to the change project. For example, in our partners in practice program, a nursing educator would be able to lead development of competencies for nursing assistants based on sound education princi-ples and her knowledge of the appropriate scope of practice for assistive personnel. A staff member from the human resources department would be valuable in writing the job description. Other approaches to those who resist change entail increased risk of failure of a current project or other planned changes in the future. These approaches include negotiation, co-optation, and coercion.

Negotiating involves finding areas in which both parties may give somewhat and both parties then gain. Negotiating with principal resisters may help move the entire group forward. This strategy has the disadvantage of alerting others to the possibility of negotiation and may leave individuals feeling that resistance pays.

Co-optation is enlisting key people from the opposition onto your side by giving them desirable roles in the process and thereby ensuring their commitment. The most frequent strategy is to co-opt the informal leaders. Care must be taken that the change agent is not seen as manipulative, thereby destroying trust and ensuring re-sistance to any future projects.

Coercion involves the threat of adverse consequences for nonparticipation in the change. Coercion should always be considered a last resort when speed is essential. Threatening job loss, lack of promotion, and other adverse consequences creates hostility, anger toward the initiator of the change, and often anger toward the entire organization as well. Active subversion of the plan may occur, resulting in its total failure.

Implementing Change

Most significant projects involving change have a specified date for implementation. Once established, those dates should be adhered to as closely as possible. A certain energy exists around any anticipated date. Changing dates or postponing actions re-sults in people becoming suspicious or critical of the process. Those who have looked forward to the change will be disappointed. Momentum is lost.

Actually implementing the change is the unfreezing process described by Lewin. Bridges (2003) discusses this phase in terms of transition. He suggests that every be-ginning is also an ending. Part of the role of the change agent is to help define those aspects that are now gone and clarify those that remain. You also treat the past with respect. Although new ways of doing things are needed, previous ways served many people well.

If you have a major role in the change, or if you are the leader on your unit, it is important that you project a positive view regarding the change and see it as an op-portunity. You need to believe that you can make a difference. Others will take their cue from you. In other words, you role model the behavior you wish to see in others.

It also is important during the process of implementing the change that good communication processes be in place. Good communication helps decrease resist-ance, lets people know what is expected of them in the process, and keeps partici-pants informed of the progress that is being made. Persons responsible for leading the change need to let participants know what is to occur and what their role will be. They need to be praised for their positive efforts. Interpersonal relationships need to be given high consideration during the change process.

According to Bridges (2003), after the ending and letting go of the old ways of op-erating, people enter what he termed the neutral zone. In this part of the transition, the new way is not working as well as it is expected to when well established; people have not yet developed the new skills they need. Some may get discouraged about the change.

Critical Thinking Exercise

On graduation from your nursing program, you seek and obtain employment in the local community hospital. You are assigned to the night shift. After working for several months, you realize that there are activities that occur among the staff at night that you believe are undesirable. For example, there has been a practice established among some of the staff members to cover for one another while they take turns napping for 1 or 2 hours. You believe this is unethical. Often, patients must wait to have their call lights answered because fewer staff members are available. You would like to change this practice. How would you proceed? What steps would you take? What would you need to consider? Of the theories and strategies discussed in this chapter, which one(s) might work best?

Monitoring and Evaluating the Change Process

Once a change has been implemented, the situation needs to be monitored and evaluated. Many questions need to be considered. Is the change achieving the goals within the allocated time and resources? Is the anticipated change occurring or is there backsliding to old behaviors? Are the participants beginning to show hope and satisfaction with the change? If the answer to these questions is no, the leader must address all the outstanding issues before proceeding further. If an RN on the new practice team cannot complete charting tasks in the allotted time, the plan needs to be reevaluated. Perhaps the nursing assistant is not yet fully trained; if so, there can be further orientation. However, if the RN is not allowing the nursing assistant to perform duties established in the plan, then the restraining force of fear of supervision will have to be readdressed. Why is the RN unwilling or afraid to allow the nursing assistant to perform to the fullest of her ability and training?

Because of all the factors that are involved in change, it is not always possible to anticipate problems in the change process. In addition, in the chaos of the health care environment today, many changes are thrust on the providers of care, leaving little time for proper planning and implementation. The key concept is to plan as carefully as conditions permit, be flexible in addressing and adjusting to problems as they arise, and reward and reinforce progress toward success.

■ SUSTAINING THE CHANGE

To be sustained, a change must be refined and standardized. This is the refreezing described by Lewin. At this point, the process can be celebrated. Participants need to be recognized for their effort and participation. Lessons learned that can be applied elsewhere should be noted. The new procedures should be documented and standardized. Lastly, it is time for the change agent to transfer the responsibility for ongoing monitoring and improvements to the participants.

Initial procedures and policies may have changed during the implementation. Actual practice must be checked to be sure that it matches final policy and procedures. A report of the change from start to finish will provide reference for others and make the same or a similar change move more quickly and efficiently in the future. In CQI organizations, this report is called a **story board** and is written at each step of the change process. Use of a story board helps everyone see progress along the way and provides motivation for team members to continue. A completed story board, in addition to serving as a report, provides evidence of success and recognizes the participants.

Critical Thinking Exercise

You are working as a new graduate on the medical unit of a local hospital. Just before you started working there, a new charting system was implemented that involved using a flowchart rather than recording everything in the nurses' notes. You believe it is a good system and find it similar to one you used in one of the hospitals to which you were assigned while in school. However, many of the older nurses disregard the flowcharts, grumble about the change, and continue to chart as they had in the past. How can you help them adapt to the new charting procedure? Why do you think they may be resisting the change? What would you do first? Are there any other persons you would involve? How would you involve them?

■ BEING AN EFFECTIVE PARTICIPANT IN CHANGE

All of us have heard the old axiom "Nothing in life is sure except death and taxes." Nothing is sure because change is a constant part of life. Our own attitude and ability to cope with change can make the difference between personal success and failure and between satisfaction and dissatisfaction with our lives and careers. In this section, we explore methods to make change work for you (Display 8-2).

DISPLAY 8-2	Being a Successful Participant in Change

Ask who, what, why, and how
Look for the benefits
Participate actively
Offer suggestions
Express concerns
Be patient with setbacks
Seek support
Remain flexible
Be a good listener
Celebrate success

Your first responsibility as a participant in a proposed change is to be sure that you understand what the change is, why it should occur, who it will benefit, and what is required for success. Do not be afraid to ask questions. Most likely, the questions you ask will reflect the same concerns that your peers have.

If you have concerns, express them in a constructive manner. For example, "I'm concerned that a nursing assistant will not be able to perform enough duties to allow me to finish my charting on time at the end of the shift." Do not focus on people or make value judgments in stating concerns. Focus your concerns on systems, organization of tasks, or behaviors.

Remember that it is natural to be uncomfortable with change because it disrupts our routine, is uncertain, and requires additional effort. Knowing that negative feelings are common, try to look for positive benefits to the change.

After you have a clear understanding of the change proposal, try to understand what the change means to you as an individual. Ask yourself the following questions:

1. Will it pay off for me?
2. Can I do it successfully?
3. Is it worth the effort it will take?
4. Must the change occur with or without my support?

If you answer yes to the first three questions, chances are that you view the change positively. You will be optimistic and well positioned for success. Understand that even with positive change there will be some uncertainty, reservations, and doubt as the process moves forward. During those times, remind yourself to stay flexible and involved and to ask for support.

If you feel that the answer to any of the first three questions is no, then your personal task will be more difficult. You may experience shock, denial, anger, and/or depression at the idea of the change. Coping with these feelings requires that you analyze your feelings and address the cause. For example, if the institution has decided to train all RNs in basic electrocardiogram (ECG) interpretation, you may want to resist the change for several reasons. Perhaps you have always thought of ECG strips as a mystery code and are afraid that you will not be able to successfully complete the training. A strategy would be to participate in setting up the training to include enough time and practice to assure success. This involvement will help increase feelings of control and decrease fears of the unknown.

Another strategy for overcoming your personal feelings of resistance is to offer alternative suggestions to achieve the same goal. You might have an idea that alters a small part of the plan but turns the proposed change into a positive one for you. For example, you might suggest that nurses newly trained in ECG readings be partnered with experienced ECG nurses for the first 6 months. That addition might transform your fear of change into excitement over learning a valuable new skill.

Participation is the essential ingredient for personal success. Changes do occur in which many nurses "go along for the ride." These nurses often feel unappreciated and dissatisfied. Nurses who become involved by asking questions and offering suggestions are the individuals who feel empowered and enjoy work. Just as success breeds success for organizations, early successes lead to future successes for individuals. Through participation, you can gain a sense of control over a planned change and influence the outcomes of that change.

Critical Thinking Exercise

You have recently accepted the challenge of serving as the charge nurse on a 36-bed unit in a long-term care facility. You see everyone working independently without volunteering to help one another. You note that even when people need help they are reluctant to ask for it because they fear being rebuffed. You would like to change the norms of working together. How would you approach this? What would be your first steps? If these were not effective, what would you do next? How would you measure success? Give a rationale for your answers.

■ FACILITATING CHANGES FOR CLIENTS/PATIENTS THROUGH ADVOCACY

Clients and families often find themselves adrift in the maze that is modern health care. From insurance and managed care companies to the actual providers, information may be difficult to obtain and even more difficult to understand when accessed. Decisions are asked of people when they are in great distress and find it hard to comprehend new information. Thus, clients and their families often need a person they perceive as being their helper in negotiating the system. This helper is formally termed the **advocate.**

Definitions of Advocacy

There are a variety of views of what it means to be an advocate. One view is that an advocate is one who plead's another's cause (Alfano, 1987). Another view of the role of advocate lies in the concept of **mediation.** Mediation involves helping two parties overcome difficulties and work out an agreement between them. The purpose of mediation is to arrive at a solution that is acceptable to all persons involved: those making the decision and those affected by it. Thus, in supporting the cause of the client, the advocate **mediates** with decision makers. This aspect of advocacy can include political action to influence public policymakers regarding issues relevant to health. Both of these views of advocacy may be significant in health care. However, still another view of the advocate as one who enables persons to speak or negotiate for themselves is growing in importance. This type of advocacy not only helps the individual with the current situation but also provides skill and confidence to face future challenges.

A central aspect of this view is helping clients to be autonomous, informed decision makers. The best interests of the client are determined primarily by the client and not by nurses or other professionals. This definition requires that the nurse and client interact as whole and unique individuals to determine the meaning of the experience for the client. Giving advice is no longer sufficient. Teaching and support are given according to client needs and choices. Advocacy moves from interceding or pleading a case for the client to actively promoting the client's rights to autonomy and free choice. We, as nurses, are required to identify and understand the client's desires and work to assure that those desires are carried out to the greatest possible degree.

Don't give advice ! →

A Background for Nursing Advocacy

For nursing, advocacy is rooted in the values of the dignity and freedom of the individual and the importance of client education. The advocacy role evolved as the nursing profession became increasingly autonomous and client centered.

As long ago as 1978, federal legislation required each state to set up an **ombudsman** program for nursing homes so that residents and families would have an advocate. Hospitals began to explore the need for a salaried position of client advocate, separate from all the service departments in the agency. Frequently, nurses were hired into these newly created positions because they understood both the setting and the problems faced by the client.

Beginning in 1991, the American Nurses Association (ANA) included advocacy in the ethical standards of clinical practice (ANA, 1991). In that same year, the Patient Self-Determination Act was passed by Congress. This act codified many patient rights into law, indicating that health care providers "who act contrary to the wishes and/or statements of their clients are vulnerable to charges of battery and offensive touching" and mandating that "anyone who attempts to avoid the legal directives of a client risks exclusion from federal funding programs for health care" (Braden & Rini, 1993, p. 1). Individuals may make their wishes known by establishing advanced directives such as a living will or durable powers of attorney for health care.

Thus, the progression of the role of advocate has increasingly involved the receiver of care in decision making and self-care. Nurses are in a unique position to be intermediaries for all persons who enter the health care delivery system. Compared with other health care professionals, nurses spend more time in contact with clients and provide more intimate physical and emotional care. Trust relationships may be built. Nurses are with clients when crisis or distress is immediate and decision making is essential. As a result, the nurse may understand client needs and values and can use this understanding to provide guidance and support in decision making. In addition, nurses are available to speak for clients. Daily interaction with other health care professionals is part of the nursing role. In the final analysis, being an advocate is part of providing care that is morally and ethically right. Being an advocate is also part of functioning as an effective leader.

 Kussman (1982) identified two approaches to the advocacy roles. One is the **responsible model,** which uses **negotiation,** compromise, and persuasion. It involves interaction with other persons associated with the situation. The second type is the adversarial, or legalistic, model. In this model, the advocate acts as an adversary to other health care professionals without regard to the rights of anyone except the client. Implementing the responsible model best serves the goals of the nursing profession.

Prerequisites to Effective Advocacy

Before being a client advocate, you must identify and define your own beliefs and values. What do you believe about advocacy, client roles and rights, professional behavior, and client–family–physician relationships? Many people in health care have difficulty moving beyond paternalism as an approach to clients and families. **Paternalism** is the restricting of an individual's liberty by making decisions for the person, in the manner of a father making decisions for his children. It usually involves withholding information and is justified because the decision maker "knows what is best" for the person. Traditionally, people credited the physician with knowing what was best, did not seek information, and allowed the physician to make choices for them.

Personal values of care providers can profoundly affect advocacy. Which do you value more: safety or freedom, obedience or the right to question, compliance or autonomy? Are you willing to take calculated risks, initiate interdisciplinary communications, address problems by considering multiple alternatives? How important to you are comfort, dignity, peace, control, and knowledge? Who receives your loyalty—the physician, health care agency, client, or all three? Who is in charge of the client's well-being? Do clients have the right to self-determination? Are you willing to give up control and give that control to the client? This is very difficult when clients do not follow the recommendations of care providers, when clients persist in taking actions that may lead to poor outcomes, and when the nurse cannot support a client's actions. Sometimes nurses put aside their own feelings and work with the client. Sometimes nurses determine that they cannot work effectively with the client and ask that the client's care be reassigned to an individual who can more effectively meet the client's needs.

Adequate education and experience produce clinical competence, which is necessary to achieve the trust and professional respect that are prerequisite to advocacy. Clinical competence gives you greater credibility with colleagues and increases your success as an advocate. You need skills that go beyond informing and supporting and that include helping the client examine and prioritize values, recognize conflicts, and consider consequences adequately. An understanding of the health care system and good working relationships with other health care professionals are essential to effective advocacy. You must be able to problem solve, negotiate, and mediate. You will need assertiveness and sound communication skills.

To be an advocate, you must believe that you have the right to speak up. Advocacy requires a commitment to view yourself in a particular way in your relation to others (Kohnke, 1982). You must accept accountability for exercising the privilege and responsibility of advocacy.

Your personal attributes can influence your ability to serve as a client advocate. Personal attributes that facilitate advocacy are objectivity, empathy, tact, flexibility, tenacity, a sense of humor, ability to cope with stress, self-motivation, power, personal autonomy, and commitment to the client.

There are increasing numbers of individuals from outside the health care system who see themselves in the role of patient advocate. This may be an individual from a support group, a family member, or someone from another advocacy group. Although their lay viewpoint can be very valuable to patients, Schwartz (2002) points out that although health providers are moving away from paternalistic approaches to advocacy, family members and other lay individuals may become paternalistic and hold their own viewpoint to be the best for all. When working with a patient who has an advocate, professionals must not abandon their own commitment to patient decision making but continue to ensure that the patient has the resources needed for decision making.

■ ASSESSING THE NEED FOR ADVOCACY

When assessing clients to identify those who may need advocacy, you will want to consider a wide variety of factors. The major categories of those who can benefit from advocacy are those who lack knowledge, those with little power, those who need to make decisions, and those who receive inadequate care.

Your assessment of the need for advocacy should focus primarily on the client. However, as you assess, you will also need to examine the situation, the options and resources, the posthospital setting, and the risks. This section focuses on client assessment. You can use knowledge gained from your clinical courses to assess the other factors.

Clients often have inadequate knowledge of the health care system and how it operates. They may be unaware of their prognosis and treatment options. They may not know the resources that are available to them or their rights as health care consumers. These gaps in the client's understanding may occur because information was not provided to them in sufficient detail or because it was not provided in terms they could understand. Clients and their families who are particularly vulnerable to lack of understanding include those who are critically, terminally, or chronically ill and those involved in research.

Clients may need an advocate because, in our complex health care system, they may be unable to verbalize needs or desires, may disagree with others viewed as too powerful to contradict, or may lack the knowledge and support to make and implement health-related decisions.

Some people are attributed less power by society and, therefore, are not heard when they speak for themselves. The poor, homeless, young, old, female, handicapped, and mentally ill may be included in the powerless. Others are powerless because they cannot speak (those who are unconscious or aphasic) or because they will not speak (those who feel powerless).

Others who need an advocate are those who are undecided about ethical dilemmas. Ethical decisions accompany many medical and nursing interventions. Decisions about restraints, feeding tubes, ventilators, institutionalization, or specific medications are based on values and, therefore, have an ethical component. Sometimes advocacy is needed to assist the client in the decision-making process. Sometimes it is needed because the client has not been given the option to make decisions or to be involved in the decision making.

Those who receive inadequate care also need an advocate. Although people who receive inadequate, unsafe, or indifferent care may take their case to various outside groups, nursing still has a responsibility to address, secure, and ensure quality client care. A nurse who acts as an advocate in this way not only will assist the client but also may assist those in the health care system to improve care.

The client has a right to choose, and health care professionals are legally obligated to comply with the client's choice. Therefore, it is important for you to know the role the client wishes to take, the role of significant others in health care decisions, and the role the nurse is expected to play (Becker, 1986). Does the client expect to make his or her own decisions? Does he or she expect the spouse or son to make needed decisions? Will he or she accept all decisions made by the doctor? Does he or she want the nurse to provide guidance in decision making?

You should be aware of the client's concerns, questions, desires, and expectations. Spiritual needs should be considered because they influence the beliefs and values that underlie decision making (Salladay & McDonnell, 1989).

In addition, you will need to assess the client's desire to know. Research by Miller (1981) showed that some individuals cope better when they have little information about threatening events, whereas others cope better with more information. You will want to know how much information your client expects in order to provide realistic, individualized teaching.

Another group whose needs are often neglected are the caregivers for the frail and disabled. In many situations, the emphasis on patients' rights to choose may fail to consider that care providers also have rights and needs (Amari-Vaught & Vaught, 1997). Many care providers see their role as to act entirely on behalf of the client. If this is problematic for the caregiver, they believe that they have no role or responsibility in the decision. One aspect of advocacy for these caregivers may be seeking the assistance of a social worker in mediating and counseling within a family.

Critical Thinking Exercise

Emily Fountain has just been admitted to Merry Haven Nursing Center directly from the hospital. She is 92 years old and was living in a retirement home until she fell, cutting her forehead and fracturing a wrist. Her son and daughter, who accompany her, live nearby. They feel that she is very unsteady and express great concern that she might fall again and be injured further. They ask that a restraint be used to "remind" her not to try to walk without help. Is this an appropriate plan? Does Mrs. Fountain need an advocate? If so, what would advocacy entail? If not, why not?

■ IDENTIFYING GOALS AND OUTCOMES FOR ADVOCACY

Broad goals for advocacy are listed in Display 8-3. Many of these relate to empowering the client and family. As you consider whether you should assume an advocacy role, review these goals and determine whether one of them fits the needs of your client. When you have identified a broad goal, you will want to determine the specific outcome for advocacy for this client.

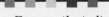

DISPLAY 8-3   **Broad Goals of Advocacy**

- Ensure that clients, families, and health care professionals are partners, especially when treatment is long, involved, and costly
- Involve clients in the decisions that affect their lives
- Provide knowledge, understanding, and suggestions for alternatives
- Promote acceptance of client choice, even when that choice is refusal of treatment or medications
- Help clients do what they deliberately choose to do
- Safeguard the interests and values of individual clients
- Help clients cope with the complex system of health care
- Provide a better quality of life for the client
- Support individualizing of health care in all settings
- Increase palliation for terminally ill persons
- Increase respectful behavior toward clients
- Prevent denial of client rights
- Leave power with the client

DISPLAY 8-4	**Client Outcomes for Advocacy**

The client will:
■ Understand the rights of patients and be afforded those rights
■ Be informed about the diagnoses, treatment, prognosis, and choices
■ Exercise responsibility for his or her own life by making personal decisions in collaboration with others
■ Have increased autonomy, power, and self-determination
■ Have decreased feelings of anxiety, frustration, and anger
■ Receive humane and just treatment
■ Have equality of opportunity
■ Have continuity of care
■ Receive effective, efficient resolution of specific problems of care

As you consider your role as a patient advocate, you will want to keep in mind what you hope to accomplish for your client. As with nursing care plans, specific, client-centered objectives or outcomes are needed. Display 8-4 lists examples of desirable client outcomes.

EXAMPLE *Accepting the Client's Values*

Mrs. Bateen is an elderly woman who has always deferred decisions to her husband. She views the physician as the authoritative expert whose advice should be unquestioningly followed. Sue Jones, the nurse working with her, has strong beliefs about women making their own decisions and not taking dependent or subservient roles. When working with Mrs. Bateen, Sue realized that she had to adjust her own planning to consider Mrs. Bateen's values and desires. Although Sue would have liked to assist Mrs. Bateen to be assertive and independent, this was not the client's desire. Sue arranged for conferences that included Mr. Bateen when all decisions were being considered. She informed the physician about Mrs. Bateen's reliance on the physician's advice and asked that the physician spend extra time explaining things to Mrs. Bateen. The outcome achieved was that Mr. and Mrs. Bateen together agreed on plans for care and discharge. Mrs. Bateen commented that the care provided was wonderful because she did not have to worry about things.

■ ADVOCACY ACTIONS

To achieve the goals of client advocacy, nurses may be required to interact with many people, individually or in groups. Those most often involved are family members, significant others, physicians, and various health care personnel. Others who may need to be involved include neighbors, employers, state agencies, third-party payers, and lawyers.

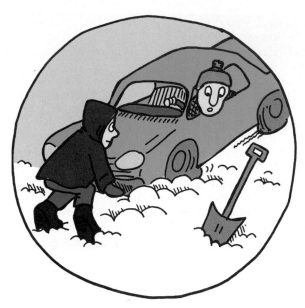

A patient advocate is not a rescuer.

You must remember that an effective client advocate is neither paternalistic nor a rescuer who usurps the client's responsibility and rights. A client advocate is one who, depending on the situation, speaks for the client, mediates between the client and other persons, and/or protects the client's right to self-determination.

Specific nursing interventions relevant to advocacy fall into the six categories listed in Display 8-5 and discussed below.

 ## Preventing the Need for Advocacy

All nurses can assist the client to gain the best possible control over the disease manifestations that interfere with thinking, feeling, and doing. We can help prevent the need for advocacy by insisting on clear, agreed-on health care goals and treatment

DISPLAY 8-5	**Actions for Advocacy**

1. Preventing the need for advocacy
2. Providing information and education to the client
3. Assisting and supporting the client's own decision making
4. Communicating with other professionals
5. Working for needed changes in the health care system
6. Being involved in public policy formulation

strategies developed by a team that includes the client or client representative. We can be knowledgeable about cultural values and practices of individual clients and communicate these to other health care personnel while emphasizing that excellent care means individualized care. We can be clinically competent, maintaining excellence in all aspects of client care. We can assist the client to find and arrange culturally appropriate and competent services as they are needed. If all these factors are operating, the client may not need an advocate. See Chapter 11 for a discussion of culturally competent care.

You should be able to cite many examples from your own experience of situations in which advocacy was unnecessary. These might include situations in which clients remained alert and were capable of thinking and problem solving for themselves. You may have seen times when patients entered the hospital well prepared for what was going to occur. You might have witnessed the admission of a person to long-term care after family and resident had all conferred as they made decisions about self-determination. When systems and procedures are set up to maximize client involvement and autonomy, there may be no need for an individual to act as an advocate.

Providing Information and Education

One of the major contributors to autonomy and thus to reducing the need for advocacy is adequate client knowledge. Therefore, education becomes a central activity of advocacy. Many clients need help in interpreting hospital policies and procedures, understanding health problems, and accessing services. Throughout your nursing education, you have acquired knowledge that you can share with your clients to assist them with informed decision making.

Before you begin to answer a client's questions, be certain of your own knowledge base. If you have the necessary information to answer questions honestly and accurately, you will want to think next about the communication itself. People working in health care often use terms that are unfamiliar to the lay public. In discussing concerns with your clients, use language with which they are familiar or take time to explain the medical terminology you are using. Also remember that how you say something is as important as what you say. Your attitude and intonation should convey caring and should encourage further information seeking and clarification.

Knowledge about current trends and about the legal and ethical implications of giving information is vital to the nurse who educates clients. Courts are holding institutions responsible for assuring that appropriate discharge instructions are provided so that the client is capable of self-care and of identifying when they need to seek additional care. Providing this essential discharge information is a nursing role. Consider the source of the information, who should provide the information and be responsible for its use, and when and how information is to be given.

Allow the client to select the information that will be received, but do not wait to be asked for information. Encourage each client to seek information from more than one source and enable selection of the information that is meaningful. It is acceptable for you to include your own views, as long as you state them as your views and do not present them from a position of power or as a persuasive or coercive force (Corcoran, 1988).

Sometimes it is necessary to teach assertiveness, which will enable the client to feel and act like an equal partner in communication, decision making, and treatment. Teaching assertiveness requires special knowledge and perhaps spending an extended period of time with the client. Remember that you empower people by giving them a means to exert personal control. You can allow and encourage a client to role play and practice assertiveness. As part of assertiveness, you can assist individual clients to present their choices to other persons involved in the decision-making process. You can help the client formulate thoughts, questions, statements, and decisions and even rehearse conversations that will be used to present his or her views to others. Trying out different ways to express themselves enables clients to be more comfortable and to feel more in control. The nurse should speak for clients only when they cannot or are afraid to speak for themselves.

Because children experience higher levels of anxiety and fear when they are uncertain about what to anticipate in relation to their care, they should be included in the information-sharing experience. Use content and age-related approaches that you learned in your pediatrics course. Family members are partners in the education process. They need information about alternative care, especially when they must choose interventions that would be acceptable to and in the best interests of a relative who is unable to make his or her own decision. If appropriate, you can remind them of the client's expressed or written wishes.

Assisting and Supporting Client Decision Making

For decision making, individuals need to know what options are available, what chance events are associated with each option, the probabilities that the chance events will occur, the outcomes that may result, and their own values assigned to the outcomes (Corcoran, 1988). The value of such information in decision making gives further credence to the need for client education, as presented in the previous section. Including the physician, other care providers, and the family in discussions adds to the information shared and to the acceptance of the information.

Critical Thinking Exercise

Gerry and Jack Haines are the parents of 8-year-old Jenny, who has severe chronic asthma. They have brought her into the clinic for adjustment of her medication. As Gerry helps Jenny get back into her clothes after an examination, Jack tells the nurse of the many difficulties they have been having in regard to Jenny's use of her medication at school. He says they received a note stating that children are not allowed to have any medicine in their possession. Just knowing she doesn't have her medicine is upsetting Jenny. The Haineses don't know what to do. How might the nurse serve as an advocate for this family? Outline a specific plan, including approaches to all relevant parties.

Communicating With Health Care Professionals

To advocate effectively, you will also need to communicate clearly on behalf of the client with other nurses and health team members. You will increase your effectiveness by establishing trust with other health care personnel. To do this, you must demonstrate knowledge and tact. Communications with other professionals will include information about the client's concerns, questions, and expectations. In this way you can assist others in honoring client rights and in showing respect. A team approach is facilitated by making other professionals aware of information regarding clients and family members. You may find it useful in some instances to work with ombudsmen and other advocacy persons and groups on behalf of a client.

Communicating with physicians is a significant part of your role as client care manager. Assuming that more than one physician is responsible for providing care, when you call a physician, be sure to choose the appropriate one. For example, call the surgeon if the problem is related to the incision or the system effected by the surgical intervention. Call the internist if the problem is related to preexisting conditions treated by the internist, complications of immobility, or other nonsurgical complications affecting the heart, lungs, or peripheral circulation. When requesting specific orders, particularly related to services after discharge or alternative care options, seek out the physician who is assuming responsibility for this aspect of care. When you approach any physician to request or discuss plans for care, present a knowledgeable, logical, concise, and accurate plan. Such presentation enhances your ability to be persuasive and therefore strengthens your role in meeting client's health care needs.

Physicians need to be maintained as allies. If differences of opinion arise, you should state disagreements carefully yet clearly, choosing wisely the time, the place, and the persons you involve. Problems should be presented directly to the appropriate colleague along with possible solutions and consequences. Negotiation and compromise are used to resolve conflicting interests between the client and provider. Advocating with a health care team member requires a thoughtful and assertive communication approach as illustrated by the following example.

EXAMPLE *Advocating for an Elderly Client*

In a 3:00 p.m. report, the day nurse stated that Mrs. Spencer, a 72-year-old woman, was admitted from a nursing home with a nasogastric feeding tube in place. The patient had pulled out her nasogastric feeding tube and indicated she did not want it replaced. Her children wanted the tube in because they were worried the patient would starve to death without it. They did not believe their mother was capable of making her own decisions. The doctor had ordered the tube insertion and tube feeding because of concern about the patient's swallowing abilities. The tube was out at the change of shift.

Mabel Wilson, the evening charge nurse, did a mini mental status assessment when she made first rounds. Mrs. Spencer's score indicated that she was mentally competent. She was alert and oriented to person, place, and time. Mabel talked with Mrs. Spencer about her health, the need for the feedings, and the reasons for the use of the feeding tube. Mrs. Spencer clearly indicated she did not want the tube to be reinserted.

When the nurse left the room, Mrs. Spencer's primary physician was standing at the nursing station. Mabel presented the patient's behavior, mental status, and refusal of the feeding tube to the physician. The physician indicated that she had ordered the tube reinserted because Mrs. Spencer's children had insisted that their mother was not mentally competent. She (the physician) stated that at the time of admission she had not had enough data to disagree with the children. She expressed appreciation for Mabel's assessments and used them to support her own decision. She ordered the tube discontinued.

Although speaking for clients does provide advocacy, encouraging direct communication between the client and the appropriate health care providers empowers the client to act on his or her own behalf. You can facilitate this process by helping clients write down questions and concerns to present to the appropriate care provider. You can arrange a convenient time for a meeting or help a client make a telephone call to set up an appointment. Setting the stage for communication between the client and others might be the primary focus of your advocacy efforts.

Critical Thinking Exercise

Joseph Mason, age 64, was admitted through the emergency department after having a cerebrovascular accident. He is aphasic and has limited motor responses on his left side only. His record shows that he has metastatic liver cancer, diagnosed 6 months ago. At home he was taking oxycodone with acetaminophen every 4 hours for pain. The admitting nurse notes that this patient has no pain medication ordered. How might the nurse serve as an advocate for this patient? Whom would the nurse approach? What specific information should the nurse have before initiating any action?

Working for Changes in the Health Care System

Working for change in the health care system is one way nurses are serving as advocates. You must know the bureaucracy in which you function. Find out about the committee structure and meet the nurse representatives who serve on the committees. It is always appropriate to challenge incorrect or ineffective policies and procedures and to work to change them. Help define current ethical issues and discuss them with the policy and/or ethics committees. Volunteer to be on or work to establish an ethics committee in your institution.

Resources should be available so that clients can select options that fit their values and choices. If a needed service or facility does not exist, assist in its creation. Clearly state the clients' needs. Know how much needed services will cost and how much it will cost not to have the service. When community services do exist, they should be well organized, so that clients can know what is available, where it is available, to whom it is available, and how to gain access.

One approach to advocacy through working within the system is described next. Your goal is to assist in making changes without making enemies. Use assertiveness along with tact and planned strategy. State expected outcomes specifically. Be sure that your behavior is consistent with your expressed values underlying the request for change. Collaborate with the responsible persons in each situation by using established channels of communication that provide the highest probability of success.

EXAMPLE   *Advocating for Family*

Community Hospital did not have a written policy about significant others being in the room during a code situation; however, they were always kept out of the room. Jeanna Brooks, an ICU charge nurse, had talked with nurses who worked in hospitals in which a significant other was allowed to be in the room during a code. The interactions and results sounded promising. When she asked about the practice at Community, she was told, "It has always been policy to keep family out and it is best that way."

She read and made copies of articles that pertained to the topic. She presented her position, with references, to her immediate supervisor and was given time to meet with the policy and procedures committee. Using the hospital policy format, she wrote a draft of her proposed policy and took it to the committee meeting. She also provided names of ICU nurses (with their permission) who had worked in ICUs that had implemented similar policies. Based on her work, the committee agreed that this appeared to be a change that would be patient/family friendly. They voted to present the proposed policy to the entire nursing staff with the committee's endorsement and to the appropriate medical staff committee for their consideration. Jeanna Brooks was pleased with the progress she had made.

Another realm of patient advocacy opens when an institution is providing substandard care or even defrauding patients and health plans through its actions. The nurse working in such a setting is faced with a decision of how to advocate for patients and whether attempts to advocate will result in adverse consequences for the nurse. Mohr and Mahon (1996) investigated the thinking and responses of nurses who worked in private psychiatric facilities that were subsequently convicted of fraud through inappropriate or no treatment and billing for unneeded care. Some nurses quietly quit their jobs in order to avoid participating in what they saw happening. Many nurses continued to work, although they were aware of what was occurring. These nurses often saw themselves as having no options in terms of other employment and, therefore, felt trapped in the situation. Taking an ethical stance in such a situation poses many problems for the nurse. Increasingly, legislative and regulatory bodies are incorporating protections for those who act as "whistle-blowers" in protecting the public.

Being Involved in Public Policy Formulation

As a citizen, each of us has the privilege and obligation to be actively involved in government and in the policies formulated by our elected and appointed officials. As a health care professional, you have the expertise to be an advocate for the health care needs of those in your community. Offer to serve on health policy task forces and committees. Contact your congressional representatives in support of legislation that benefits health care consumers or makes needed services available to them. Be actively involved in nursing organizations that work for programs and services for clients, and network through professional organizations, alumni groups, friends, and coworkers.

The ANA has expressed concern that when the media addresses health issues, the viewpoint of nursing is often missing from the discussion. To combat this, the ANA is encouraging nurses to step forward as the experts they are to speak to the media. Wallace (1998) provides suggestions and help in formulating an approach for those who would be interested in this avenue of advocating for health care. The following example shows how a nurse might be an advocate for clients in the policy arena.

EXAMPLE *Advocating for Public Policy Changes*

Jeremy Zinc had worked with in-home elderly for 3 years. He knew that several of his previous clients could have remained at home if the home health agency had offered, through their own department or by referral, part-time daily companion services. He had worked with a local task force to create the service, but the administrative expenses involved made it too expensive to implement. Knowing that the state nurses' association was concerned about this need and was planning to approach legislators about introducing a bill to address it, he asked to be involved with the district and state legislative committees of the association. He worked with a subcommittee to prepare a comparison of the cost of this program with the cost of institutionalization. He actively recruited other nurses and concerned persons to contact their legislators in support of the bill, which would create the needed service as an expansion of the state health program.

 ### Critical Thinking Exercise

A nursing student has been volunteering at a shelter for the homeless. She has become increasingly concerned about the plight of the mentally ill in this setting. She believes that they are often exploited by others in the homeless population. She would like to see volunteers with special training in mental illness work with these clients. She would also like to see some way of separating some of the mentally ill from the general population at the shelter. How could this student become involved with policy and decision making in this shelter? How might she begin to influence the planning of this agency? What information does she need before attempting to advocate for these mentally ill clients?

■ BECOMING AN ADVOCATE FOR OTHER STAFF MEMBERS

Nurses' practice of collaborating with and supporting other nurses in multiple professional activities has increased greatly during the past few years. Your collaboration with and support of nurses who are functioning as advocates is another part of your own advocacy.

Nurses also may be effective advocates for other staff members. The first-line manager frequently represents the staff in meetings with other departments and upper management. Managers must address staff needs, requests, problems, and rights. A sensitive, effective leader consistently advocates for his or her group and for individual staff members whenever the need arises. This requires careful judgment relative to the staff member's situation and the needs of the agency. The same approaches to advocating for clients are appropriate when advocating for staff.

EXAMPLE *Advocating for a Staff Member*

Juan Sanchez was the evening charge nurse on the skilled nursing unit of a small nursing home. As report ended, one of the regular nursing assistants, Tina Hall, entered the conference room. She was obviously upset but only asked about her assignment for the evening. When Juan asked if she wanted to discuss whatever the problem was, she stated that the director of nursing met her coming in late for the third time this week and "chewed her out." She wondered whether she should just quit before getting herself fired. Because of her home situation, Tina sometimes has had to seek a ride with a neighbor at the last minute, which caused her to be late. Juan knew that Tina was an excellent, efficient, and caring nursing assistant. She consistently did her share of the evening work and performed better than many of the other employees.

Juan knew that lateness must be discouraged. However, because of his concern for the well-being of the residents and his concern for the staff person, he talked with the director of nursing. He stated his assessment of the situation, emphasizing Tina's value to the residents. He suggested that mutually acceptable ways could be negotiated to compensate for her lateness when it occured and offered to work on solving this problem. Thus, he advocated for a staff member. This advocacy was helpful to the individual employee, but also resulted in positive care outcomes for clients and increased the morale of all the nursing assistants.

Critical Thinking Exercise

You are employed as a staff nurse in a long-term care facility. You work with a team of nursing assistants and a licensed practical nurse (LPN). Several of your colleagues have made negative comments about the nursing assistants and do not treat them as equal members of the nursing team. You want to see this attitude changed. How would you begin? Of the strategies mentioned in this text, which do you believe would work best for you? Why? Which ones would you be hesitant to try? Why? How would you go about building trust with both the nursing assistants and with your colleagues?

■ CONSTRAINTS AND SUPPORTS FOR THE ADVOCACY ROLE

Constraints on advocacy exist in many forms. There can be conflict for the nurse between the interests of an individual client and the duty to serve other clients, self, the profession, and/or the institution. Often, there is a lack of support for the advocacy role from institutions or other professionals. The nurse may also feel that he or she does not have the necessary knowledge or judgment to advocate.

Nurses may perceive a greater obligation to the employing institution and the physician than to the client. Advocacy may be viewed as bucking the system, which creates undesirable risks for the advocate. There is the risk of being caught in the middle when all involved believe they know what is right for the client. Based on their knowledge or previous experience, nurses may fear legal or social consequences of advocacy and find it more appealing to do only what is ordered.

Nurses may believe that being a team player and presenting a unified, competent team image are more effective in building client trust and confidence and are therefore more desirable than advocacy. They may concur with a public perception that the physician is the sole authority and decision maker in health care, or they may perceive themselves as lacking authority and power.

Clients who have control and practice self-determination may be threatening to individual nurses. There may be fear of noncompliant clients who ask too many questions. A nurse may disagree with a decision made by a client and not want to assist in the implementation of the decision.

The major support for the advocacy role is the legal mandate to acknowledge client rights and comply with client decisions, but another compelling support is the reward the nurse receives from knowing that clients are receiving high-quality care in accordance with their rights and without sacrificing their dignity. The personal growth of clients—in goal setting and achievement and in accepting responsibility for consequences—adds to the nurse's satisfaction and encourages future advocacy.

If advocacy is approached in a professional manner, collegial communication and cooperation are improved. Positive interdisciplinary experiences increase feelings of self-worth and contribute to pride in team accomplishment.

With the advent of consumerism, feminism, and the shift in power to the health care consumer, the risks for the client advocate are decreased. The advocacy position is strengthened by the increasing support for the belief that the interests of both health care providers and health care consumers are best served by effective consumer participation at the decision-making level. The legal mandate for client self-determination and informed consent supports the educational component of advocacy.

■ KEY CONCEPTS

- Change is occurring in the health care field at an astounding rate and is driven by many economic, political, and technological forces.
- Lewin's force-field analysis is a theory of change that examines the driving forces for change and the restraining forces that would limit change. Reducing restraining forces is usually more effective in accomplishing change than is increasing the driving forces.
- A number of other theories of change exist, which include recognizing emotional responses to change, identifying factors that determine successful planned change, specifying phases of the change process, and listing elements in the process of planned change.
- The three most commonly used change strategies are the empirical-rational strategy, the power-coercive strategy, and the normative-reeducative strategy. In real-life situations of change, all three strategies may be operating.
- A change agent seeks to facilitate the processes of change. An effective change agent uses an understanding of the change process to plan and implement any change.

■ The process of change includes unfreezing the current status, changing, and then refreezing to fix the changes in place. In unfreezing, the change agent works to alter the driving and restraining forces.

■ Enabling the change requires the development of new values, new attitudes, and new behaviors. To refreeze, new norms must be adopted, and there must be recognition and reward for those who participated in the change.

■ An effective participant in change seeks to understand the proposed change, why it should occur, who will benefit, and what is required for success. In addition, the effective participant expresses concerns in a constructive manner and focuses on the goals.

■ Building a sense of trust is perhaps the most critical aspect of all change processes. Unless a sense of trust prevails, most planned change projects fail.

■ Good communication is essential to the change process. Looking for ways to communicate clearly and frequently will make a difference in how the change progresses.

■ To effectively negotiate change, the situation must be thoroughly assessed, a detailed plan must be made, and then the planned change must be implemented, evaluated, and monitored for effectiveness. Sustaining a change requires ongoing monitoring for effectiveness.

■ Advocacy may involve speaking on behalf of the client, mediating between the client and another person, and protecting the client's right to self-determination.

■ Nurses are in a unique position to be effective advocates because of their ongoing contact with clients and families, their knowledge of the system, and their communication skills.

■ The primary goal of advocacy is to ensure client rights by providing information and power as needed by the client to increase feelings of respect, control, and partnership.

■ Actions for client advocacy include preventing the need for an advocate, communicating with other health care professionals, providing information and education, assisting and supporting the client decision making, working for change, and becoming involved in public policy formation.

■ Because of their knowledge of the system and skills in communication, nurses may also act as advocates for staff within the health care system.

■ There are both constraints and supports for the role of client advocate. You will want to consider these before accepting the advocacy role.

■ Although the major support of the advocacy role is the client's right to involvement in decision making, nurses often receive feelings of satisfaction and self-worth as a result of functioning effectively in the role.

REFERENCES

Alfano, G. J. (1987). The nurse as patient advocate [editorial]. *Geriatric Nursing, 8*(3), 119.

Amari-Vaught, E., & Vaught, W. (1997). Don't I count? *The Hastings Center Report, 27*(2), 23–25.

American Nurses Association (ANA). (1991). *Standards of Clinical Nursing Practice*. Washington, DC: Author.

Asprec, E. (1975). The process of change. *Supervisor Nurse, 6*, 15–24.

Becker, P. H. (1986). Advocacy in nursing: perils and possibilities. *Holistic Nursing Practice, 1*(1), 54–63.

Benne, K. D., Bennis, G., & Chin, R. (1976). Planned change in America. In W. G. Bennis, K. D. Benne, R. Chin, & K. E. Corey (Eds.), *The Planning of Change.* New York: Holt, Rinehart and Winston.

Braden, R. N., & Rini, A. G. (1993). Advanced directives: an update. *MAIN Dimensions, 4*(4), 1–4.

Bridges, W. (2003). *Managing Transitions: Making the Most of Change* (2nd ed). Cambridge, MA: Perseus Publishing.

Corcoran, S. (1988). Toward operationalizing an advocacy role. *Journal of Professional Nursing, 4,* 242–248.

Foley, E. J. (1993). Leadership. *Emphasis: Nursing, 4*(2), 5–6.

Jick, T. D. (1993). *Managing Change: Cases and Concepts.* Homewood, IL: Irwin.

Kohnke, M. F. (1982). *Advocacy: Risk and Reality.* St. Louis: CV Mosby.

Kussman, J. (1982). Think twice about becoming a patient advocate. *Nursing Life, 6,* 46–50.

Lewin, K. (1951). Field theory in social service: selected theoretical papers. New York: Harper Brothers.

Miller, S. (1981). Predictability and human stress: toward a clarification of evidence and theory. *Advanced Experiments in Social Psychology, 14,* 203–255.

Mohr, W. K., & Mahon, M. M. (1996). Dirty hands: the underside of marketplace health care. *Advances in Nursing Science, 19*(1), 28–38.

Perlman, D., & Takacs, G. J. (1990). The ten stages of change. *Nursing Management, 212*(4), 33–38.

Salladay, S. A., & McDonnell, M. M. (1989). Spiritual care, ethical choices, and patient advocacy. *Nursing Clinics of North America, 24,* 543–549.

Schwartz, L. (2002). Is there an advocate in the house? The role of health care professional in patient advocacy. *Journal of Medical Ethics 28*(1), 37–40.

Thomas, J. M., & Bennis, W. G. (1972). *The Management of Change and Conflict.* Baltimore: Penguin.

Ventura, M. J. (1998). Can these nurses make a difference? *RN, 61*(7), 47–48.

Wallace, B. C. (1998). Be a voice for nursing. *RN, 61*(6), 31–33.

9

The Nurse as Conflict Manager, Negotiator, and Mediator

Learning Outcomes ■ ■ ■ ■ ■

After completing this chapter, you should be able to:

1. Describe situations that nurses encounter in which they will fill the role of negotiator or mediator.
2. Compare and contrast the early views of conflict with how conflict in organizations is viewed at present.
3. Identify five positive outcomes of conflict.
4. Examine at least four factors that can result in conflict within organizations.
5. Outline five modes or styles the nurse could employ when dealing with conflict.
6. Analyze situations that result in a win–lose situation, a lose–lose situation, and a win–win situation.
7. List the steps to be considered in conflict resolution.
8. Outline guidelines to be followed when involved in negotiation.
9. Describe how the negotiation process can be used to resolve a conflict situation.
10. Discuss other situations in which the role of the nurse might involve negotiation or mediation.
11. Outline briefly the history of collective bargaining in nursing and sketch the role of the American Nurses Association in the process.
12. Discuss four issues related to collective bargaining in nursing.

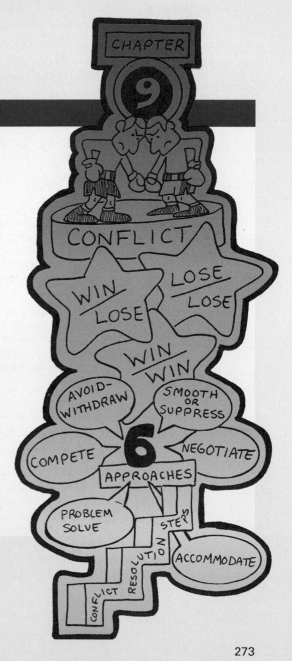

273

Key Terms ■ ■ ■ ■ ■

accommodating

agency shop

avoiding

collaborating

collective bargaining

competing

compromise

conflict

consensus

dominance power

forcing

grievance process

integrative decision
  making

intrapersonal conflict

lose–lose

mediation

mediator

negotiation

problem solving

role ambiguity

role conflict

scarcity of resources

smoothing

win–lose

win–win

withdrawing

T wo of the major responsibilities you will assume as a manager in the health care environment are that of negotiator and mediator. Why are they key roles? Because managers are expected to maintain a positive working relationship among the various personalities that form the health care team. Whenever we bring together people having a variety of different beliefs, values, lifestyles, ethnic backgrounds, and goals, some conflict is inevitable. The remarkable number of changes that have occurred in the delivery of health care along with the economic impact the area is experiencing leave it vulnerable to conflict as professional values and competition for resources peak. Conflict is one of the most challenging of managerial responsibilities, because when conflict is left unresolved progress stops. This chapter is devoted to the role of the nurse as manager of conflict, as a negotiator of differences, and as a mediator for other parties in conflict.

■ UNDERSTANDING CONFLICT, NEGOTIATION, AND MEDIATION

In a very broad sense, **conflict** is the dissension that occurs when two or more individuals with different values, interests, goals, or needs view things from different perspectives. In other words, conflict arises when there is a disagreement in points of view. Working from this general definition, we examine conflict as a situation that exists when there are differences of opinion or opposing points of view among persons, groups, or organizations. When conflict occurs, it often needs to be resolved. One way in which this can occur is through negotiation and mediation.

Negotiation, very broadly defined, is "communication between two or more parties to determine the nature of future behavior" (Volkema, 1999, p. 2). Although many view this as synonymous with bargaining, he differentiates negotiating from bargaining by observing that bargaining describes the process of determining the final price of a purchase or sale.

Mediation "is a negotiation moderated by a neutral party to resolve a conflict and address related concerns in ways that meet the parties interests" (Phillips, 2001, p. 7). This process is a friendly or diplomatic intervention intended to settle disputes between people. When a conflict situation arises, it may be resolved through the process of mediation in which the mediator helps the involved parties to negotiate toward a solution. Thus, in the process of mediating disputes or issues, the mediator assists the parties to reach decisions and settlements and to agree on arrangements.

■ CONFLICT SITUATIONS AND NURSING

In fulfilling your role as a professional nurse you will need to possess skills that will enable you to manage conflict situations. The opportunities for conflict in the health care environment abound. Nurses may be required to deal with verbal abuse, authority figures, assignments they would prefer to decline, expectations that are difficult to fulfill, role conflicts, colleagues whose practice is suffering because of physical problems with chemical dependence, and a work environment that encourages disharmony. Working in crowded spaces, such as critical care units, leads to stress and increases the potential for conflict. In addition, because health concerns strike at core abilities and at life itself, feelings and emotions of patients and families set the stage for potential conflict. The nurse serves as a representative of the system, and families may focus their anger toward the nurse.

 ## Conflict Between Members of the Health Care Team

The potential for conflict with members of the health care team is great. Conflict that can exist between physicians and nurses is very stressful to nurses and can play a significant role in job satisfaction. Historically, the physician has been trained to exercise authority over nurses. Nurses have moved into more professional roles requiring critical thinking, decision making, and accountability. They spend more time with the patient than does the physician. As a result, nurses sometimes have suggestions for alternative ways of managing a patient's care. When the physician discounts these suggestions or is unwilling to listen to them, conflict can result. On occasion, physicians display verbal abuse or other inappropriate behavior. A study reported by Rosenstein (2002) looked at how such behavior negatively impacted nurse satisfaction and retention.

Conflicts can also occur between departments that are providing services to the client. For example, a patient may be scheduled for a physical therapy (PT) session. Members of the PT department arrive to take a patient to therapy before the nurse has had the opportunity to complete the morning care that needed to be given. The nurse feels the PT department should adhere to a schedule for their patients and the PT workers think the nurses are oblivious to anyone's work other than their own. Or there may be conflict with the pharmacy about the time that medications are delivered to the unit. Members of the housekeeping department may be at odds with the nursing staff about the lack of timeliness in the provision of housekeeping services. And it is not unusual for a staff member from the Emergency Department (ED) staff to arrive unannounced on the unit with a new patient during a time when all the unit staff is busily involved in patient care and find it challenging and frustrating to devote additional time to a new admission. The nurses are upset because the ED did not call first; the ED staff member is distressed because other patients were waiting for the ED bed and he believes the nursing unit is being unreasonable. These represent but a few of the potential types of conflict nurses encounter on a daily basis. Conflict can occur in the workplace because of the differing values of the members of the workforce. This may be particularly true in situations in which English is a second language and often results from misunderstandings regarding expectations. As mentioned in Chapter 2, groups that are in the minority often are represented through the informal organization. If concerns are focused on dissatisfaction with the leadership (which may be steeped in a middle-class value system), it may disrupt the quality of care provided. As nursing strives to bring more representatives of minority populations into the profession, each nurse needs to be senitive to the values of the various cultures and to understand both verbal and nonverbal behavior of different groups.

Swansberg and Swansberg (2002) include defiant behavior by coworkers among causes of conflict in nursing, because it violates the acceptable protocols for adult interaction. Behaviors that are cited as defiant include refusing to work (individuals who scowl and walk away), those who do their work but do it mockingly and with contempt, and those who avoid commitment and participation. You can probably think of times when you have observed such behavior in one form or another. It represents a real challenge to the busy manager (see Chapter 12).

Critical Thinking Exercise

It is a busy morning on the unit you manage, and one of the nursing assistants is absent because of illness. As you adjust assignments, you ask Melody to assume care for Mrs. Wrangler, a patient who has a history of belligerent and complaining behavior. When you give this assignment to Melody, she becomes upset and says she will not take care of that patient and that she has had her turn at having to deal with Mrs. Wrangler's complaints. How would you feel if this happened? What would be the first thing you would do? What other actions would you take? How much time do you think you could devote to the issue? Would you employ any type of follow-up? Why or why not?

Conflict With the Patient's Family

Because nurses occupy a primary role in the provision of care and have ongoing contact with patients and their families, they may be the targets of conflict. Emotions and feelings often are frayed during the stress of illness and hospitalization. Anger, which is a normal and healthy reaction to situations and circumstances over which people have little control, may be directed toward the nurse. When this occurs, it is important for the nurse to recognize what is occurring and develop ways to deescalate the emotions.

Health care as a whole has its own culture and language. As students study for their career, a type of professional socialization occurs regarding the newly learned information on health and illness and they move farther away from some of the values, beliefs, practices, and habits they had when they began their studies. It is not unusual to hear a patient state, "They speak a foreign language and I have no idea what they are talking about." Because of this nurses may be viewed as possessing different values and beliefs than those for whom they care. Often the only methods of healing considered appropriate are those that are scientifically proven to work. As nursing as a profession moves toward evidenced practice, nurses need to be sensitive to the alternative approaches that may be of particular significance to their clients, thus avoiding some of the conflict that can occur with a patient and the patient's family. The values and beliefs of the health-care provider should not be forced on the client.

Conflict Between Nurses

Nurses may also be involved in conflicts with other nurses, such as differences of opinion regarding the philosophy of care delivery, the best treatment modality to be used for a patient, the desired forms to be used in charting, work-shift assignments, time off at the holidays, the most efficient way to organize supplies in a storage cupboard, or a myriad of other issues that arise when people work together closely. Differences in educational levels can give rise to conflict among nurses as a professional group. In these situations, it is especially important to recognize that conflict exists, that it can be dealt with positively, and that the end result can be constructive.

Conflict Related to Values and Beliefs

The health care environment is rife with opportunities for differences of opinion related to personal values and beliefs. Ethical issues such as abortion, stem cell treatment, gene therapy, orders to withdraw or withhold treatment, and do-not-resuscitate orders are just a few of the areas in which personal values may come into conflict. On another perspective, the nurse's personal goals may be in conflict with those of the organization. The organizational climate may not be one in which the nurse is comfortable. Any change being implemented by the organization, such as downsizing, restructuring, or changing policies and procedures, may cause conflict in what the nurse sees as important (see Chapter 8). Discrimination practices with regard to age, culture, or gender—if present in the work situation—may give rise to conflict.

■ EXAMINING THE VIEWS OF CONFLICT

Like so many other things in our society, our view of conflict has experienced change. Once viewed as negative, conflict is now seen as having positive attributes.

Early Views of Conflict in Organizations

A review of literature in the area of management reveals that the early writers and theorists (called traditionalists) held a negative view of conflict. They perceived conflict to be a disruptive and destructive force within any organization. The "good" manager was the individual who administered a unit free from conflict. In some early situations, the "troublesome" employee may have been dismissed from his or her job.

In the 1940s, this view of conflict began to change. A new breed of theorists (identified as behaviorists) began recognizing the positive aspects of conflict. They accepted it for what it is—inevitable—and looked for ways to either reduce it or to make it work positively for the organization. Some would say that this changing view of conflict, which occurred toward the end of World War II, was related to this country's involvement in nuclear strategies, a situation that compelled us to recognize conflict and find positive means to address it.

Organizational literature of the 1970s was replete with the examination, explanation, and positive application of conflict in the workplace. New theorists (called interactionists) emerged who viewed conflict as a creative force.

Present-Day Views of Conflict

Today we are inclined to view conflict as inevitable, and, if recognized and properly managed, capable of contributing positively to the operation of an organization. Improperly managed, conflict may be detrimental to the organization. Different writers and researchers have described conflict in a variety of terms. As you read through their various approaches, you will note that they often use different terms to describe similar phenomena.

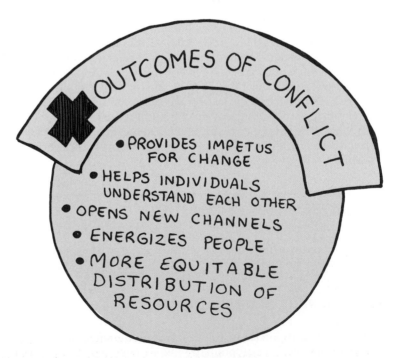

Properly managed conflict can contribute positively to the operation of an organization.

DISPLAY 9-2	**Types of Conflict**

Intrapersonal: Conflict that occurs within the individual.
Interpersonal: Conflict that occurs between two or more people.
Organizational: Conflict that occurs between two or more people in an organizational setting.

Intrapersonal Conflict

It is difficult for any one of us not to experience some intrapersonal conflict in a particular week. An **intrapersonal conflict** occurs within an individual in situations in which he or she must choose between two alternatives. Choosing one alternative means that he or she cannot have the other; they are mutually exclusive. For example, we might internally debate whether to complete an assignment that is due the next day or watch a favorite television program. Or we might argue with ourselves about accepting an extra serving of our favorite pie versus politely declining because of the additional calories it contains. Intrapersonal conflict, like other forms of conflict, may be rather insignificant or may take on sizable proportions within our lives.

Critical Thinking Exercise

Identify intrapersonal conflicts that you experienced this past week. How did you deal with them? What are some of the significant intrapersonal conflicts with which you have struggled over the past year? How have you set about resolving those problems? Could any of the techniques that you used be applied to your role as a health care provider?

Interpersonal Conflict

Interpersonal conflict is conflict between two or more individuals. It occurs because of differing values, goals, actions, or perceptions. For example, when you have a weekend free from studies, you might want to go to a science fiction movie, but your partner may prefer to attend an opera. Interpersonal conflict becomes more difficult when we are involved in issues relating to racial, ethnic, and lifestyle values and norms. As we struggle to address these issues, we can come into additional conflict regarding sensitive ways to approach multicultural values.

Certainly, conflict over ideas and approaches to problems can be a big source of controversy. As nurses move into roles requiring greater autonomy, as they learn to use assertiveness skills to achieve desired outcomes, as they grow in their ability to advocate for themselves and their clients, conflict will result. When individuals are educated to think critically and develop new beliefs, general approaches suggested by others or mandated from above may not be welcomed.

Organizational Conflict and Its Causes

Conflicts also occur in organizations because of differing perceptions or goals. Organizational conflicts may be intrapersonal or interpersonal, but they originate in the structure and function of the organization. Typically, aspects of the organization's style of management, rules, policies, and procedures give rise to conflict (Huber, 1996). When conflicts occur within an organization, it is important that the conflict be resolved in a constructive way in order to maintain the team's motivation. The leader's role takes on special significance. Leaders not only model the behaviors related to conflict and the resolution of the conflict, but also choose the methods of intervention and the timing that will follow.

ROLE AMBIGUITY AND ROLE CONFLICT

Two areas responsible for conflict in organizations are **role ambiguity** and **role conflict.** Dove (1998) refers to this concept as ambiguous jurisdiction, meaning that the authority or legal power is unclear or vague. Well-written job descriptions and clear communication about expectations take on importance in these situations.

Role ambiguity occurs when employees do not know what to do, how to do it, or what the outcomes must be. This frequently occurs when policies and rules are ambiguous and unclear. For example, a sexual harassment policy may not clearly explain what steps should be taken when sexual harassment occurs. This leaves those who have the responsibility of seeing that the policy is followed in a confused state, not knowing what should be done or how it should be carried out.

Role conflict occurs when two or more individuals in different positions within the organization believe that certain actions or responsibilities belong exclusively to them. The conflict could relate to competition. For example, in some hospitals, conflict has existed between the nurses and the social workers about the responsibility for providing discharge planning. Both groups see discharge planning as an important aspect of their own care of the patient.

Another type of role conflict occurs when a person's position in the organization requires assuming a number of different roles. An example is the unit manager who must be a skilled caregiver, a teacher, a negotiator, a patient advocate, a manager, and a motivator. The requirements of giving care may conflict with requirements for managing the unit. As you can easily surmise, the individual experiences role conflict and much intrapersonal stress; consequently, productivity and job satisfaction are reduced. This type of role conflict is a major cause of burnout. As more and more facilities move toward shared governance, in which the role of the supervisor or manager changes to encompass many of the activities listed previously, we might anticipate more of this type of conflict.

ORGANIZATIONAL STRUCTURE

An organization's structure may be another source of conflict. Often this is seen as a conflict over territory (often referred to as turf or less frequently as fiefdom). Everyone tries to protect his or her current territory or area of responsibility and perhaps expand it. This type of conflict increases as organizations grow. To minimize it, organizations use job descriptions, organizational charts, and other such mechanisms (see Chapter 2).

The size of an organization may also relate to the degree of control individuals have over their jobs. In a large organization, an individual may have less control over the work site. When individuals have little control in planning their work, the opportunity for conflict becomes greater.

EXAMPLE *Conflict in Proceeding With Work*

Mary Brown, the staff nurse on a medical unit, wants to begin the patient's morning care. However, she cannot do this until the patient has had breakfast. The patient cannot have breakfast until a fasting blood sugar has been drawn. The personnel from the laboratory are delayed in coming to the unit because one of the technicians called in ill and no replacement could be found. When Mary called the lab to see why the technician was delayed, her impatience was interpreted as criticism, the laboratory representative became upset and replied, "Cool your jets!"

All persons in this conflict feel the stress of the situation. This type of conflict is most apt to occur within an organization when units depend on one another for assistance, information, and other types of coordination.

SCARCITY OF RESOURCES

Conflict also results from a **scarcity of resources,** which Dove (1998) refers to as conflict of interest. When budgets are established, managers of various departments may be in conflict because each has priorities but not all priorities may be funded. Each one advocates for personal department needs. Even within a unit, there may be conflict among staff when priorities are determined. Some individuals may believe that the highest priority is a mechanical lifting device whereas others think that the unit is much more in need of additional computer stations for documenting care.

As mentioned earlier, resources are not only monetary. Resources may also refer to employees, space, or other elements critical to the operation of any unit within an institution. When funds are available for increased staffing, conflict may revolve around the question of whether to hire more unlicensed assistants or more registered nurses (RNs) and thus fewer people. Among surgeons, prime operating times are valued and sometimes there is conflict over the growth of one surgical specialty that is requesting more use of the valued times—the scarce resource. Some common sources of conflict within all types of organizations include the size and location of one person's office or the number of people required to share an office or a telephone line. Such conflicts may relate to an individual's perceived status and power within the group.

■ PERSONAL STYLES FOR DEALING WITH CONFLICT

Individuals use a wide variety of approaches to manage conflict. Any one of them may be useful in a given situation. Factors that influence the decision as to which approach is best include relative importance of the issue, potential for positive outcomes, and energy and time available. Several researchers interested in learning more about conflict believe that individuals possess behavioral predispositions or personal styles for handling and resolving conflict (Barton, 1991; Berkowitz, 1962; Blake & Mouton, 1964; Mallory, 1985; Thomas, 1976). These styles tend to fall into one of five different categories.

Avoiding or Withdrawing From Conflict

Avoiding or **withdrawing** from conflict occurs when the individual involved chooses not to address the issue at hand. This response may also be referred to as denying conflict, believing that if the conflict is not acknowledged, it doesn't exist or will go away. It is generally seen in people who are made very uncomfortable by conflict situations. Most students can think of a time during their schooling when they were aware of cheating or plagiarism by a classmate and struggled with deciding what to do. Many people faced with this avoid the conflict by saying nothing.

Avoiding conflict is most appropriate in certain situations. These situations include times when there is more to be lost by directly addressing the conflict than there is to be gained, when there is not time to gather adequate data, when the problem is only a symptom of a larger concern within the organization, when there is nothing you can do about the problem or it is not your problem, or when the situation will take care of itself if you wait it out. For example, the staff nurse disagrees with a decision by the unit manager but says nothing because the staff person does not believe that her views will make any difference.

Sometimes avoiding a conflict with others can create internal conflict with your own values. Do you report a colleague whom you know is taking supplies from the unit? What if you know that an individual is charting assessments he or she has not done?

Those who routinely employ avoidance as their primary tactic for dealing with conflict often do not see any positive attributes in conflict. They tend to cope well in situations in which there is harmony but will not become involved in conflict. Think for a minute. Do you know someone who fits this description? Perhaps you are such a person. Do you prefer to remain neutral when a conflict occurs, avoiding situations that might require you to take sides? Although avoiding conflict may produce less upset, it may also result in the loss of important information. Each of us brings special skills, abilities, and perceptions to a work environment. These should be shared in bad times as well as good times.

EXAMPLE *Avoiding Conflict in the Cafeteria*

Cheryl Maybee, RN, was in line in the hospital cafeteria and had only 20 minutes for lunch. The area was very busy. The clinical nurse specialist who has been visiting Cheryl's mastectomy patients prior to discharge crowded in front of her in the salad line. Rather than challenge her boldness, Cheryl just stepped back. Cheryl had had a particularly hectic morning and, in addition, she was counting on a recommendation from this individual for a merit increase. She decided to avoid the conflict inherent in this situation because there was more to be lost than there was to be gained.

Accommodating or Smoothing

Accommodating or **smoothing** a conflict involves trying to eliminate anger and expressions of difference without addressing the issue itself and usually involves giving in to the wishes of another to preserve harmony or build up social credits. It is often seen in situations in which one individual has more power than the other. It is an appropriate approach if you are wrong and the other individual is right, if the issue is unimportant to you, or if you can gain more later by giving in on this situation. It also may be appropriately chosen when the conflict and anger are disrupting the work setting or interfering with the immediate needs of patients.

Those who deliberately choose accommodating or smoothing must also plan another approach to solving the problem at a later time if it is to be resolved. For example, a unit manager hears two of the nursing assistants arguing over who should take coffee break first. Patient's families are observing the dispute. The manager approaches the assistants and tells them they may both go on break at the earlier time. This settles the dispute but does not address the inappropriate behavior of the nursing assistants or plan for coverage on the unit when both are gone.

People who have a pattern of choosing to accommodate or smooth over conflict are often described as having a strong need to be liked and are concerned for the welfare and needs of others. If a conflict threatens how others will perceive them, or if it presents too many challenges to someone important to them, they try to smooth over the problems. In striving to maintain a peaceful environment, they must sacrifice personal goals and values. Thus, this is often described as a self-sacrificing mode of conflict resolution.

Accommodators can fill a positive role in a conflict by providing support to others involved in making tough decisions. However, in accommodating the situation, the individual may be abandoning responsibility for providing valuable input to problem resolution. For example, if a physician approaches the nurses' station and rudely demands the vital signs of her patient, the problem of inappropriate behavior on the part of the physician is not resolved by the accommodating action of the unit manager who graciously rushes to provide them. It is yet to be resolved.

EXAMPLE *Smoothing the Situation by Accommodating a Physician*

Connie Evener was at the desk charting. Several visitors and one patient were standing near the desk. Dr. Bellows came out of a room and shouted, "What kind of incompetents work here? I said I wanted everything in the room for that dressing change when I got here!" Connie believed his actions were disruptive to those present, and the patient needed to have the dressing changed now. Therefore, she got up immediately. She said, "I'm sorry things were not ready. I'll get them immediately, and you can go back in to see Mrs. Brown while I am doing that." Connie smoothed over the existing situation and accommodated Dr. Bellows's demands to preserve harmony. However, she planned to speak with him privately about the inappropriateness of his expression of anger.

Forcing the Issue or Competing

Competing or **forcing** the issue in a conflict involves working for your particular desired solution exclusively. You might choose this strategy if you believe that you have more information or greater expertise than others or when your values are such that you believe no compromise is possible. People who routinely address conflict in a competitive manner emphasize personal goals and desires, failing to consider the needs and opinions of others. These individuals have a strong need to come out of any conflict as the winner. Although this aggressive approach may serve to move issues that are deadlocked, it can prevent good problem solving and results in a win–lose situation. Despite all the attention conflict has received in workshops, conferences, and material in the literature, health care providers are concerned that this mode of dealing with conflict is too often the one of choice.

(handwritten margin note: win/lose)

Competitors win by outtalking their colleagues, by discounting the good ideas presented by others, or by personally attacking others through name-calling or threats. Sarcasm is often used as a strategy during the conflict. We can all think of an example of a conflict that was resolved with the competitive approach—possibly something as simple as deciding with a friend whether you would go to one movie or another. You will want to develop the ability to know when a competitive approach to a problem is desirable and when another method should be employed.

EXAMPLE *Forcing the Adoption of a Position Through Competition*

> At a meeting of the procedure committee, the technique for cleaning a tracheostomy is being reviewed. Sarah Boxer understands that several approaches have always been considered correct, but she has just read a new article on this topic. She is convinced that the hospital should switch to the new procedure recommended in the article. Sarah has excellent verbal skills and outlines her argument well. Whenever anyone else suggests a different approach, she quickly interrupts with more strong reasons why her idea should be accepted. She talks at some length about the findings of the research study she read. Others stop presenting different ideas and Sarah's suggestion is adopted.

COMPROMISING OR NEGOTIATING

The approach to conflict that employs **compromise** or **negotiation** involves give and take. A compromise is a resolution of conflict in which each gets something of what he or she desired. Negotiation is a process used to come to a compromise acceptable to both parties. To arrive at compromise, one factor in the situation is balanced against another. This method of conflict resolution works because it minimizes the losses for all parties while providing some gains for each. Some view this approach as a win–lose strategy for each individual, because each gains something but at the same time gives up something. It is an appropriate approach to conflict when the goals of both sides seem incompatible, when the conflict has time constraints, and when a settlement is needed and earlier discussions have stalled.

(handwritten margin note: win/win per theory)

Both this approach and the problem-solving approach discussed next require that you be willing to confront the person with whom you disagree. Confrontation in this respect does not mean that you attack someone or are aggressive, but rather that you are direct in identifying your view of the conflict to the person involved (see Chapter 5 on communication). Being direct may be uncomfortable, which is one reason that many people choose avoidance. Another difficulty with an approach that involves compromise is that the problem often resurfaces. In deciding to use compromise to resolve a conflict, you need to assure yourself that this is the best way to deal with the situation.

Compromise involves a settlement of the issue that involves each side giving up some demands or making concessions. Compromise may also involve taking responsibility for your part in the conflict and offering to change your own behavior. In this way, you set the stage for the other person to take responsibility for his or her own behavior. Identifying a common goal may also help to facilitate compromise.

EXAMPLE *Compromising Regarding Holiday Time Off*

Jonathan Barter, the evening charge nurse on a busy medical unit, very much wished to take off both Christmas Eve and the evening of Christmas day to spend with his family. However, Tim Baxter, who replaces Jonathan, is expecting company and wants both days off also. Jonathan decided to discuss the matter with Tim. After a few minutes of discussion, it is clear that Tim was not willing to work both shifts, although he had less seniority on the unit than Jonathan. Jonathan explored his plans with Tim and learned that Tim's family's dinner and gift opening usually take place on Christmas day. On the other hand, Jonathan's family prefers to celebrate on Christmas Eve. Jonathan offered to work on Christmas day if Tim would work Christmas Eve. After some thought, Tim agreed. Both gained something and gave up something.

Problem Solving or Collaborating

Many studies of conflict resolution advocate **problem solving** or **collaborating,** while acknowledging that it may be the most difficult to achieve. This method encourages the individuals involved in the conflict to work toward common goals. Thus, it is considered a win–win situation and is usually the best one, especially when the issue is one requiring consensus. The solution may be one that neither party has considered. However, this approach has the drawback of being more time consuming; thus, decisions may be delayed.

The collaborative approach requires that all participants come to the discussion table willing to examine issues thoughtfully and work in a task-oriented fashion to solve the problem. This approach requires a commitment on the part of all persons to be supportive and considerate of one another, to listen to one another, and to try to understand the other person's point of view. It demands awareness and sensitivity, open and honest discussion, and a noncompetitive stance on the part of all participants.

EXAMPLE   *Collaborating on the Work Schedule*

Willard Merger was working on a unit in which different nurses were assigned to various management activities. The one for which Willard was responsible was the scheduling of hours. Much dissension occurred on the unit with regard to the scheduling of weekends off. Willard decided to call all unit staff together to discuss the problem and establish the criteria by which weekends off would be rotated among staff. The goal was to involve everyone in the decision making. The unit staff met together and was able to develop guidelines for rotating weekends off.

■ CONFLICT WITHIN A GROUP

Groups are affected by conflict and by the outcomes of conflict. Winning tends to increase cohesiveness among members and to create a more relaxed climate in which to function. Concern for the members' needs increases and, at the same time, concern for task performance declines.

Similarly, groups are affected by losing. There is a tendency to deny the reality of losing, excusing it as the result of bad luck or misunderstanding. Internal conflicts may occur as members blame one another for the defeat. Members may also work harder and reorganize in order to be more effective. When working with groups, one should consider certain characteristics. First, there is a common tendency to decide issues by majority vote. Certainly, that is how our political leaders are selected and how motions are decided in formal meetings. Somebody (or one group) wins and somebody (or one group) loses. In the situations mentioned, that is the most orderly way in which to conduct activities.

However, when a unit or department is trying to achieve common goals, working toward consensus (agreement among group members) may provide for greater harmony than deciding issues through the majority vote. Consensus building takes more time and requires more interpersonal skills on the part of the leader, but it results in easier implementation because of group acceptance. This method avoids some of the "we–they" positions taken in both the win–lose and the lose–lose strategies. It allows both sides to look at conflict as a problem needing resolution, tends to depersonalize the issues, and emphasizes outcomes.

There are times in a conflict situation when the needs or desires of the involved individuals or groups become polarized. That means they are diametrically opposed, or at opposite ends of a continuum. In these instances, focusing on the means for resolving the problem rather than on the outcomes may be desirable. This approach is known as **integrative decision making.** The people involved spend time identifying their needs and values, search for all possible alternatives, and then select the one that works best. This method tends to bring attention to the problem rather than to the persons involved.

■ THE NEGOTIATING ROLE

As mentioned earlier, negotiation involves the exchange of ideas with the purpose of coming to a mutual decision regarding changing a situation. Negotiation is often a part of the mediation process. It also occurs on a day-to-day basis as we work with others. Shell (1999, p. 6) reminds us that we all negotiate many times a day; often we are not aware of doing it. He views negotiation as a "basic, special form of human communication." When negotiating, compromise is essential. Negotiation is used when individuals do not initially agree but want to achieve at least part of their goal.

Negotiation, therefore, is not a new process to you; you have used it all your life. You may have negotiated with a friend to pick up a book at the library for you this week and you would return the favor later. You might have negotiated with a teacher for more time for an examination. In nursing, you might find yourself negotiating with staff members about sharing responsibilities, with a manager about assignments, with a client about adhering to certain health care expectations. As a client advocate you may find yourself negotiating with a physician about options available to your client.

Planning for Negotiation

Having sufficient information before beginning to negotiate helps you be more effective and successful. Volkema (1999, p. 28) states that the three most important elements of negotiation are "information, information, information." Remember that information is power and you want to arm yourself with as much of this type of power as you can. You will want to ask yourself: What are the constraints in the system? Who are the other affected parties? What policies are in place that might impact the situation? What would be an acceptable compromise—in other words, what is the bottom line for which I am willing to settle? What are the interests that are served by the other person's position?

Negotiation works best when it is limited in its scope. When possible, consider only one issue at a time. If several items must be negotiated, prioritize them in your own mind. Which are most important to you? On which would you be most willing to yield your position? Negotiation will be more successful if you have a clear view of your own position first.

Implementing Your Plan for Negotiation

Some of the things that affect negotiations are perceptions of power (see Chapter 1), the time available for negotiating, and the adequacy of information available. As you move into a situation requiring negotiation, you will want to convey the image of a self-confident, capable person. Your verbal communication should be clear, direct, and decisive. Avoid tentative or uncertain language. Use your assertive communication skills (see Chapter 5). If you are confronted with something totally unexpected, ask that the negotiation session be delayed until another time. Simply stating that you are not prepared to discuss that issue now and asking for another meeting after you have had time to consider the information should adequately handle the situation.

While negotiating, you will need to listen carefully to understand the other person's position and viewpoint. Use all your active listening skills to encourage that individual to clearly explain his or her viewpoint to you. Try to understand the other person's position. The better you understand, the more likely you will be able to discern a common ground or identify the aspect on which the other person might yield a position. Keep an open mind and consider alternatives.

Watch carefully for nonverbal clues of feelings such as anger or defensiveness. Pay attention to your feelings and intuitive perceptions. Consider patterns of behavior more than a single, isolated response. By altering your response, you may be able to avert an unpleasant interaction and maintain a businesslike approach. Some individuals perceive that changing a position or yielding reflects an inappropriate weakness. Try to find a way that the person can save face when changing position. Avoid making anyone feel backed into a corner. People who feel they have no way out frequently become more defensive or aggressive.

Volkema (1999) suggests that the successful negotiator also asks questions. Questioning serves several purposes in the negotiation process. First, it helps in the effort to gather data about the other person's position or thinking. It can also assist in controlling the discussion and keeps the other individual busy while you have time to consider a response. It also helps avoid direct disagreements. Although you know how much time you can give to negotiating and when you must come to a decision, you do not know the time constraints of others involved. Ask questions to help you analyze the deadlines that may be present. Do not assume that an initial statement of a deadline for a decision is absolute. Often, deadlines are flexible and this is one area in which compromise may occur.

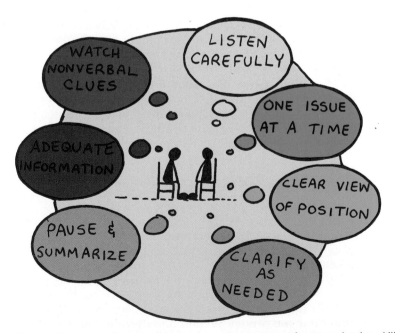

Conflict negotiation requires careful planning and expert use of communication skills.

When you believe that you have reached a conclusion in negotiations, always pause and summarize the decisions that were made, including any time frames for action that were agreed on. This clarifies where you are and helps to avoid the problem of an individual continuing to change positions after agreement has been reached. Be certain that you understand what the other person has agreed to and that he or she understands your position. Finally, make every attempt to close the negotiations on a friendly note with appropriate social, good-natured remarks.

Negotiating When the Sides Are Not Even

In 1994, a book by Phyllis Kritek titled *Negotiating at an Uneven Table* was published. In this book, she discusses the positions in which nurses often find themselves when involved in negotiations. Although the situation is gradually changing, nursing historically has been predominately a woman's profession. When working with other health care providers such as physicians and pharmacists (many of whom are male), nurses have not always been viewed as equals.

It is important to be able to recognize situations in which you may be at a disadvantage. The negotiation process will be weakened if some of the others at the table view you as powerless or weak. Kritek discusses **dominance power,** which is described as possession of control authority or influence over others and expands it to include such qualities as physical might, mental or moral efficacy, and political control or influence (Kritek, 1994, p. 45). In negotiating with individuals who are viewed as having dominant power, those without this quality may be seen as naïve as opposed to compelling and sentimental rather than substantive.

If you believe that you will be negotiating in this type of environment, it is even more important that you adhere to the suggestions offered previously. Increase your self-awareness, be honest, listen closely to what others are saying, be kind and considerate of others, know what you are willing to accept in the process, be creative, recognize your limitations, and stay with the process.

Critical Thinking Exercise

You have worked on the medical unit of a community hospital for just 3 months. The current policy regarding staffing is that each staff member receives every other weekend off, a standard valued highly by all employees. You have just had your weekend off when you learn that an old friend is arriving in town the coming weekend. You want to ask a colleague who will have that weekend off whether she would change her time so that you can be free to spend time with your friend. How would you begin the negotiation? What factors should you consider? What problems can you anticipate in the process?

■ MEDIATING CONFLICT

Given the inevitability of conflict and the fact that it can have positive outcomes within an organization, we are challenged to find the most effective ways of resolving it. One of the methods through which this can be accomplished is to enlist the skills of a mediator. As previously stated, a **mediator** is an individual who acts as an intermediary or conciliator between persons or sides who disagree or are in conflict. Working to resolve conflict and serving as mediator with a group can be challenging. Kheel (1999) identifies five roles of the mediator: (i) housekeeper of the proceedings, (ii) ringmaster of the negotiations, (iii) educator of the negotiators, (iv) communicator between the disputants, and (v) innovator of creative approaches on substantive as well as procedural issues. Although he was referring more to the role of a formal mediator, some aspects apply in all situations requiring settlement. These are a lot of roles for the novice to the management role in nursing to consider.

Steps in the Mediation Process

As you approach a conflict situation with the goal of seeking an equitable resolution, there is a series of steps you will want to follow. The approach that one uses depends on the nature of the conflict, the characteristics of the individuals involved, and the personal skills of the individual responsible for seeing that a resolution occurs. Some people are intimidated by conflict and associate it with unpleasant feelings and a sense of threat. Others are all too ready to "take on the world." The steps in the mediation process are summarized in Display 9-3.

ASSESSING THE CONFLICT

Before beginning any mediation regarding an issue, a conflict assessment should be completed. Not unlike the data collection you complete when planning patient care, this process involves gathering as much information as you can about the issues involved. What are the issues? Whom do they affect? Why are they a concern? Who will benefit one way or the other? Are there other things that impact the situation? Is there a time frame in which decisions must be reached? This means that the issues are identified and the needs and concerns discussed.

ANALYZING THE INFORMATION

Do you have a complete understanding of the problem? What factors limit your understanding? Is your perception accurate? Where can you gain additional information? Can the problems be easily resolved by adjusting a condition that led to the conflict? Are the parties involved amenable to talking and resolving the issue? What facts are obvious? What issues may be hidden? What goals should be established? While conducting this analysis, it is wise to determine which individuals need to be

---

DISPLAY 9-3	**Steps in the Mediation Process**

- Assessing the conflict
- Analyzing the information
- Planning the process
- Implementing the planned strategy
- Evaluating the outcome

involved in the process, the investment of each, and an understanding of desirable outcomes. On occasion, thorough analysis of a problem will provide quick resolution with the need for further mediation.

EXAMPLE *Analyzing a Conflict Regarding Coffee Breaks*

The nurses on a particular unit were in conflict because the time allowed for all employees to take a 15-minute morning coffee break extended from 9:15 to 10:00, an insufficient period to allow all employees a break. Employees began to challenge one another over who could go first, second, third, and so forth, with the last group often not having time for a break. Much energy was being invested in trying to remember or track who had the first break the day before and the day before that. When the situation, rather than the conflict itself, was analyzed and reviewed, adjusting the time allowed for the coffee break easily solved the conflict. An additional time period was added; some employees were permitted to take their 15-minute break at some point between 8:15 and 8:45.

PLANNING THE PROCESS

One of the roles of the mediator is to design the process for mediation and the strategies that will be used. During this phase, you will want to consider the timetables for resolving the issues. Is the issue urgent and therefore requires immediate settlement? Should discussion be delayed to allow emotions to become less heated? How will the discussions be conducted? Where will they be held? How will people that need to be involved know about the meetings? How will the outcomes be communicated?

An important step in planning for mediation is reviewing and adjusting your own attitudes. It is difficult to maximize insight, compassion, awareness, and common ground when our own attitudes get in the way. Assess your emotional involvement. If you find that you have certain biases regarding a person or situation, the biases must be adjusted before you begin to resolve the conflict. Our attitudes provide the screen or sieve through which we receive and give information. They can serve to distort or warp data being provided to us. We need to discriminate between situations in which we are dealing with facts and those in which we are dealing with feelings and then put each in the proper perspective.

IMPLEMENTING YOUR PLANNED STRATEGY FOR MEDIATION

Having completed these initial steps, you are ready to move on to more tangible aspects of conflict resolution. The next steps are those in integrative decision making or problem solving, which were discussed earlier.

Arrange a Meeting of Involved Persons. At this point, the persons involved in the conflict are called together to work on the problem. People should be notified in advance of the meeting, the time, the place, and the issue to be discussed. Although advance notice may initially create some anxiety among participants, it lessens the emotional impact, eliminates the discomfort of a surprise meeting for which they cannot psychologically or mentally prepare, and results in greater trust. The meeting should occur on neutral ground, and privacy and confidentiality should be assured. Sufficient time should be allotted to permit full discussion of the issue.

Encourage Expression of Individual Viewpoints. At this meeting, the mediator wants to encourage expression of individual viewpoints. Each individual should be encouraged to express his or her views, perceptions, needs, and goals. A climate must be created that will encourage and support a free exchange of ideas and attitudes. This step in the resolution of the conflict will result in the identification of the problem. It is important that the problem be fully defined before solutions are outlined. There are times when the full magnitude of the conflict is not brought out because of personal tensions or the desire to get things over with as quickly as possible. It is important to continue active questioning until all issues are identified. All participants should be encouraged to share both positive and negative thoughts. It is also important that the person responsible for providing leadership to the group be able to discourage behaviors that are destructive to this process. All points of view should be accepted and all perceptions taken seriously.

Look at All Alternatives to Solving the Problem. Once all sides are set forth and the problem is identified, there is a psychological lift. Now it is important to look at all the alternatives to solving the problem, even those that may seem to have little relevance, merit, or impact on the situation. All persons should be encouraged to supply solutions to the problem. Just as they are involved in the conflict, they must also be involved in finding the solution. It may be appropriate at this point to seek outside help or information. Use of outside resources is common in integrative problem solving.

Narrow the Choices for Action. After alternatives to solving the problem have been identified, the choices for action need to be narrowed. Identification of solutions concludes with a narrowing of choices for action. Criteria for evaluating the merit of the various alternatives must be established. Different approaches to the problem should be discussed and the best solution identified. Again, all persons must be involved; such involvement results in a commitment on the part of all individuals to see that the solution is implemented. The solution may require that some members of the group change their behavior. Members of the group are most likely to do so if they have exercised an instrumental role in identifying the solution. If solutions are suggested that some members of the group cannot support, discussion should continue until alternative methods are identified.

Plan the Implementation of the Decision. The last part of this step involves planning to implement the decision that has been reached. Before attempting to implement the solution or the activities it necessitates, you should clearly understand and communicate who is to do what and in what time frame. It may be useful to prepare a written plan for implementation or an implementation table and distribute copies to all. This plan or table should also deal with the timelines. During this process, criteria for evaluating the outcome should be defined. Group members need to know how they will monitor the process and how they will assess whether it is working.

EVALUATING THE OUTCOME OF THE MEDIATION

By using the criteria established in the previous step, the outcome of the decision needs to be evaluated. If the situation lends itself to doing so, this information should be given to members who were involved in discussing the conflict. This will help build in accountability and ownership for the successful completion of the plan. If the plan that was designed is not working, another meeting may need to be called and new strategies planned. Through the evaluation process, as with the nursing process, we are able to determine those actions that work best so that we can use them again in the future. We can also identify those actions that we may not want to use again.

Qualities That Facilitate Mediation

Stiebel (1993) describes the three ingredients of resolving stubborn disputes as trust, clear communication, and willingness of the parties to negotiate. As Stiebel points out, it is difficult to trust someone you don't know or someone with whom you disagree. At this point it is important for the two parties to place trust in the mediator. Often, mediation is successful because both parties trust the mediator although they may lack trust in one another.

Certain behaviors will help build trust. Phillips (2001) emphasizes the importance of intensive listening because it is a profound communication of respect, a cornerstone to peacemaking. She also encourages speaking honestly. Clarifying issues and recognizing and accepting divergent points of view will also build trust. Allowing and encouraging open discussion helps create a supportive climate that tends to energize people and results in creative thinking. It is important that peaceful resolution be stressed and that the individuals involved work toward understanding the other person's point of view. Emphasizing shared values and interests is often helpful. Discussion should be steered toward an exchange of ideas and should avoid personal references. Encouraging the use of "I" (versus "you") statements is important. It encourages participants to deal with the issue and not with personalities. By focusing on the problem at hand and not the characteristics of the persons involved, each party is able to maintain his or her self-respect and self-esteem. You can go a long way toward mitigating an unpleasant state of affairs by encouraging all participants to accept responsibility for being a part of the problem rather than blaming others. Blaming is viewed as a control strategy and defeats the goals of mediation.

Let people know that they are appreciated. Give positive feedback when good ideas are presented. Keep the discussion open and the atmosphere accepting. It is more important for all views to be heard than it is to have a peaceful meeting. Give all participants an equal opportunity to be heard and assure that their statements are listened to actively. For example, in one meeting in which some participants had a tendency to do more than their share of talking and occasionally tried to talk at the same time, the leader distributed poker chips. Blue chips were worth 5 minutes of time, red chips were worth 3 minutes, and white were worth 1 minute. Chips were distributed equally to all participants, who bought time by throwing a chip to the center of the table. This helped to lend some degree of order to the discussion and encouraged all participants to think about what they were going to say before using up their time. It also helped those who had a tendency to talk too much to recognize their own behavior. Perhaps most importantly, it added a degree of tension relief to the discussion.

It is helpful to clarify positions presented by others by restating them or rephrasing them. When the listener rephrases a statement, he or she provides assurance that it was heard as intended. In the feedback loop, this would be similar to correct decoding of the message by the receiver. When the meeting promises to be a volatile one, it is important to think of ways to limit the damage that can be done. A highly structured, formal type of meeting with an explicit agenda may be desirable. It is also important to establish game rules before beginning. Be certain that all participants understand what behavior is acceptable during the session and what is not. Once rules have been established, be certain that they are followed. Let us say, for example, that it is decided that dehumanizing behaviors such as laughing at or verbally discrediting an individual's description of feelings will not be allowed. If halfway through the discussion one member says to another, "I can't imagine why you would feel that way!" it is important for the leader to stop the discussion and remind participants of the rules.

During the mediation process, it is important that the mediator remain professional and in control of his or her own feelings. This is a time to be very patient and unemotional. No part of or person involved in the mediation should be considered unimportant or insignificant. Often, the process is as important to a lasting solution as the outcome members decided to adopt.

Stumbling Blocks to Effective Mediation

Phillips (2001) describes a number of stumbling blocks that deter effective mediation. Included among these are the following.

The *need to control others* can significantly affect negotiations. People who have a need to control also often feel they must make the final proposal and in the process alienate others. In such a situation, it may be helpful to have it appear as though the mediator originated all proposals, thus eliminating ownership and allowing the proposals to be considered on their own merit.

The *need to be right* will also deter effective mediation of disputes. It is often difficult for individuals to acknowledge that they were in error. It is not easy for many to say, "I am wrong, you are right." Many of us need to work at the ability to let go.

The *need of participants in the conflict to keep fighting* even when they achieved most of what was desired hampers good mediation. Phillips (2001) recommends recognizing when this loop is starting as a good way to stop the behavior. Agreement is more important than power. The need for vindication also plays a negative role in mediation. When the desired goal is achieved, everyone in the process needs to be gracious.

Critical Thinking Exercise

Maria and Josephine have worked as nursing assistants on the unit you supervise in a long-term care facility for almost 6 months. During that time, more conflict has come into their relationship. They disagree about who should have first lunch, who should have first access to the shower, and the distribution of time off during the holidays. This morning, they have come to you arguing about workload. Maria believes she is being asked to do more than Josephine. You have assigned Maria seven moderate care patients, and Josephine two heavy care patients and three moderate care patients. Of the approaches suggested in your reading, which do you believe would work best? Why? How would you begin to work with the situation? What must be done first? To what degree would you involve them in the conflict resolution? Why? If your plan for resolution is not successful, what would be an alternative?

■ COLLECTIVE BARGAINING

One of the common situations in which nurses find themselves negotiating is in the collective bargaining process. **Collective bargaining** involves a set of procedures by which employee representatives and employer representatives negotiate to obtain a signed agreement (contract) that describes conditions of employment, especially wages, hours, and benefits. In nursing, conditions of employment may also include defining the practice committees that will be in place, their memberships, and similar issues. The goal of the negotiations is to reach agreement about these issues, resulting in a contract that spells out in writing the decisions that have been reached.

Collective Bargaining and Nursing

Some employers have long chosen to engage in collective bargaining with their employees. In many states, the state governmental authorities were required to bargain with their employee groups. However, many private employers did not engage in collective bargaining until 1935 when the National Labor Relations Act (NLRA) was passed that required certain employers to negotiate with employees who chose that option. The majority of nurses did not have this option until 1974, when this legislation was amended to require that nonprofit hospitals engage in collective bargaining with duly elected employee groups. At that time, health care facilities and their employees were brought under the jurisdiction of the National Labor Relations Board (NLRB), a group created to ensure proper enforcement of the conditions of the NLRA.

As early as 1931, the American Nurses Association (ANA) was publicly recognizing its obligation to advocate for the general welfare of its members and developed within the organization a legislative policy that addressed this concern. Through the years, the ANA has worked constantly to provide leadership and support to nurses as they negotiated salaries, working conditions, benefits, and governance issues. This culminated in 1999 with the formation of the United American Nurses, an autonomous arm of the ANA that supports state organizations that bargain for nurses and provides a bargaining agent for those whose state does not have a collective bargaining agency. Table 9-1 highlights the activities of the ANA related to collective bargaining.

At one time collective bargaining by nurses was considered unprofessional, and in 1950 the ANA established a no-strike policy because it was concerned about the image of nursing. The thought of withholding needed services was abhorrent to many. This policy was rescinded in 1968 as the concept of unionism by professional groups became more accepted throughout the United States.

There are many reasons nurses chose to bargain collectively for working conditions and benefits. Although salary issues and benefits were important considerations in choosing to bargain, other critical issues included establishing a procedure for reporting poor or unsafe nursing care and assuring protection for those who report it. Staffing concerns, improper skill mix of care providers, floating without orientation, the use of temporary personnel and unlicensed personnel, mandatory overtime, and lack of input to the governance structure are also reasons nurses have felt the need to come together in a common voice. Although some of these issues might be addressed in employer-sponsored shared governance policies, only collective

TABLE 9-1	AMERICAN NURSES ASSOCIATION (ANA) ACTIVITIES RELATED TO COLLECTIVE BARGAINING
Year	**Activity**
1931	Addressed the general welfare concerns of its members through a legislative policy developed within the organization.
1945	Appointed a committee to study employment conditions.
1946	Established the ANA Economic Security Program as an outcome of a 1945 study. State nurses' associations were encouraged to act as bargaining agents for their memberships.
1947	Collective bargaining between nurses and hospital administrations implemented in several states with negotiated contracts in effect.
1950	No-strike policy officially adopted by ANA due to concern about the image of nursing.
1967	ANA identified as the bargaining agent for nurses in Veterans Administration hospitals.
1968	No-strike policy rescinded.
1991	ANA embarked on a Workplace Advocacy Initiative to improve the work environment of nurses. This led to the formation of the Commission on Workplace Advocacy.
1999	United American Nurses established as an autonomous arm of ANA to bargain for nurses
2003	ANA restructured to allow United American Nurses/AFL-CIO and Center for American Nurses (CAN)—formerly the Commission on Workplace Advocacy—to function independently of the ANA. Nurses allowed to pay dues to only Constituent Nurses Associations (CNA) or only the ANA.

bargaining results in a legally enforceable contract to require the employer to carry out decisions reached.

Contracts also contain language regarding reasons and processes for termination or disciplinary action and spell out the steps to be followed in a grievance procedure. A grievance is a circumstance or action believed to be in violation of a contract (or of policies if a contract is not in place) (Ellis & Hartley, 2004). The **grievance process** spells out an orderly method to be used in mediating the grievance between parties. Typically, this is a series of steps to be taken and the timeline for accomplishing the steps. These policies usually are included in a personnel handbook as well as the contract if one is in effect.

 ## Issues Related to Collective Bargaining

Collective bargaining by nurses is not without its concerns. Essentially there are four. We have already alluded to the first one: is it professional for nurses to bargain collectively. Nursing's history of altruism and selflessness along with its strong religious influence carried with it the ethic that it was unprofessional to consider issues such as salary and working conditions. The fact that nursing was and still is a profession comprising predominantly women often contributed to this view. However, over the years, many have come to believe that the collective action of nurses provides an unparalleled approach to achieving professional goals and exercising control over nursing practice. As nurses have become more sophisticated with regard to the manner in which the bargaining is conducted, more and more nurses are uniting through union activities.

Another topic at issue with regard to collective bargaining among nurses relates to the group that will represent nurses at the bargaining table. Although the ANA through its state nurses' associations has been a strong force for a number of years and currently represents more nurses than any other organization, there has been a strong push from other organizations to occupy this role. In 1977, the National Union of Hospital and Health Care Employees was formed. The Service Employees International Union (SIEU) has united with this group to form something of a "superunion" to negotiate contracts for health care workers. The Teamsters and the American Federation of Teachers are two other groups that might negotiate for nurses. Nurses face a difficult decision when trying to decide which group should represent them. Some believe that the ANA will be the strongest organization because it is composed of individuals who best can understand nurses and nursing. Others believe that organizations that are devoted entirely to collective bargaining activities will be most effective. Choosing a nonnursing organization would answer the concern of those who believe that it is not realistic for one group to work with the professional aspects of nursing as well as with the issues of wages, benefits, and working conditions. If two groups are chosen, one to represent nurses professionally and one to bargain for salaries, the cost of membership to both groups is a consideration. Paying dues to two organizations when those fees per year exceed $350 each may be more than some nurses choose to afford.

This brings us to the third major issue: whether to join a union. Some nurses still believe that unionism is unprofessional and have chosen not to join a collective bargaining group. However, more often it is the cost of membership that impedes individual participation. In response to this concern, many contracts now include **agency shop** clauses, which specify that all persons covered by the contract must pay dues for membership. Nurses who belong to the union often seek this provision, because the costs of negotiating and enforcing a contract are considerable. If everyone does not belong, then the costs are borne disproportionately by those who do join. The law requires that those who are not members have all the same rights and protections of the contract as those who are members. This includes the defense by the union if they should have a grievance. When an agency shop is in place, if, because of religious or philosophical beliefs, an employee is unwilling to pay dues to the bargaining group, an amount equal to the dues can be paid to a charitable group, such as a foundation.

The final issue related to collective bargaining relates to the role of the supervisor. The NLRA does not apply to individuals working as supervisors or in administrative positions within organizations. Debate has occurred regarding what is considered supervision. When a nurse's role requires providing direction to others, should this be considered supervision? In 1994 and again in 1996 this issue was before the Supreme Court. In the latter instance, the Supreme Court ruled that the essence of the nurse's role was judgment, and further explained that the authority that arises from professional knowledge is distinct from the authority of a frontline manager ("NLRB to the Supreme Court: Labor Law Protects Nurses," 1996). Therefore, the ruling supported the view that staff nurses in hospitals are not supervisors and are therefore eligible for collective bargaining. This ruling does not extend to nurses in settings in which the staff nurse may have authority for evaluation and hiring and firing recommendations, such as what occurs in some nursing homes.

In 2003, the U.S. Labor Department proposed a new rule that would change many professional workers from an hourly category eligible for overtime pay to a salaried category not eligible for overtime pay. If this proposed rule had been approved, nurses who did not have negotiated contracts could have been switched in their category. Many labor groups vigorously opposed this rule change. In September 2003, the House of Representative passed legislation prohibiting the Labor Department from establishing this new rule. Labor issues will continue to offer many challenges in health care.

Critical Thinking Exercise

As a new graduate you have been offered equally desirable positions by both the hospitals to which you applied. One of the hospitals has a union with the State Nurses' Association serving as the representative. The other hospital is not unionized. What arguments can you make for accepting employment at the unionized facility? What are the arguments in favor of accepting employment at the other hospital? What factors will influence you? Why?

■ KEY CONCEPTS

- Conflict occurs when individuals, groups, or organizations hold differing values, goals, or perceptions. Nurses experience conflict in their professional roles in many forms and situations and must know how to manage conflict situations. Although people hold a variety of views of conflict, it is inevitable in our society and can have positive outcomes if managed appropriately.

- Many conflict situations occur in nursing. There may be conflict between members of the health care team, with the patient's family, between nurses, and conflict related to values and beliefs about nursing practices.

- Our views of conflict have changed over the years. Once viewed as an indication of poor management and a circumstance to be avoided, conflict is now viewed as inevitable and potentially having positive outcomes.

- When looking at positive outcomes, conflict provides an impetus for change, helps individuals understand one another's jobs and responsibilities, opens new channels of communication, energizes people, and may result in a more equitable distribution of resources within an organization.

- The outcomes of conflict resolution can be viewed as creating a win–lose situation, a lose–lose situation, or a win–win situation. Win–win situations most often result when integrative decision making is used.

- Conflict can occur within the individual, between individuals or groups, or between organizations or the organization and the environment.

- Within organizations, conflict occurs because of role ambiguity or role conflict, the structure of the organization, or scarcity of resources within the organization. The manner in which the leader deals with conflict will influence the organization. Several different styles may be used for managing conflict.

- A number of personal styles of dealing with conflict exist. These include avoiding or withdrawing, accommodating or smoothing, competing or forcing, compromising or negotiating, and problem solving or collaborating.

- Problem solving may represent the best approach to conflict and may also be the most difficult to achieve.

- Conflicts also occur with a group. Groups are affected by the outcome of conflict. Winning tends to increase group cohesiveness; losing can result in blaming, denial and internal conflicts.

- Nurses may be required to mediate conflict. The steps in the mediation process include assessing the conflict, analyzing the information, planning the process, implementing the planned strategy, and evaluating the outcome. Using interpersonal skills adroitly is an important part of conflict resolution.

- A number of qualities facilitate mediation. Among these, the development of trust is critical.

- Stumbling blocks to effective mediation include the need to control, the need to be right, the need to keep fighting, and the need for vindication.

- When involved in negotiations it is important to plan your actions. Gaining as much information as possible prior to initiation of the negotiations is critical.

- Successful negotiations involve active listening, asking questions, maintaining an open mind, watching for nonverbal cues from your opponent, and summarizing the decisions that have been reached at the conclusion of the negotiation.

- During the negotiation process, it is important to recognize which party has the dominant power or influence over others. When lacking it, special strategies should be employed.

- Collective bargaining is one of the important occasions when nurses are engaged in negotiations. Collective bargaining has not always been viewed as appropriate for nurses, but such thinking has changed over the years.

- Collective bargaining provides nurses the opportunity to have a voice regarding professional issues of staffing and practice patterns as well as wages, benefits, and working conditions such as evaluation, termination, and grievance.

- Collective bargaining concludes with a written contract that includes all the issues agree on in the negotiation process.

- Four major issues surround collective bargaining in nursing: whether it is professional, which organization should represent nurses at the bargaining table, whether to join the union, and the role of the supervisor in relationship to the right to bargain collectively.

REFERENCES

Assael, H. (1969). Constructive role of interorganizational conflict. *Administrative Science Quarterly, 14*(4), 573–582.

Barton, A. (1991). Conflict resolution by nurse managers. *Nursing Management, 22*(5), 83–86.

Berkowitz, L. (1962). *Aggression: a social analysis.* New York: McGraw-Hill.

Blake, R., & Mouton, J. (1964). *The Managerial Grid.* Houston, TX: Gulf.

Dove, M. A. (1998). Conflict: process and resolution. *Nursing Management, 29*(4), 30–32.

Ellis, J. R., & Hartley, C. L. (2004). *Nursing in Today's World: Trends, Issues, & Management* (8th ed.). Philadelphia: Lippincott Williams & Wilkins.

Filley, A. (1975). *Interpersonal Conflict Resolution.* Glenview, IL: Scott, Foresman.

Huber, D. (1996). *Leadership and nursing care management.* Philadelphia: W.B. Saunders.

Kheel, R. W. (1999). *The Keys to Conflict Resolution: Proven Methods of Settling Disputes Voluntarily.* New York: Four Walls Eight Windows.

Kritek, P. B. (1994). *Negotiating at an Uneven Table: Developing Moral Courage in Resolving Our Conflicts.* San Francisco: Jossey-Bass.

Lewis, J. (1976). Conflict management. *Journal of Nursing Administration, 6*(10), 18–22.

Mallory, G. (1985). Turn conflict into cooperation. *Nursing 85, 15*(3), 81–83.

"NLRB to the Supreme Court: Labor law protects nurses." (1996). *American Journal of Nursing, 96*(4), 67, 72.

Phillips, B. A. (2001). *The Mediation Field Guide: Transcending Litigation and Resolving Conflicts in Your Business or Organization.* San Francisco: Jossey-Bass.

Rosenstein, A. H. (2002). Nurse-physician relationships: Impact on nurse satisfaction and retention. *American Journal of Nursing* 102(6): 26-34.

Shell, G. R. (1999). *Bargaining for Advantage: Negotiation Strategies for Reasonable People.* New York: Viking.

Stiebel, D. (Presenter). (1993). *Resolving Stubborn Community College Disputes* [Interactive video presentation]. Washington, DC: American Association of Community and Junior Colleges.

Swansburg, R. C., & Swansburg, R. J. (2002). *Introduction to Management and Leadership for Nurse Managers* (3rd ed.). Boston: Jones and Bartlett.

Thomas, K. (1976). Conflict and conflict management. In M. Dunnette (Ed.), *The Handbook of Industrial and Organizational Psychology.* Chicago: Rand McNally.

Thomas, K., & Kilmann, R. (1974). *Thomas-Kilmann Conflict Mode Instrument.* Tuxedo, NY: Xicom, Inc.

Volkema, R. J. (1999). *The Negotiation Tool Kit.* New York: AMACOM (a division of the American Management Association).

3

EVOLVING ISSUES
IN NURSING PRACTICE

Unit 3 addresses topics that will touch on your career as a professional nurse. It begins with a chapter that relates to advancing your career. Many aspects of planning your career, mapping your future, and identifying areas of nursing in which you wish to work are discussed. Techniques for seeking desired positions in nursing and resigning those positions as you advance your career are presented. A sample resumé, letter of inquiry, and a cover letter, along with a sample letter of resignation, are provided to guide you in the process of developing these important documents. Information regarding the interview and the interview process are intended to facilitate that experience. The chapter concludes with a discussion of entrepreneurship in nursing.

The importance of attaining and maintaining competence spurs the discussion in Chapter 11. Cultural competence, interpersonal competence, and technical competence are requirements of the nurse who will function effectively in today's health care environment. As you move forward in your career and assume increasingly greater responsibility for directing the activities of others, you will encounter those individuals who offer a challenge to your interpersonal and management skills.

Chapter 12 discusses some of the problems commonly met in the workplace, including the chemically impaired individual, the individual who is clinically incompetent, and nonproductive and marginal employees. Seeking out and using new information resources are significant aspects of our daily existence, and they play an increasingly important role in our professional lives. Knowing where to look for information and how to access it will significantly impact your skill in using basic research to advance your own knowledge and to be involved in evidence-based practice. Although you will not be expected to understand or implement sophisticated research techniques, the ability to read and comprehend basic research information can make a difference in your performance. This chapter also discusses the use of computers and informatics in the health care arena.

The book concludes with an exploration of activities that will affect the future of nursing. Cast against a brief history of nursing education, approaches to differentiated practice are outlined. The work that has been done on developing a universal language for nursing is described as well as its purposes in the profession. A discussion of violence in the workplace, a concern receiving greater attention among nursing leaders finalizes the chapter. Thus, this book brings you full circle, from introducing you to leadership behaviors and management skills, through discussing roles that you will perfect throughout your career, to concluding with content that involves looking toward your professional future and the aspects of nursing you can anticipate in the future.

Advancing Your Career

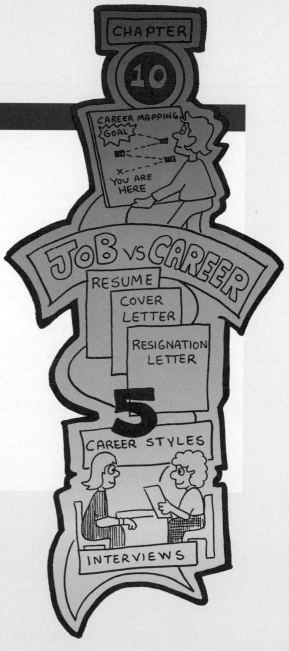

Learning Outcomes

After completing this chapter, you should be able to:

1. Differentiate between the terms *job* and *career*.
2. Analyze the various concepts of career styles, comparing and contrasting the focus of each, and relate them to your personal situation.
3. Discuss career mapping and the general components that might be included in a personal career map.
4. Identify factors that should be considered in your self-analysis of your professional needs and development of goals.
5. Describe the purpose of the resumé, and identify important aspects of it.
6. Discuss ways by which information can be gained about prospective employers.
7. Describe the critical elements of an interview, specifying why each is important.
8. Compare and contrast the various continuing education opportunities available to you.
9. Analyze the various entrepreneurial opportunities available to nurses and outline the skills needed for success.

Key Terms ■ ■ ■ ■ ■

career	cover letter	job
career counselor	entrepreneur	letter of inquiry
career development	exit interview	mentor
career mapping	formal education	promotion
career styles	goals	recruitment
clinical career ladder	interview	resumé
continuing education		

Y ou are about to embark on a career in nursing. It is the realization of goals you established for yourself several years ago when you decided to enter the nursing profession. In reaching this decision, you may have been motivated by a number of different reasons. Perhaps you chose to pursue a nursing career because of job security or the flexibility the job offered. Maybe you perceived that the profession carried status and prestige with others in the community. Or perhaps you started your schooling for altruistic reasons, such as the unselfish concern for the welfare of others. Maybe you chose nursing because the skills and aptitudes required of its professionals corresponded to attitudes and abilities that you possessed. Whatever the basis for your decision, you made a career commitment. A career commitment is different from a commitment to a job. In this chapter, we present content that hopefully will assist you to find the position in nursing that is best for you and will keep you motivated and enthusiastic about the profession.

■ DIFFERENTIATING A JOB FROM A CAREER

If you are like many other individuals, you have held a number of jobs in your life. A **job** is a specific task or work that one has agreed to do for pay. Many jobs require no formal education. Beginning jobs may be as simple as delivering newspapers or bagging groceries at the local supermarket. Other jobs such as waiting tables, retail sales, or manufacturing are full time and serve to support oneself and one's family but without an expectation of lifetime commitment and involvement.

By contrast, a **career** may be defined as a profession or occupation for which one trains and pursues as a lifework (Neufeldt, 1996). In nursing, we have veered away from the word *trains* in favor of the concept *educate,* because of our desire to move nursing from its early history of apprentice-type preparation. However, nursing is viewed as a profession and is pursued as one's lifework as opposed to being a stepping-stone to another venture. When we choose a career, it is usually a process of identifying a line of work that allows us to fulfill personal goals. When that career involves a profession, we can anticipate that it will only be reached after several years of formal education that, in the case of nursing, involves both theoretical and practical applications of knowledge. A career commitment speaks of one's attitude toward a profession and the motivation to make that profession one's life work (See Table 10-1). When we plan to make a career commitment, to make a profession our life work, we also need to think about the direction that career should take. The process of planning and implementing career plans is referred to as **career development.**

Prior to the 1970s, organizations did little to assist employees to plan or develop their careers. However, in the last two decades, many organizations have looked at the positive aspects of career development programs. During the late 1980s and early 1990s, a number of individuals began studying and writing about the various aspects of career development (Kramer, 1974; Peters and Waterman, 1982; Vogel, 1990; Henderson & McGettigan, 1994; Swanson, 1994). Among factors they considered were the employee's role in career development and planning and the organization's response to that process of career planning. In health care, job satisfaction was a major issue because when employees were satisfied in their positions, staff turnover was reduced. Staff turnover can represent a significant financial issue to organizations. Swansburg and Swansburg (2002) indicate that the annual national turnover rate among hospital nurses is between 20% and 70%. People leave jobs when they believe the positions are no longer rewarding or fulfilling or if there is too much associated stress. In addition, nurses became concerned about how, within the profession of nursing, we assist new graduates to develop expertise without suffering from disillusionment or burnout.

Friss (1989), in studying career development, identified five distinctive **career styles.** No style is better than another; they are simply different. The first style Friss identified as the steady state. It is characterized by a long work history often in the same area. An example might be the nurse who chooses to care for clients and families in the birthing center, then expands that to patient education of new mothers, working on specialty committees or organizations, and perhaps earning certification. Notable is the fact that the individual remains in the same area and becomes increasingly competent.

The second style is referred to as linear and is demonstrated by a steady climb to jobs of increasing responsibility, authority, and usually compensation. An example of this style would be the staff nurse who moves into a charge nurse position, is promoted to unit supervisor, becomes a hospital supervisor, and eventually reaches the

TABLE 10-1   COMPARISON OF CHARACTERISTICS OF JOBS AND CAREERS

Characteristic	Jobs	Careers
Personal commitment	May have little dedication	Lifetime commitment
Educational requirements	Characteristically none or very few	Requires a special amount usually at the college level and typically culminating in a degree or certificate
Identification	Little group identification	Members share a common identity and subculture
Goals related to position	Financial	Lifetime involvement as well as financial

position of vice president of patient care service, thus moving up the hierarchy of the organization.

The third style is entrepreneurial and is manifest in individuals who choose to go into business for themselves. These persons are often very creative and prefer to operate away from the restrictions that might be imposed by an organization and in a more flexible environment. An example would be seen in the independent nurse practitioner or the nurse who opens a consulting service. We discuss entrepreneurial roles in nursing at the end of the chapter.

The transient style is the fourth career style. It describes the individual who holds a series of unrelated jobs of relatively short duration. The best example of this style may be the nurse who is employed as a "traveler," moving from one facility to another as the need arises. It might also occur if a nurse is required to relocate frequently because of the demands of a partner's job responsibilities, as might be seen with a nurse married to someone in the armed forces.

The final style is referred to as spiral. It is characterized by a 5- to 7-year period of intense employment, followed by a period of nonemployment or a different type of employment. This might describe the nurse who is actively involved in nursing, then reduces to part-time or complete retirement to raise a family, and then returns to the profession, seeking once again opportunities for self-development.

The studies by Friss clearly provided for a time in a nurse's career when family needs would be considered. If your career must revolve around a family and family demands on your time, you will have an appreciation for the different styles he identifies.

EXAMPLE   *The Career Spiral*

> Janey Mosher accepted a position on a busy medical unit of a large urban hospital immediately following her graduation. She married 3 years later, and 1 year following that she and her husband decided to start their family. Janey worked full time until the seventh month of her pregnancy and then decided to resign. Her husband worked for a large computer firm and his salary allowed Janey the opportunity to be a full-time mother. Two more children joined their household over the next 5 years. When the youngest child started to school, Janey decided she wanted to return to nursing on a part-time basis. She missed the stimulation she found in nursing.

Benner (1982) examined work with respect to levels of proficiency. The five levels she defined are novice, advanced beginner, competent, proficient, and expert. These increments were based on both education and experience. It encouraged the nurturing of nurses at all stages of career development, resulting in better utilization of skills and greater job satisfaction.

This last statement is of particular importance. As a discipline, nurses are often accused of being critical of one another. A more nurturing attitude will provide a climate in which nurses, whether new to the profession or to the role, will feel comfortable during the period of time they are becoming familiar with expectations. Older, seasoned nurses often express frustration and impatience with those who are inexperienced, thus creating anxiety, uncertainty, and eventually lack of personal fulfillment, resulting in job dissatisfaction in those inexperienced individuals. All nurses can benefit by remembering how it felt when just beginning a new position.

Thinking about these various approaches to career development may assist you as you take charge of your career in nursing. As a student about to complete your program of study, you probably feel you have your hands full just reaching graduation day. You may feel like saying, "Just let me get through with this and then I can think about planning my career!" However, time moves quickly, and as you start thinking about securing a position in nursing, you need to give some thought to what will result in nursing being a fulfilling career for you. The conclusion of giving this no thought could well be that you wind up someplace that you prefer not to be or involved in activities from which you derive little satisfaction.

■ CAREER MAPPING

Career mapping is a process by which you develop a master plan for career advancement. Much like the strategic plan developed by an organization, or the route that you would plan for a vacation by car to a certain area of the country, career mapping provides a systematic and methodical approach to your future or to where you are going. A career in nursing is more satisfying if it is properly planned. Planning will help you understand the work environment in which you plan to practice and reduce the uncertainty and anxiety that can result in burnout. Without career mapping, you will find yourself reacting haphazardly to opportunities for career advancement and to job offers.

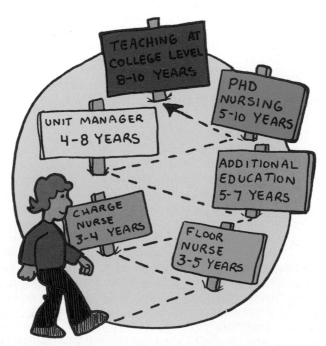

Career mapping is a process by which you develop a master plan for career advancement.

Mapping your career, even if it is a fairly general plan, will tell you whether you need more education to reach your personal goals. Planning of this nature will help you identify the types of experiences you will need, give some direction to where you will want to seek employment, and indicate the type of networking that will result in moving toward your goals. For example, if your goal on graduation is to work in a coronary care unit within 2 years of graduation, you will want to seek employment in an acute care facility that has such a unit. You will want to plan to take courses on managing arrhythmias, either at a local college or through the hospital, and you may want to become involved with the American Heart Association, the American Association of Critical Care Nurses, or the Society for Vascular Nursing.

Critical Thinking Exercise

Assume that your goal after graduation is to work with the elderly. Develop a career map for yourself that would lead you to this type of care. Think about where you will want to be 1 year and 5 years from now. Identify the activities that should take place for you to reach the goals that you have set for yourself. What should be done first? What additional education would be appropriate? Where would you seek initial employment? What organizations might you join?

Planning for a career is not always an easy undertaking. Goals may not mesh with reality. Opportunities arise that may interrupt a well-developed plan. Personal situations change and may impact the career direction one is pursuing. However, given these constraints and realities, a general plan will result in a more satisfying career and greater self-actualization on the part of the individual involved. In the following sections, we discuss the steps that facilitate the development of an effective career map.

Complete a Self-Assessment and Self-Analysis

Whether you are moving into nursing as a new graduate and applying for your first position or reexamining where you are going in nursing, it is wise to begin with a self-assessment and self-analysis of your values and goals. This self-assessment and self-analysis will help you to determine what is important to you and which of the many opportunities available in nursing will most help you realize your goals while bringing the greatest sense of satisfaction. Self-assessment and analysis will also help you identify the steps you must take to achieve those goals.

Begin by examining your own values and beliefs. What is important to you? What is your philosophy of care? What religious or spiritual beliefs or practices are important to you? How do you perceive the role of the nurse? What aspects of nursing challenge you the most? Which ones bring you concern? In which situations do you feel most empowered? Which ones make you feel most powerless? It is important that there be an appropriate match between the things that you value and which are important to you and the manner in which you use your skills as a nurse. For example, if you believe it is wrong to place patients at risk, you would probably not be comfortable working in a research hospital where research protocols required nurses to administer treatments that could pose potential threats to patients. Similarly, if you believe all patients should have access to all treatment available, you may find your values challenged if you are working in a situation involving a double-blind study in which some patients receive the treatment and others receive a placebo when both patients would benefit from receiving the treatment. To you, the importance of safeguarding the health and well-being of the patient would take precedence over the outcomes of a study in which patients may be used as sources of data. You can use the knowledge of what is important to you to guide your selection of employment opportunities.

When you look at your personal goals, you will want to ask yourself a number of questions. Your career map will be helpful here. Where do you want to be in 5 years? In 10 years? Would you prefer a career track in clinical nursing, administration, or some other role in nursing? Is nursing education a possibility? Does the position you desire require additional education? Is that formal or informal preparation? You will want to look at your own strength and weakness because matching goals with abilities is very important. What are your current skills? Do you have limitations that must be considered as you move forward in your career? Personal issues also need to be considered. Where do you find challenges and satisfaction in nursing? What aspects of nursing leave you frustrated or dissatisfied? Are there others whom you must consider in your decision making? Do you need to take into consideration the effect any change will have on a partner or on children? Is the timing right for making any changes?

Once you feel you have done a complete self-assessment and analysis and have answered all the questions appropriate to guiding your career, you will want to set your goals. Personal goal setting is much like the goal setting with which you are already familiar with regard to your patients.

Set Your Goals

Career **goals** help you plan your future constructively and should be both short and long term. Short-term goals will include those activities that you want to accomplish in the next month and the coming year. For example, as a new graduate you may have the short-term goal of securing a beginning nursing position on a medical unit in a community hospital. Short-term goals are ones that you will want to review in at least a year's time.

Long-term goals reflect your professional aspirations 5 or 10 years from now. The individual who was seeking a beginning nursing position on a medical unit in a community hospital as a short-term goal may have the long-term goal of working as a unit manager on a medical unit, or perhaps of returning to school for an advanced degree or certificate in nursing.

You may also have intermediate-term goals. For example, your short-term goal may be securing a position on a medical unit in a community hospital and your long-term goal may be to work as a unit manager in that facility. An intermediate goal may involve working as a charge nurse in that facility or it might include gaining some special expertise by completing courses on management at a local college or university. In all cases, it is wise to have alternative goals and to keep your goals as broad and as flexible as possible.

EXAMPLE *Application of Career Mapping*

James Justin looked forward to completing his nursing education in 2 months. As a part of a course preparing students for transition into the world of employment, James was required to develop an initial career map. After examining his values and beliefs, James decided he really wanted to work with a disadvantaged population because he received a great deal of satisfaction from helping with the less fortunate. He determined that his own needs were not great; thus, salary was not a major concern. His goal was to find employment in a community outreach program serving the needs of those who could not afford health care. Thus, his job search began by exploring community resources that would identify sources of employment. Ultimately, he thought he would like to work with Doctors Without Borders.

 ## Seek a Mentor or Career Counselor

When possible, it is very desirable to seek the assistance of a career counselor or a mentor. Typically, a **mentor** is a more experienced nurse who is willing to provide time, advice, and assistance to one with lesser experience. This should be someone whose behavior you admire and whom you wish to emulate. It should be an individual who will be straightforward in giving you both positive and negative feedback and who will help you build self-confidence. This individual should be able to help you stretch and grow and provide insight into issues and approaches that you have not considered, both in your nursing practice and in your career development. In a sense, the mentor can empower you. In studying factors that will help attract and keep nurses in nursing, Campbell (2003) notes, "The nursing profession must assume responsibility for mentoring and bringing those behind them 'with them'."

As mentioned elsewhere in this book, the nursing profession is striving to attract and retain more members of minority races among its ranks. The need for a culturally diverse workforce to assist in reducing the health disparities that exist among the nation's population is well documented. It is also important that the members of minority groups that are being recruited into nursing have mentors from their own cultural or ethnic group to assist them in role transition. One of the goals of the National Advisory Council on Nurse Education and Practice (NACNEP) is to increase the use of mentors for students and those nurses who are young in their careers.

A **career counselor** is a professional with skills in helping people explore their interests and abilities and setting career goals. Some health care organizations are now employing career counselors, or there may be such an individual available to you at your college or university. In health care organizations, the career counselor may be employed in the staff development or human resources area. In addition to planning work experiences, the career map that is developed would include off-duty activities such as conferences, workshops, courses, professional activities, and similar actions that will help further the goals established. A career counselor should assist in the assessment of interests, skills, and values and aid in establishing career plans that take these into consideration.

Establish a Plan for Employment

Seeking employment involves putting you in the best possible position and light to be offered the job that you aspire. This takes some forethought and planning. One of the first things you will want to do is develop a **resumé** that can be shared with a potential employer.

PREPARING THE RESUMÉ

A resumé is a brief overview of your qualifications for a position. Its purpose is to let the prospective employer know whether you have the knowledge, skills, and qualifications for the position for which you are applying. You will want this resumé to be viewed positively by the potential employers such that it will create the impression that you can successfully do the job. You want to sell yourself to the employer as a desirable team member. Nurse recruiters view the resumé as an important instrument. They use the resumé as a screening mechanism for hiring. Resumés also are used for important promotion decisions; therefore, they should be kept current once they are developed.

Appearance. The overall appearance of your resumé is important because it says something about you to the prospective employer. Is it neat and free from smudges and stains? Is it easily read? Is it free from errors? A resumé should not be longer than two standard-sized (8.5 by 11 inches) white or off-white pages on good-quality paper; one page is better. It should be in typed format and easy to read. (Many computer programs now provide templates for resumé formatting.) It should focus on your accomplishments, skills, and results. Statements should be short and concise, and use action verbs to describe each accomplishment. Resumés should emphasize your strengths and minimize your weaknesses. You may want to place bullets before items that you consider important to draw special attention to them. Underlining is discouraged because many organizations scan resumés into computers and underlining sometimes does not scan. Avoid fancy fonts that often are difficult to read. It is better to use fonts such as Arial, Times Roman, or Tahoma.

Format. There are many acceptable formats for resumés. The most important thing is that the resumé gives a correct and positive reflection of you and your abilities. You should tailor any recommended resumé format to meet those criteria. The recommended formats for most resumés suggest that your name, address, and a telephone number at which you can be reached be listed first. If you will be moving, indicate when that move will take place and provide a contact where you can be reached. E-mail addresses are helpful, but if you have an e-mail address that could be viewed as less than professional (such as *cutiepie* or *bigboy*), set up an e-mail address for business use. Using your own name or a derivation of it gives a more professional impression.

Following this personal data, it is desirable to state your personal objective, such as "To secure a beginning position as a registered nurse on a challenging surgical unit that will provide an opportunity for professional development." Be certain that your objective is realistic and reflects the skills and abilities that you can bring to the position. For example, if you state that you wish to work in the operating room but have no experience in the area, your application may be set aside.

Include information regarding your licensure and other appropriate information regarding your credentials. If you have received your license or temporary permit, the number should be listed. If you have not received your license, indicate the date that you anticipate having it. If you are licensed in more than one state, the license number from each jurisdiction should be included.

You will want to include a section that focuses on your education. You should identify the school from which you received your preparation for nursing and the year of completion. If you have completed additional course work that is relevant to the position you are seeking, this is a good place to include that information. For example, if you have completed a course in basic arrhythmias or if you have completed a special preceptorship, this could be listed here.

Another section of the resumé should emphasize your work experience. This would include all relevant and meaningful jobs you have held. You should identify the position, the dates you were employed in this job, and the duties associated with it. If you have had only two or three jobs, each can be listed. However, if you have had a number of jobs, it is wise to group them. For example, you might list, "a variety of jobs to help finance education, including clerk, wait staff, and babysitting." The overall dates relative to the time you had these jobs should also be included. Create a fresh impression on your resume by varying the verbs that you use to describe your past activities. Delete the personal pronouns "I" and "me," because they may give the impression that you are thinking only of yourself. This would be especially true if that impression is reinforced in your personal interview. Statements that you are available for day-shift work only or that you need every other weekend off, or a detailed listing of personal achievements, will not help you secure a position. Although it is important to be proud of your accomplishments, you want to think ahead to the position for which you are applying and build the impression in the employer's mind that you will make a valuable contribution. Avoid the use of clichés such as "self-motivated," "patient-centered," or "self-starter," that tell little about your actual abilities.

If you have received special honors or recognition, the information can be included in another section. Likewise, if you have special experiences or have been heavily involved in volunteer activities in your community, a section can be added to provide that information. You should not include a listing of your hobbies, marital status, age, race, or past salary history.

Personal References. Personal references should not be listed. References are typed on a separate sheet of paper that can be given to the prospective employer if requested and usually include at least three names. If you are a student about to graduate, potential employers will expect that one of your references is an individual who has been one of your instructors, preferably in the clinical area. Some facilities will request two references from instructors. It is desirable to have a reference come from a former employer, an individual who can address you work habits, skills, and effectiveness as an employee. Another reference should be someone who has known you for a fairly long period of time, such as a pastor or priest, professional colleague, or neighbor who can speak about personal attributes such as honesty and your ability to relate to others. Some employers do not request this personal reference and may specify the references they want. Be prepared with names, addresses, and telephone numbers so that the employer can contact these individuals easily.

Before listing someone as a reference, you should ask that individual's permission to do so. Seeking this permission provides the opportunity for you to outline what you would like that individual to emphasize. For example, you might say, "If they contact you, I would appreciate your comments on my work ethic and effectiveness as an employee."

A great deal of information is available that gives direction to the preparation of a resumé. Local community and college libraries will have reference material and books that provide good advice. You can also access the Internet for assistance. Typing in the words *nursing resumé* into the "search" section of your browser will provide a long list of potential sources. The University of Pennsylvania's School of Nursing (www.upenn.edu/careerservices/nursing/jobhandbookindex.html) provides an excellent resource with helpful instructions for writing a resumé that includes a variety of examples. Another helpful source is found at www.careerjournal.com. A sample resumé is given in Display 10-1.

SELECTING A PROSPECTIVE EMPLOYER

Once you have a resumé in hand, you will want to make a decision regarding potential employers. Again, doing your homework pays off. Learn everything you can about potential employers. What kind of a facility is it? What type of clients does it serve? What types of services are offered at the facility? Is there an internship for new graduates? If so, how long does it last? Are the employees unionized? If so, who represents them at the bargaining table? Are employees promoted from within the organization? What type of staff development program is in effect? Does the facility have a clinical ladder? If you are applying to a facility to which you were assigned as a student, you might talk with hospital employees or your former instructors. The facility's Web site will provide basic information on its size, structure, areas of interests, and key contacts. Local libraries also carry directories from organizations that provide useful information. Some additional information can be gathered at the time you interview for a position.

Coccia (1998) has identified six implicit signs of an organization's culture that you might want to consider before seeking employment with that organization. If time allows, the questions might be answered during the interview session. If there is not adequate time, or if you want the answers to these questions before the interview, the answers should be researched through community resources. The questions and the reason why each is important are as follows:

1. How many layers exist in the organizational structure? The chain of command may provide information about the rigidity of the organization.
2. Is it possible to talk with people on the organizational chart? The wider the picture you can gather of the organization, the better informed you will be.
3. How frequently are policies updated? How are they developed and implemented? The administrative manual provides a snapshot of the organization's personality.
4. Is a walk-through during off-hours possible? Much can be learned from talking with people who work for the organization, such as perceptions of staffing patterns, organizational support, and personal recognition and value.
5. How do the nurse managers dress? Dress codes will speak volumes about the organization's culture and perceptions of the nurses' role.
6. Do nurse managers attend medical staff meetings or other important administrative sessions? Communication among administration, medical staff, and the nursing department is essential.

DISPLAY 10-1	**Sample Resumé**

Carol J. Schooner

Current Address
6676 Cactus Flower
Indian Wells, CA 92260
(760) 886-2354

Address After June 1, 2004
4016 Eldorado Drive
Manhattan Beach, CA 90266
(310) 489-7760—cjschooner@juno.com

Objective:
To secure a beginning staff nurse position in a large urban acute care hospital that offers opportunity for professional growth and stimulation.

Education:
Associate Degree in Nursing
College of the Desert
May 2004

Licensure/Certification:
California RN License # 556832
Health Care Provider CPR through the American Heart Association

Skills:
■ Bilingual in Spanish and English
■ Experienced in multicultural community
■ Strong work ethic

Experience:

1998–present   Master's Care Center, Indio, CA
Certified Nursing Assistant
Provided care and assistance to elderly clients, focusing on the dignity of the individual. Required strong interpersonal skills and understanding of Hispanic culture.

1994–1998   Various jobs to provide funds for school, including clerking at 7-11, delivering newspapers for the *Desert Sun*, and babysitting for next-door neighbor.

Honors and Awards:
Outstanding graduate of the A.D. Nursing Program, 2004.

Personal References:
Available on request

At the present time, the job outlook for new graduates is bright. Organizations that are struggling to fill empty job slots are bringing back internships, and it is likely that you will receive more than one job offer. Recruiters may approach you. **Recruitment** is the activity of seeking out or attracting applicants for existing or anticipated positions. Some experts believe the health and effectiveness of an organization rests in their recruitment practices. Nurse recruiters often are employed in the human relations department of the hospital or health care facility and may not be nurses. They will bring information about the facility they represent to job fairs, conventions, workshops, or perhaps to your school. You can learn a great deal about nursing opportunities, salaries, and benefits by spending a few minutes talking with a recruiter.

APPLYING FOR A POSITION

Once you have decided the facility or facilities to which you wish to apply, you should contact the human resources department and request application materials. Frequently, this is done with a **letter of inquiry.** This letter may be called a **cover letter** because it is sent with your resume. The letter should focus on your special qualifications but should not duplicate information presented in the resume. If you think of the resume as merely a set of facts that provide little opportunity to convey how you would fit within a particular organization, you will see the opportunity provided by a cover letter. For example, if you have seen the position you are seeking advertised and you possess many of the qualifications listed in the advertisement, your cover letter can focus on those. The letter's general appearance, as well as its content, provides the employer with the first impression of you. You will be judged on grammar, spelling, neatness, and clarity. Therefore, you will want to give your letter of inquiry the same careful scrutiny that you used when developing your resume. A sample letter of inquiry is provided in Display 10-2.

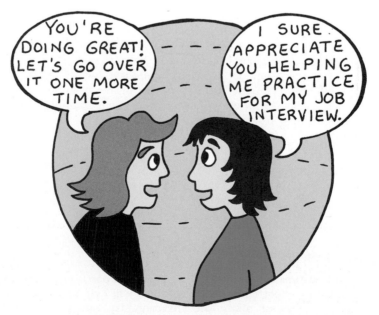

An experienced friend can help you practice for an interview.

DISPLAY 10-2 **Sample Letter of Inquiry**

Juan Lopez
1286 14th Ave. N.E.
Seattle, WA 98105

June 10, 2004

Mary J. Higdon
John Bright Medical Center
3619 Boyleston Avenue
Seattle, WA 98760

Dear Ms. Higdon:

I am interested in working as a registered nurse in the Emergency Department at John Bright Medical Center. Prior to entering the nursing program at Shoreline Community College, I worked on weekends as an EMT I for the Seattle Fire Department. We often brought patients to your emergency department and I have always been impressed with the care and organization that we encountered there. During the last semester of our nursing program, I spent four weeks in a preceptorship in your emergency room. This convinced me that I wanted to seek employment at John Bright.

I completed my licensing examination three weeks ago and have received my registered nursing license. I am available for employment within two weeks of notifying the Seattle Fire Department of my resignation.

As a registered nurse in your employ, I believe I can combine my past experience in prehospital care with the sound foundation in basic nursing that I received at Shoreline Community College to benefit clients that come through your Emergency Department. I am enclosing my resumé. If you wish to contact me, I can be reached at the number on the resumé. An answering machine will take messages when I am away from the telephone. I will contact your office if I do not hear from you within two weeks.

Sincerely,

Juan Lopez, RN

PARTICIPATING IN THE INTERVIEW

The first time you formally interview for a position, the **interview** can be an anxiety-provoking experience. Preparing for it will help to reduce your anxiety. If you are especially nervous about the situation, try rehearsing specific questions to ask or points that you want to make. Anticipate questions that you think might be asked of you and think about how you would answer them. If you have an experienced friend, perhaps that individual would be willing to set up a situation in which you can practice the interview.

EXAMPLE   *The Practice Interview*

> Emily Johansen was petrified at the thought of the job interview she had scheduled for the following week. She shared her concern about the interview with a fellow student Maybeth, who suggested that they meet the following evening and conduct a practice interview; Maybeth would take the role of interviewer and Emily would be the interviewee. Although still somewhat doubtful that this would provide help, Emily agreed. Maybeth prepared her interview questions well, fashioning many of them after questions she had encountered when she interviewed for a nursing position. She asked Emily about her philosophy of care and her goals for herself. Among other questions and other exchanges they had, she asked Emily to describe a nursing situation she had encountered as a nursing student in which she believed her actions had made a difference. A week later when Emily completed her interview, she called Maybeth to share the news that she had been offered a position. Emily reported she felt she had done very well on the interview and attributed much of the success to the practice session she had had with Maybeth.

Your appearance and behavior are critical. You should arrive on time looking neat, clean, well groomed, and professional. In other words, you want to dress for success. Although a suit is not always necessary, a professional look is. Long painted fingernails, flashy clothing and jewelry, ragged beards, obvious tattoos, dirty shoes, and wrinkled clothing convey a message of unsuitability for a professional position. A suit may appear inappropriate if the skirt is especially short or if it has a long slit up the side. Despite all that is being said about being oneself and changing social mores, you are seeking to advance your career. You will be judged against professional standards. Some facilities are refusing to talk to candidates who don't dress appropriately for the interview.

Be polished and polite. Courtesy and respect go a long way to creating a good first impression. Your attitude, enthusiasm, and motivation are important qualities in the eyes of recruiters. Be flexible, respectful, and focused. Abide by the time frame established for the interview and do not push to extend that time.

During the interview, be willing to share information about yourself. Hellinghausen (1998) states that you want to "showcase your talents, compassion and intellect." Rather than simply listing the things you are able to do, tell a short story about what you have accomplished as related to your skills. For example, you might briefly describe a very stressful situation in which you were involved and then discuss how you managed the situation. Communicate enthusiasm and excitement about nursing and patient care and a willingness to learn.

You will want to remember that an interview is a two-way proposition; an interviewee can be gathering just as much information as does the interviewer. Both participants should be making judgments as they move through the interview so that if at the interview's conclusion the position is offered to the interviewee, that individual is prepared to accept, decline, or do further exploration. Do not be afraid to ask big questions such as, "Is the hospital a part of a larger system?" "What impact does that have on the employees?" "Is it possible (or required) that an employee move from institution to institution?" "What are the responsibilities of the position?" "What are the possibilities for advancement?" or "Where does the employer see the organization (or the job) going in the future?"

It is helpful to have your questions written down. This will allow you to remain attentive and to the point and is an indication to the interviewer that you cared enough to come prepared. If you have your major thoughts written down, you will find it easier to relax in the interview and project a positive image because you won't be struggling to remember the points you want to ask.

After the interview is over, whether it has gone well or poorly, it is always gracious to write a note thanking the interviewer for the time that person gave to you. The note should be short and genuine. If you have been advised to contact the organization again within a given period of time, this is a good opportunity to remind them that you will be doing so. Display 10-3 gives an example of an interview follow-up letter.

If your interview goes well, you may want to be prepared for a second interview. In large organizations, a nurse recruiter or an individual working in the human resources office often conducts the interview. If that goes well, a second interview with a unit supervisor, head nurse, or clinical manager may be the next step. At this point you will know that you are probably one of three or four other individuals being considered for the position. Although you should be patient regarding the lapse of time between interviews, it is also wise to check back to determine whether you are still under consideration. Tact and diplomacy are important when making these contacts.

At some point in the interview process or shortly thereafter if you are to be offered the position, you will want to be prepared to show a copy of your license, any special certificates you possess (such as a CPR card), and identification documents that establish your eligibility to work in the United States. (In the majority of situations, showing a copy of your Social Security card and a driver's license satisfies this latter requirement.) You may have to document current immunizations, have a physical examination, and perhaps be fingerprinted. Different agencies have different employment practices, and you should not be surprised at information or data that you may be asked to provide. With the problems we have experienced as a society with regard to abuse of drugs, many health care facilities are including drug testing as part of their employment screening and continuing random drug testing of employees after they are hired.

ACCEPTING A JOB OFFER

If you are offered the position for which you have interviewed, you have one final step to complete. You need to decide whether you wish to accept the position. There are a number of questions you will want to ask yourself with regard to your answer. The first of these questions will be guided, to a large extent, by the career map that you previously developed. "Am I currently prepared to accept the responsibility associated with this position?" or "Will the job train me for or advance me toward the position I want in the future?" Other questions will be directed toward the working setting itself. "Is there a job description for the position?" "Were the responsibilities associated with the position clearly explained?" or "What type of orientation will be provided?" "Are nurse–patient ratios realistic?" Some questions

---

DISPLAY 10-3	**Sample Interview Follow-Up Letter**

■ ■ ■ ■ ■

Alice Duckworth
8490 Mobile Lane
Chico, CA 92746

June 18, 2004

Mary Heller, RN
Medical/Surgical Clinical Supervisor
Bradley General Hospital
176 Stone Way
Chico, CA 92748

Dear Ms. Heller:

Thank you for the time you spent with me in an interview for a registered nurse position at Mary Grace Hospital. I understand that I am to follow-up on that interview by contacting your office within the next two weeks to schedule a second interview with the unit manager.

I was particularly impressed with the tour through the hospital. The strong sense of collegiality that I felt existed among the people that I met on that tour convinced me that Mary Grace was a hospital whose staff I would be proud to join.

I will contact your office as directed in two weeks.

Sincerely,

Alice Duckworth

---

will be focused on the organizational climate and culture that exists in the facility. What is your gut feeling about the job and the persons you have met so far that are associated with the organization? Do they leave you with an inclusive feeling or do you feel like a stranger? Do you think you will have a harmonious relationship with your immediate supervisor? And finally, you will have practical questions that will need to be answered. Does the job offer you a salary that is reasonable and the benefits that you need? Are you willing (or can you afford) to live in the neighborhood or community where the facility is located or is commuting to the facility a practical option? What about parking and security? Only after you have acceptable answers to these questions should you decide to take the job offered to you. Having to resign and relocate is expensive and disheartening and should be avoided if at all possible.

Critical Thinking Exercise

Joan Callon wants eventually to work in a birthing center. After 4 years in school, she has depleted her financial resources and needs to find a job in nursing. The position she has been offered is in a hospital that does not offer obstetrical care. What questions should she ask herself with regard to accepting the position? What alternatives are available to her? What would be the disadvantage(s) of taking the job? What would you do if you were in her position and why?

■ RESIGNING FROM A POSITION

All of us have had the experience of resigning or leaving a position. In most instances, one resigns because of changes that are occurring in life that preclude the possibility of continuing in the job that you have. For example, you may have worked as a nursing assistant in a local long-term care facility on weekends to help finance your nursing education. As you graduate, you may wish to accept a beginning position as a registered nurse in an acute care facility, thus requiring that you resign from the nursing assistant position.

Other times, you will need to leave a position because of relocation, additional schooling, the offer of a better position, or because you are truly unhappy in the job that you have. Leaving a position, especially if it is preceded by circumstances that are less than desirable, is equally as important as moving into a new position. The process should always be professional and well thought out.

As you seriously consider resigning, check on the policies of the organization. How much notice are you expected to give? To whom should your letter of resignation be written? What are the procedures to be followed for severance? Are there any accrued benefits that should be considered, such as a buyout of unused sick leave or financial investments in the organization? Is there a particular time when it would be more beneficial to you to leave than another, assuming that your reason for resigning is not based on time-compelling constraints? Are there ethical standards you should consider in planning your resignation?

As you write your letter of resignation, find positive statements to make, if at all possible, or, at the very least, do not make negative ones. This is no place to unload all the unhappiness or dissatisfaction you may be feeling about the organization or people in it. Your letter of resignation may go in your personnel file. Remember, the people you are leaving are the ones who will be called for a recommendation for your next position. Therefore, it is never wise to offend the individuals you leave behind you, regardless of how tempted you may be to do so. In almost all situations, the organization will continue to function after you have gone elsewhere.

If you feel you absolutely must share some of your concerns, this is best done through an **exit interview.** Arrange to meet with the appropriate person to discuss the reasons you are leaving. During that interview, be fair and unemotional. Use "I" statements as opposed to "You" statements (see Chapter 5 on communications).

Your letter of resignation should be neat, in typed format, and, like other letters you have written regarding employment, should be free of spelling and grammatical errors. It should identify the last day that you will be available for employment and how you wish to handle any unused vacation. Finally, it should express appreciation

DISPLAY 10-4 **Sample Letter of Resignation**

Dana M. Schmit
5703 Walnut
Carson City, NV 47863

January 26, 2005

Albert J. Jones, Vice President, Patient Services
Community Medical Center
8840 12th Street
Carson City, NV 47860

Dear Mr. Jones:

   This serves as notification of my intent to resign from my position as staff nurse
on the medical unit at Community Medical Center effective February 14, 2005. I
have decided to pursue a baccalaureate degree at California State Domingues Hills
and will be relocating to the Los Angeles area to begin those studies.
   I wish to express my thanks and appreciation to you and the staff on Medical
III for the support and experience I have gained in my three years at Community Medical Center. I will miss the collegiality I have come to enjoy.

Sincerely,

Dana Schmit, RN

cc: Janice Jones, RN, Unit Manager Medical III

to any individuals or areas that have played a significant role in your professional
growth while an employee of that organization. Display 10-4 provides an example of
a letter of resignation.

Critical Thinking Exercise

After 3 years on a medical unit of a community hospital, you feel frustrated,
stymied, and unable to make any professional advances. You believe that the hospital fails to provide adequate opportunity to its new graduates. You are afraid you are
beginning to experience burnout. What can you do to regenerate your enthusiasm
for nursing? What individuals could provide you counsel? How can you communicate to your supervisor the information that you are feeling caught in a job for which
there is no advancement? What are the risks you would take if you were to resign
from the position?

■ SEEKING A PROMOTION

As you established your career plan you may have built into that plan some type of **promotion.** Most often, this involves a vertical move up the organizational hierarchy. Promotions also involve moving outside the organization to a better position with another group. Either way, moving ahead with your career represents a time in life to which most people look forward.

Seeking a promotion involves all the same processes that were employed in seeking your first position. You will need to submit a resumé, fill out an application, interview, and compete for the job. Once again, you will find yourself in the position of marketing yourself, projecting positive values and attitudes, enthusiasm, and self-confidence. If the position is internal (a promotion within the organization with which you are employed), you should not assume that because people know you, you could neglect promoting yourself as an excellent candidate. You may find yourself competing with peers and colleagues as well as people from outside the organization. And, although organizations will be looking for the best candidate for the position, you may find yourself involved with interpersonal relationships often referred to as office politics.

You should anticipate that people with whom you have worked might interview you. Many individuals find it more difficult to interview with a group of peers than with persons they do not know. If you are extended an invitation to interview, be certain to prepare for the interview carefully. Because some of the members of the interview team know you and your work, you must be very careful about the manner in which you present your accomplishments. Be certain to share credit for accomplishments with others in the organization who had a role in that accomplishment; this is an ethical commitment all should make to their coworkers. If the interview includes a discussion of problems to be solved within the organization, avoid the appearance of placing blame on or criticizing others. Focus instead on the problem itself and possible solutions. A common failing of internal candidates is to assume that others know your work and that you do not need to expand on questions asked. Be sure to answer questions completely.

You should also remember that new jobs involve new job requirements. Simply being employed by an organization for a number of years is no credential for advancement. If the position you are seeking requires additional education, it is important that you have completed it. If it requires specialized job knowledge, you also will have to demonstrate that you are skilled in that area. Once again, the importance of having a career plan becomes increasingly evident. We do not always know when an opportunity will come our way and it helps to be prepared.

■ ADVANCING ON A CLINICAL CAREER LADDER

A **clinical career ladder** is a system of advancing nurses developed around specific criteria that are used to evaluate and promote nurses who wish to remain at the bedside as opposed to pursuing different jobs in nursing, such as administration, teaching, or research. These systems work similarly to other promotion systems. For example, a basic model might include a Clinical Nurse I, a position filled by a new graduate;

a Clinical Nurse II, filled by an advanced beginner; on to Clinical Nurse V, a position represented by someone considered an expert in the area. Fortunately or unfortunately, many systems are based on seniority. Ideally, this will not be the major or only criterion. A reasonable pay differential between levels should also be in place. Specific job descriptions should be developed and in place for each level. Performance criteria for the clinical ladder should be spelled out for each level, based on the job descriptions. Evaluations should include input from more than one individual.

■ ADVANCING YOUR CAREER THROUGH CONTINUING EDUCATION

If you are pursuing any type of career plan, **continuing education** will be critical to realizing your goals. That education may take the form of on-the-job training, workshops, or conferences. In fact, many states require evidence of continuing education for license renewal.

Regardless of whether continuing education is required for license renewal, it is required to maintain competence in practice. A tremendous number of programs, workshops, seminars, lectures, classes, and home study programs are available to nurses. Many health care agencies help reimburse the costs of attending workshops or seminars and some agencies provide for "professional days" in the contract to allow individuals to attend without taking a day off. As the field of nursing informatics has grown, programs have become available over the Internet. (See Chapter 13 for more discussion about the Internet and chat rooms.) Professional journals have articles that, when read and posttests are completed and mailed in, provide continuing education credit.

It is important to your continued growth that you select, subscribe to, and read at least one professional journal. Journals, while often providing information about the latest technologies and treatments, also have the benefit of providing a national look at nursing. Almost all nursing specialties publish a journal focusing on that particular area of nursing. In addition, there are journals that are general in nature that address areas such as clinical nursing, nursing administration, and nursing education. Regular reading of these journals will help you maintain up-to-date information about nursing practice.

■ SEEKING FORMAL EDUCATION

Making the decision to pursue higher education and an additional degree takes on a more serious perspective. Many nurses feel they are too busy with professional obligations and family to think about adding the addition stress of formal schooling. However, it does not have to seem like an impossible dream.

Like all other aspects of career development, pursuing another degree requires careful planning. There are many reasons nurses should continue their **formal education.** Personal satisfaction is a major reason and should not to be discounted. The need for more educationally prepared nurses is well documented. One of the serious threats to the nursing profession is the shortage of nurses prepared with higher degrees in nursing. This is particularly noted in the area of nursing education but prevails in clinical nursing also. Higher degrees increase job security and job opportunity. Many of the doors that are opened by additional education are the ones that result in jobs that operate on a Monday-to-Friday schedule or have greater flexibility in scheduling, thus making them more compatible with family life. Jobs requiring additional educational preparation usually carry higher financial remuneration because they typically represent advancement in position or standing.

If you are thinking about returning to school, it is important that you are clear about your desires and motivations. What are the reasons you are considering this step at this time? Is the timing right? Is it financially possible? Are there other persons that need to be considered as you make this decision? The education you seek must also match with your nursing interests; a higher degree will not be rewarding if it takes you away from a fulfilling role in nursing practice. It is important that you are clear about your desire to return to school. Lyon (1998, p. 28) recommends the following five steps to help with your decision making.

1. Envision five years into the future: Is the present role and work going to be marketable and meaningful in 2009?
2. Write down and examine personal values, passions, and motivations for pursuing a higher degree in nursing.
3. Clarify the specific results you expect from the degree.
4. Develop an education plan with goals and objectives.
5. Clarify specific outcomes expected from obtaining more education, such as a new job, more money, or expanded knowledge and skills. Evaluate how realistic and clear the outcomes are and adjust them as necessary.

As with other aspects of career development, it is advisable to make a plan. You will want to gather information about continuing your education. Budget considerations will need to be a part of your plan. What will be the financial obligation? Tuition? Books and fees? Automobile expenses? Additional help at home? Child care? Increased food budget? Loss of income? With regard to financial matters, you will want to learn what scholarships or loans are available. Does your employer support formal education either fully or partially?

What will be your specialty focus? Do you want to become a clinical specialist or nurse practitioner as a part of the educational program you pursue? Most states now require a master's degree for these positions. Would certification in a nursing specialty, which is less costly and quicker, meet your goals or allow you to pursue the position you desire? Is flexibility important? Talk with friends or colleagues who have returned to school and get their perspective of the challenges and rewards it brings. Explore with them the lifestyle changes you should anticipate. It is always helpful to have a mentor.

Finally, you will want to make a decision regarding the school you attend. Although the prestige of the university or the credentials of the faculty may seem very important to you, in reality the decision often rests with which school is most geographically and practically accessible. This is particularly true for individuals who have a family and for whom relocation is not a possibility. Recent years have witnessed the emergence of programs leading to higher degrees in nursing that are available via distance education in the form of video conferencing, CD-ROM, the Internet, or e-mail. Although the cost initially appears expensive, because relocation and travel can be largely avoided, the cost may be comparable or not significantly more than attending a traditional college or university. As you select a school, you will also want to learn whether that college or university gives recognition for the work you have completed previously. Policies regarding the granting of previous credit vary greatly among schools.

Whatever your decisions, whether your plans are pursued now or later in your career, you can be assured that you will be more satisfied with the outcomes if you have taken the time to think critically about managing your career.

Critical Thinking Exercise

Develop a plan for yourself for formally continuing your education. Make a list of the factors that you will need to consider. What approaches do you have to the financial aspects? What will be important to you when you select a school? If you have to make a compromise on any aspects of your plan, when would that compromise best occur? Who else should you consider as you make your plans? What are your ultimate goals in pursuing more education? How will additional education help you realize those goals?

■ NURSING AND ENTREPRENEURSHIP

One of the opportunities opening for nurses is that of entrepreneurship. What is a nurse **entrepreneur?** Very simply, it is a nurse who owns a business. The business is typically related to a specialty in which the individual who is the owner has worked and developed skill and expertise but is not necessarily limited to that. A nurse who has been working in a particular area of nursing will see the opportunity to create a related service or product and puts together the resources necessary to build the business providing this service or product. Operating a business appeals to individuals who like autonomy, independence, and unlimited income opportunities and who are self-motivated. It requires expertise in nursing as well as in business.

Numerous examples of entrepreneurship in nursing can be cited and in almost every nursing specialty. Three common examples seen today would be the travel nurse who supplements staffing in health care facilities and operates as an independent contractor; the advanced practice nurse or nurse practitioner; and the legal nurse consultant whose primary role is to evaluate, analyze, and render informed opinions on the delivery of health care. A legal nurse consultant may be self-employed, providing services to attorney and others seeking such consultation or they may be employed by health care facilities in risk management, insurance companies, and defense legal firms. The American Association of Legal Nurse Consultants has been formed to serve the needs of individuals pursuing this avenue of practice.

Other areas of entrepreneurship abound. A nurse who has worked with patients with breast cancer may open a store that sells special bras and prostheses to patients who have had breast cancer. A nurse with background experience in labor and delivery might establish a business that rents breast pumps and/or offers lactation consultation. A nurse who has worked with nephrology patients may establish a dialysis unit, or offer continuing education, seminars, and certification review courses to nurses. A nurse with a background in cardiology might open a fitness center aimed at offering cardiac rehabilitation services. A rehabilitation nurse may own and operate a day care center or an inpatient assisted care facility or operate a business that rents or sells equipment to those with a physical handicap. Informatics nurses work with computerized data and hardware used to improve efficiency, reduce risk, and improve patient care. The informatics nurse may be employed by the health care facility but also may work as an independent contractor. Nurse recruiters may establish businesses that bring nurses to health care facilities who are seeking employees. This is particularly true for upper management positions in nursing. Forensic nurses have specialties that include death investigators, nurse coroners, correctional nurses, and domestic violence and sexual assault nurse examiners. They may contract with an agency or provide private investigation services (Business Career Options in Nursing, 2003). These examples reflect but a few of the many options available. The independent nurse contractor will contract with a health care facility to provide the unique services that person can offer. Usually, this is on an hourly basis but might be structured otherwise. This would not be unlike the emergency physicians who contract with hospitals to provide emergency department coverage.

Why do nurses seek such employment? The reasons vary. For some this offers an opportunity to escape the frustration and stress that some find when working as a staff nurse. For others it gives vent to creative ideas and emerging opportunities while offering independence and the potential for making more money. Duffett-Leger (1996) makes the point that many of the skills needed in the nursing process are also required for success as an entrepreneur: assessing the market, planning your actions, implementing your strategies, and evaluating results. It is estimated that over 5000 nurses throughout the United States are in a business (Business Career Options in Nursing, 2003). Starting as a newsletter for business-minded nurses in 1985 and later adopting the name National Nurses in Business Association (NNBA), this organization encourages the growth of nurse entrepreneurs. The Web site for the NNBA is http://www.nnba.net.

Critical Thinking Exercise

Identify additional examples of opportunities for nurses to develop entrepreneurial businesses in connection with a particular area of nursing practice. To whom would the services be marketed? What actions would need to be taken to establish the business? What other factors would need to be considered? How would you monitor success other than by financial rewards?

■ KEY CONCEPTS

- ■ Differences exist between careers and jobs. Careers imply lifetime commitment and professionalism. Jobs are tasks to be completed for a stated salary.
- ■ Career development has been studied by a number of individuals, some of whom have developed theories around the process. Attrition and job satisfaction are critical elements to be considered by employers who are concerned about the cost of staff turnover, which may be increased by dissatisfaction with the job or job-related stress.

■ Examining the focus of these studies may help you identify your own career status and seek employment in a health care facility that supports the career path you are pursuing.

■ Before seeking your first position in nursing, or before making a change from your present position, it is wise to do a self-analysis that will help put you in touch with your values, goals, and aspirations.

■ The development of a resumé is requisite to applying for a position. A number of formats can be used for resumés; whichever is used, it should present you in a positive light.

■ When seeking a position, you will want to learn as much as you can about the organizations to which you plan to apply. Informational interviews are one method by which information may be gained.

■ A letter of inquiry should accompany your request for an application. Letters of inquiry should focus on the special qualities you would bring to a position.

■ An interview is an important step in securing a position. It is wise to prepare for the interview and to remember that it is a two-way process.

■ After the interview, a brief thank-you letter to the person or persons who interviewed you reinforces the impression that you are thoughtful and skilled in interpersonal relations. A second interview is often conducted.

■ If you are offered the position for which you applied, you will need to make a decision about whether to accept it. Your decision can be guided by more critical analysis.

■ Resigning from a position also requires thought and consideration. If you are leaving under less than desirable circumstances, it is important not to offend those you are leaving behind. An exit interview will provide the opportunity for you to share any messages you think are important.

■ Clinical career ladders provide the opportunity for nurses to advance within an organization while remaining at the bedside. Clinical ladders need to be well developed and implemented.

■ When seeking a promotion, remember that you will need to go through all the processes you did when initially seeking a job. If it is considered a new job, it is a new job interview. If the promotion is internal, some additional stresses may be involved, including consideration of colleagues in the workplace and interviewing with peers and colleagues.

■ Career management typically involves additional schooling, either formal or informal. It is important that decisions to pursue formal education be preceded by careful analysis of your motivations and goals and thoughtful planning.

■ Many nurses are establishing businesses related to nursing and are viewed as nurse entrepreneurs. The businesses reflect all areas of nursing practice as well as nursing forensics, information, and legal consulting.

REFERENCES

Benner, P. (1984). *From Novice to Expert*. Menlo Park, CA: Addison-Wesley.

Campbell, S. L. (2003). Cultivating empowerment in nursing today for a strong profession tomorrow. *Journal of Nursing Education, 42*(9), 423–426.

Coccia, C. (1998). Avoiding a "toxic" organization. *Nursing Management, 29*(5), 32–33.

Business Career Options in Nursing. (2003). [Online]. Available at www.nnba.net/job_options_within_nursing.htm.

Duffett-Leger, L. (1996). Looking to the future: nursing and entrepreneurship. In *CNSA April 1966 Connection* [Online]. Available at http://www.cnsa.ca/publications/connection/1996april/article10.php

Friss, L. (1989). *Strategic Management of Nurses: A Policy Oriented Approach.* Owings Mills, MD: National Health Publishing.

Hellinghausen, M. A. (1998). Dream come true: how to wow recruiters and get the job you crave. *NurseWeek, 11*(17), 6.

Henderson, F. C., & McGettigan, B. O. (1994). *Managing Your Career in Nursing* (2nd ed.). New York: National League for Nursing Press.

Kramer, M. (1974). *Reality Shock: Why Nurses Leave Nursing.* St. Louis: Mosby.

Lyon, M. (1998). The ABCs of pursuing higher education. *NurseWeek, 11*(17), 28–29.

Neufeldt, V. (Ed.). (1996). *Webster's New World College Dictionary* (3rd ed.). New York: Simon & Schuster.

Peters, T. J., & Waterman, R. H., Jr. (1982). *In Search of Excellence.* New York: Harper Row.

Swansburg, R. C., & Swansburg, R. J. (2002). *Introduction to Management and Leadership for Nurse Managers* (3rd ed.). Boston: Jones and Bartlett Publishers.

Swanson, E. (1994). Career development: its status in nursing. In McCloskey, J., & Grace, H. (Eds.), *Current Issues in Nursing* (4th ed., pp. 549–558). St. Louis: Mosby.

Vogel, G. (1990). Career development: an integral process. *Holistic Nursing Practice, 4*(4), 46–53.

11

Attaining and Maintaining Competence

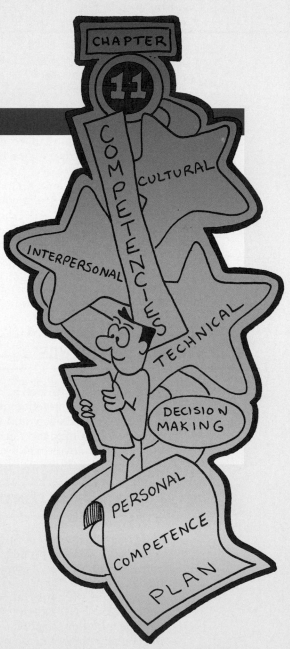

Learning Outcomes

After completing this chapter you should be able to:

1. Discuss the current health care emphasis on continued competence for all health professionals.
2. Describe the various approaches to maintaining continued competence of registered nurses.
3. Identify the various aspects of competence that are identified as essential for registered nurses.
4. Identify aspects of interpersonal competence that contribute to effectiveness in nursing.
5. Identify the various types of technical competence that are expected of nurses.
6. Consider how competence in decision-making may be assessed.
7. Explain how individuals and institutions can assure culturally and linguistically appropriate services.
8. Assess yourself in relationship to multiple competencies.
9. Establish a plan for maintaining and enhancing your own competence.

Key Terms ■ ■ ■ ■

competence

cultural competence

cultural desire

culturally appropriate
decision-making
competence

interpersonal competence

linguistically appropriate

psychomotor (technical)
competence

Every member of society would agree that all health care providers in practice should be competent. What does it mean to be a competent nurse? How does competence as a nurse relate to competence in managing and coordinating nursing care? Certainly, every nurse has both a legal and an ethical obligation to maintain and increase competence over time. How can that be determined? Are there different aspects of competence? Could an individual be competent in one aspect and not in others?

Although the idea of competence has always been with us, the publication of the Pew Health Professions Commission (1998) report "Strengthening Consumer Protection: Priorities for Health Care Workforce Regulation" created impetus for a wider discussion of what it means to be competent and how the public can be assured that its health care providers are competent. That report identified that the current system was not adequate to keep up with the many changes taking place in health care. They were particularly critical of the lack of any mechanisms to assure that health care professionals continued to be competent throughout their professional lives.

■ DEFINING COMPETENCE

"**Competence** is defined as the application of knowledge and the interpersonal, decision-making and psychomotor skills expected for the practice role, within the context of public health, safety and welfare" (NCSBN, 1996). Thus, we see that competence in nursing is complex and needs to be addressed from multiple perspectives that would include areas involving knowledge, skills, and attitudes.

 ## ■ APPROACHES TO CONTINUED COMPETENCE

The National Council of State Boards of Nursing (NCSBN), the American Nurses Association, various specialty nursing organizations, and government agencies have addressed the issue of competence in nursing. Each of these different organizations has approached competence from a different point of view. Although almost everyone is united on the importance of assessing for continued competence as a matter of policy, Glazer (1999) points out that the practical realities of establishing a system become a matter of politics. Various states are examining different options for assuring competence of practicing nurses (deVries, 1999).

Regulatory agencies such as the state boards of nursing began examining how they might assure continued competence in the 1980s. In 1996, a national commission on health manpower recommended that physicians undergo periodic reexamination. Other health care professions saw this as the initial suggestion in a move to use testing as a means of assuring continued competence. This approach drew opposition from the health professions. As individuals practice in a specialty or particular focus, the type of examination that addresses broad entry-level competence no longer seems to have relevance. An individual is more likely to be expert in a narrower area of practice. For example, at the time of graduation, all nurses who are licensed possess basic understanding and competence in care of the postpartum mother and baby. However, if that nurse works for 3 years on an oncology unit, she will likely lose some of the knowledge she once possessed regarding mother and baby care and will have gained a great deal more knowledge about patients requiring oncology services.

Continuing education (CE) was then suggested as an alternative mechanism of assuring continued competence. Health professional regulatory agencies began to require continuing education for licensure renewal. Although CE is clearly a method for monitoring competence, there is no research evidence to demonstrate that attendance at CE programs assures competent practice. Both Colorado and Washington instituted CE as a requirement for relicensure of registered nurses and later retracted the requirement, in part because of this conclusion. Currently, 26 states require CE for relicensure of nurses (NCSBN, 2003a).

There continues to be a concern from regulatory agencies about the ongoing competence of health care professionals. In several states, pilot projects have been initiated to assess competence through testing. The Province of Ontario has developed a program to examine competence through different avenues. The first avenue is competence evaluation followed by remediation if needed. From this perspective, an individual who demonstrates problems in practice would be assigned specific, targeted strategies to improve knowledge and ability to practice with the appropriate standards. The second avenue is self-assessment and peer evaluation followed by the implementation of a learning plan. From this perspective, the professional is expected to be accountable for self-evaluation, and those within the profession are expected to assume responsibilities for helping assure competence in the entire profession. This perspective places accountability for competence in the hands of the professional. The third avenue involves a project to assist employers to develop organizational patterns that support quality practice. Because nurses are employees in health care agencies, they require the support of those agencies to maintain competence. There must be avenues for education, opportunities for evaluation, and support for developing institutional policies and procedures that reflect competent care. (Whittaker et al., 2000).

EXAMPLE *An Institution Demonstrating Support for Maintaining Competence*

Waverly Hospital determined that to meet its goals for excellent patient care, they needed to standardize care based on the best available evidence. The nursing administrator convened a series of committees that wrote policies and protocols for a wide variety of nursing care situations. To implement these policies and protocols, education events were held throughout the hospital. After the education events, nurses were asked to come to the education department at specifically designated times to demonstrate competence in a selected group of these policies and procedures. Each nurse was tested by having him or her move to a set of stations. Each station represented a different patient situation requiring the appropriate application of policies and protocols. If a nurse failed to meet the standard, that nurse was scheduled for remedial education and then was asked to retest. This process continued until each nurse was able to demonstrate competence in the required behaviors.

The NCSBN (1996) suggested that boards of nursing have the responsibility of assuring competence in order to meet their mandate of protecting the public. It has identified standards for competence (Display 11-1) along with indicators of the achievement of the standards. It further developed a framework that identifies how competence will be assessed. Within that framework, the NCLEX RN examination assesses for competence of the new graduate. It suggested that ongoing effective practice might be verified through peer review, professional certification, or a professional portfolio for a randomly selected number of nurses. When an individual has been out of practice, assurance of competence would be through a mandated refresher course. For those who had disciplinary action taken, the assurance of competence would be through an individualized plan. A recent summit was held by the NCSBN in which state boards examined the various alternatives to ensure competence (NCSBN, 2003a). All states have implemented the assessment of competence for the new graduate through the NCLEX RN and for the person who has been subject to discipline through an investigation and hearing with subsequent remediation and monitoring of practice as indicated. Many states require refresher courses for those who have been out of practice for a specified period of time. CE verification continues to be the primary method of assessing ongoing competence. In its latest model nursing administrative rules (NCSBN, 2003b), the NCSBN suggests that continued competence be a requirement for relicensure.

DISPLAY 11-1   Standards for Competence

The nurse is expected to
1. Apply knowledge and skills at the level required for a particular situation.
2. Demonstrate responsibility and accountability for practice and decisions.
3. Restrict and/or accommodate practice if cannot safely perform essential functions of the nursing role due to mental or physical disabilities.

From NCSBN. (1996). Assuring competence: a regulatory response. *National Council Position Paper* [Online]. Available at http://www.ncsbn.org/public/resources/ncsbn_competence.htm, accessed November 20, 2003, with permission.

EXAMPLE   ***Competence Assured Through
a Refresher Course in Nursing***

> James Ohlne had worked as a registered nurse in a hospital for 5 years after gradua-
> tion. After that time, he had an opportunity to work for a medical supply company as
> a sales representative. His nursing background gave him the foundation to under-
> stand the needs of the nurses and the institutions, and he had the interpersonal skills
> gained in nursing to enable him to do well in this new role. James worked for this
> company for 8 years and expected that he would never go back to nursing. However,
> he continued to keep abreast of nursing changes through regular journal reading.
> Then as the economy changed, he found himself laid off from the medical equipment
> company after it was sold to a competitor. He decided that he would like to return to
> nursing practice. He contacted the state board of nursing and was directed to take a
> nursing refresher course that included supervised clinical practice. When he had sat-
> isfactorily demonstrated competence and completed this course, the state board re-
> instated his license and he was able to apply for a position in a residency program
> designed for new graduates and that included nurses returning to practice.

In the regulation of advanced practice nurses, most states require that the individual
maintain specialty certification. They rely on the requirements for certification to assure competence. The American Nurses Credentialing Center has been studying the
effect of certification and preliminary results would support the value of certification
in maintaining competence (Trossman, 2000).

EXAMPLE   ***Competence Assured Through
the Maintenance of Certification***

> Amelee Woo is a family nurse practitioner in Washington State. In Washington,
> nurse practitioners are licensed as advanced registered nurse practitioners (ARNPs)
> and required to maintain certification in their specialty for licensure renewal and
> must show evidence of specific CE in pharmacology related to their area of practice
> in order to maintain prescriptive authority. To maintain her certification through the
> American Nurses Credentialing Center, Amelia must show evidence of a minimum
> number of hours of practice in the role of nurse practitioner. In addition, she must
> document CE hours related to her specialty. Amelia assumes the responsibility for
> maintaining her own records of the CE she has taken, keeping track of her clinical
> hours, and making sure that she has completed all paperwork needed to maintain
> her certification and her licensure. When the time for license renewal arrives, she
> has the necessary information to be able to process her renewal in a timely manner.

Competence in nursing is clearly a complex phenomenon. Some of the most important aspects of competence in nursing are those identified in the NCSBN definition:
interpersonal relationships, decision making, and technical or psychomotor skills.

Working with individuals from many different cultures requires the use of both interpersonal skills and decision-making abilities. This is often referred to as **cultural competence.** The development and enrichment of each of these require a different focus.

Interpersonal Competence

Interpersonal competence refers to having the ability to relate effectively with coworkers, clients, family members, and members of the community. Interpersonal competence is essential to every other aspect of the nursing role. To provide direct care through assessment, analysis, planning, implementation, and evaluation, the nurse must communicate effectively with the client and family. In addition to offering clients the same acceptance and courtesy that would be extended to another human being, the nurse must be able to elicit information; respond to feelings and concerns; serve as a resource person to provide specific answers to specific questions; teach both formally and informally; offer direction to the client, family, or group; and counsel so as to promote experiences leading to greater health for the client. All these require definitive interpersonal skills and competence.

To manage care given by others, the nurse must communicate with nursing staff, direct their work clearly, maintain ongoing communication with them to monitor progress, and provide them with feedback about their performance. Without interpersonal skill, relationships deteriorate and the nurse is unable to draw others into the development of a culture of excellence.

Critical Thinking Exercise

Identify the ways in which you demonstrate your interpersonal competence. How might you evaluate your own interpersonal competence? Suggest a variety of ways that an employer might evaluate your interpersonal competence. What mechanisms might be used for a licensing authority to evaluate interpersonal competence?

Technical Competence

Another aspect of competence that has been identified in the NCSBN definition is technical or psychomotor competence. **Psychomotor (technical) competence** refers to the ability to carry out psychomotor skills effectively, safely, and efficiently. There are many technical skills used in the field of nursing. However, the technical skills used by nurses vary greatly based on their area of practice. A nurse may be very technically competent with the skills used in a critical care unit but not have the technical skills used in the operating room. Even at the time of graduation from a basic program, new graduates vary greatly in their technical skills. Competence in technical skills required for entry into practice is determined by requiring that schools of nursing be approved. The approval of the school is contingent on clinical practice and the development of psychomotor skills in the student.

Based on the Joint Commission on Accreditation of Healthcare Organization's (JCAHO) standard that requires accredited agencies to assure the competence of

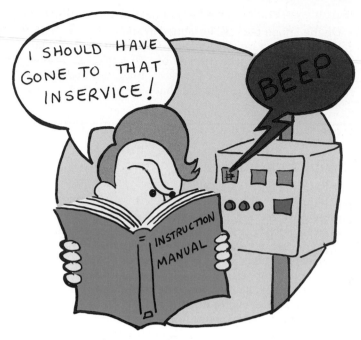

Clinical agencies have developed plans for competency assessment of technical skills.

their employees (JCAHO, 2003), many clinical agencies have developed very extensive plans for competency assessment in the area of technical skills. This is frequently done by competence check-offs in which specific skills must be demonstrated accurately. The individual who fails the competence examination is provided with remedial education and then retested. Competence examinations may be differentiated based on the area of practice. Thus, all the nurses practicing in the childbirth unit must pass competency testing in newborn resuscitation whereas nurses practicing in the coronary care unit may be required to pass competency testing related to interpreting cardiac rhythms. In many hospitals, nurses performing some highly technical skills such as the insertion of peripherally inserted central catheters (PICC) must complete a prescribed inservice education program along with supervised practice to be "certified" by their institution to perform this skill. Thus, employers assure the ongoing technical competence of nurses.

EXAMPLE *Skills Testing for Critical Care*

Enrique Vasquez works in the critical care unit at Mercy Hospital. Each year, Mercy Hospital requires that all critical care nurses participate in a skills competency test process. On January 24, Enrique was scheduled to come into the education department for skills demonstration. Before that time, he picked up the study booklet that outlined the skills to be checked and provided review material. He reviewed each skill and spent extra time on some of the skills that he had used only infrequently.

On the appointed day, he signed in at the education desk and began going from station to station. At each station he completed a written quiz, demonstrated the required skill, and was checked off. If he had not passed a particular skill, he would have been given more educational materials and an opportunity to work with someone on his unit to improve that skill. After that he would have been required to schedule a time for retesting.

Decision-Making Competence

Decision-making competence refers to the ability to use critical thinking in solving patient care problems. Chapter 6 discussed the concept of decision making and the many important aspects of making appropriate decisions. How decision-making competence can be evaluated is the subject of much discussion.

New graduates have been evaluated in their decision making in their clinical experience as students. The expectation is that during this experience they will have the opportunity for decision-making and the faculty member will have the opportunity to observe decision making in actual practice. Not all educators believe that this is the most effective environment in which to evaluate competence. Therefore, some educators use specifically scheduled performance testing in the clinical area for the evaluation of decision making.

Decision-making competence is one aspect of the competency outcomes and performance assessment (COPA) model developed by Lenburg (1999a). This model was developed for use with students in nursing programs as a method for assessing competence for clinical practice. The COPA model is based on clearly identifying the specific competence to be learned and then structuring an effective method to evaluate it. Competency performance examinations sample behaviors in a systematic manner, using situations and simulations that allow for standardization (Bargagliotti et al., 1999).

Decision-making competence is also tested in the NCLEX RN examination. Situations requiring decision making are included in the questions. Because of the structure of the computerized adaptive test, each individual receives a unique but equivalent examination that tests this skill.

Evaluating decision-making competence in the practicing nurse is much more difficult. In some instances, this is part of the performance evaluation. However, performance evaluations are based on convenience samples of behavior that may not be representative. Although nursing has supported the importance of competence assessment in regard to decision making, no consistent method has been shown to be effective.

Critical Thinking Exercise

Analyze your own nursing education program in regard to teaching and evaluating decision making. What strategies were used to teach you decision making? What strategies were used to evaluate your decision-making competence? What suggestions would you make for change or enhancement of the strategies used for teaching and evaluating decision-making competence?

Cultural Competence

Many countries of the world are composed of people with a variety of ethnic, racial, and cultural backgrounds. The United States and Canada are no exception to this. Culture refers to "integrated patterns of human behavior that include the language, thoughts, communications, actions, customs, beliefs, values, and institutions of racial, ethnic, religious, or social groups" (National Standards for Culturally and Linguistically Appropriate Services in Health Care, 2000, p. 2).

"Cultural and linguistic competence is a set of congruent behaviors, attitudes, and policies that come together in a system, agency, or among professionals that enables effective work in cross-cultural situations" (National Standards for Culturally and Linguistically Appropriate Services in Health Care, 2000, p. 3). As you will note, the National Standards definition is very complex; however, the Cultural Diversity Organization has a much simpler approach. It defines cultural competence as "obtaining cultural information and then applying that knowledge." This straightforward definition can guide the individual in a continuing quest for information and the development of skills to effectively apply that information.

Cultural competence is not identified separately in NCSBN's definition. Cultural competence is composed of multiple aspects such as basic knowledge, interpersonal skills, and ethical beliefs. Cultural competence is also characterized by effective decision making in regard to clients from different cultural backgrounds.

When persons with different cultural orientations meet in any type of association, the likelihood of a mutually satisfying relationship developing is improved if all parties in the relationship try to learn about each other's culture. This is especially true in health care environments, in which culture has a significant impact on health care beliefs, perceptions of health and illness, disease prevention, self-care practices, selection and compliance with treatments, and identification within the family structure of who makes the decisions regarding health care.

Meyer (1996) suggested that individuals attempting to become culturally competent health care providers face four challenges. The first challenge is one of simple knowledge about clinical differences in health patterns of different groups. Knowledge of these differences can help guide assessment and interventions. The second challenge is of communicating effectively across differences in language, understanding, and willingness to discuss personal issues. The third challenge lies in ethics. A belief that one's own way of being, doing, or acting is the best way stands in the way of acknowledging and accepting the values and strengths of others' belief systems. The last challenge is that of trust. When differences between provider and patient exist, there are many barriers to trust. Class, status, and racial differences may make patients feel that providers will not act in the patient's best interest. These challenges can be overcome but do require an ongoing commitment to education and effort by health care providers.

ASSESSING FOR CULTURAL COMPETENCE

Most nursing education programs include content relative to multicultural issues. This may include general education courses available to all on campus and specific nursing classes that address multicultural content. Many programs include the infusion of multicultural issues into all areas of the curriculum. Assessing students for cultural competence based on this education preparation is challenging. To meet this challenge, Rew et al. (2003) developed a research instrument that can be used to measure cultural awareness in nursing students. Their research in the development of this tool led to the conceptualization of five categories within the cultural awareness scale: general educational experiences related to cultural awareness, cognitive awareness of cultural beliefs, research issues related to cultural awareness, individual's behaviors toward and comfort with people from other backgrounds, and cultural issues in patient care and clinical issues. This scale is new, but it has potential for assisting nursing education programs in assessing their own effectiveness in developing cultural competence in their students.

The National Standards for Culturally and Linguistically Appropriate Services (CLAS) in Health Care (2000) include standards related to culturally competent care. These standards relate to what the entire organization should provide rather than the competence of the individual health care provider. One standard is "Health care organizations should ensure that patients/consumers receive from all staff members effective, understandable and respectful care that is provided in a manner compatible with their cultural health beliefs and practices and preferred language." What does this standard mean for the organization? How can it assure this respectful behavior from all employees? How can it assess to determine whether this is occurring? This standard reflects on the need for each person to develop an awareness of one's own thoughts and beliefs, to increase understanding of each client's culture, to accept and respect cultural differences, and adapt care so that it as aligned to the client's beliefs as possible. How the organization can evaluate this poses serious challenges.

For the individual nurse, the question of what this standard means personally may be answered by honest self-appraisal. To accomplish the goal of **culturally appropriate** care, the nurse will want to use respectful language, to have assessed the client and family in order to understand their cultural health beliefs, and to obtain translation services when those are needed. The nurse should incorporate cultural differences in care planning and in personal communication strategies. The individual nurse can look at his or her own behaviors, personal relationships with clients and families, and the plans for care developed as part of self-assessment.

LINGUISTIC CONCERNS IN CREATING CULTURALLY APPROPRIATE CARE

Perhaps no aspect of culturally competent care is as challenging as the domain of communications, because it is interrelated with all other areas of health care and involves nonverbal as well as verbal skills (see Chapter 5). One should be particularly attentive to paralanguage variations, such as voice volume, tone, intonations, and reflections. Loud tones may be interpreted by some cultures as anger. Hierarchical relationships, gender, and some religious beliefs may affect communication among individuals from some groups. Effective communication for health care purposes also requires the willingness of individuals to share their thoughts and feelings. In cultures in which members are expected to be publicly shy, withdrawn, and reserved, this may be difficult.

Health care requires clear and accurate communication between care providers and clients at all levels and in all settings. However, those with limited English ability may not have adequate vocabulary kills to communicate in situations in which strong verbal skills are needed or in which highly abstract levels of verbal skills are required, for example, in psychiatric settings. Several of the CLAS standards relate to the need for translation services. Translation services need to be provided by individuals with language skills that include medical terminology and understanding in both languages. Family should not be used for translation services unless the client specifically requests that this be done. Patients may feel that revealing personal information to a family member is inappropriate for many reasons, such as age differences, gender differences, and relative position in the family. However, they may be reluctant to express this concern, and, as a result, there may be limited communication of important information. Further, families may lack understanding of medical terminology and may be unable to explain processes and procedures effectively. In some instances, family members may not understand the concept of informed consent and do not value communicating the information. Staff members without medical background also are not a good choice for translation services. Some of the same barriers are present in nonmedical staff, such as lack of understanding of the language and different values around information and its importance (National Standards for Culturally and Linguistically Appropriate Services in Health Care, 2000). This highlights the need to increase the variety in the cultural composition of persons involved in providing health care.

Within an organization, there may be other health care professionals who know the patient's language. When it is possible to have the provider speak directly with the patient, this is the most desired situation. In areas with many Spanish-speaking clients, having health care providers who are proficient in Spanish is the most effective way to enhance communication. An individual health care provider may also serve as a translator for other health providers. For example, a nurse with language skills may communicate with the patient in the patient's language but also translate for the physician, the lab technician, and the physical therapist.

When no translation services can be provided by personnel engaged in care, a translator is needed. Many major health care agencies provide a list of appropriate medical translators for various languages. In some instances, a telephone language bank can be used. Although not ideal, this is particularly helpful when working with someone whose language is not common and translators are few.

Working with translation services requires skills from the individual health care provider. Some of the following actions will make this easier. Because a major challenge is to assure that you are speaking to the client or patient and not to the translator, always face the patient so that nonverbal communication can occur between provider and patient. Choose words carefully for clarity and check with the translator to assure that the translator understands what you are trying to communicate. Display 11-2 outlines suggestions for working with a translator.

| DISPLAY 11-2 | **Suggestions for Working with a Translator in Health Care** |

1. Face the patient while speaking, not the translator.
2. Address your remarks to the patient.
3. Ask for validation that both the translator and the client understand what you have said.
4. Use gestures, demonstrations, and pictures to communicate information as well as using words.
5. Avoid the use of idiomatic expressions (e.g., "The doctor is going to sit on this problem until morning," by which the physician means that he or she is going to wait to make a decision until morning and not that he or she will be "sitting" on anything).
6. Avoid raising your voice volume when someone does not understand.

HEALTH SYSTEMS AND CULTURALLY AND LINGUISTICALLY APPROPRIATE SERVICES

Cross and others wrote about organizations and institutions in relationship to culturally competent care. They identified five elements they believe demonstrate cultural competence when seen at every level of the organization. These five elements are identified in Display 11-3. These elements emphasize values, self-assessment, and systems of service delivery with the agency (Cross et al., 1989).

An institution's commitment to **linguistically appropriate** care includes posting signs in languages other than English when that would serve an identified population group. Another aspect is reflected in patient education materials in languages other than English. Written documents for consent in a person's own language provide greater autonomy for the individual. Notices in regard to patient rights and processes for assuring that rights have been supported are useful only if the individual can read those notices (National Standards for Culturally and Linguistically Appropriate Services in Health Care, 2000).

Personal Competence

Nursing organizations at every level place the responsibility for maintaining competence on the individual nurse. The code of the International Council of Nurses (2000) includes, "The nurse carries personal responsibility and accountability for nursing practice and for maintaining competence by continued learning." The American Nurses Association (2001) Code for Nurses includes, "The nurse owes the same duties to self as to others, including the responsibility to preserve integrity and safety, to maintain competence, and to continue personal and professional growth."

Self-Assessment of Competence

Each nurse has the responsibility for maintaining her or his own competence. As you strive to do this, your first step will be to assess your own abilities. Consider the areas of competence identified previously.

How will you assess your own interpersonal competence? Looking at one's own communication patterns, ways of relating to others, and skill in enhancing commu-

---

DISPLAY 11-3	**Essential Elements for Institutional Cultural Competency**

1. Valuing diversity
2. Having the capacity for cultural self-assessment
3. Being conscious of the dynamics inherent when cultures interact
4. Having institutionalized cultural knowledge
5. Having developed adaptations of service delivery reflecting an understanding of cultural diversity

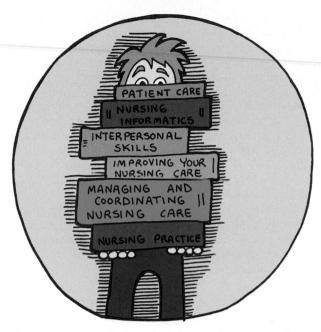

Individuals are accountable to maintain personal competence in nursing.

nication of others may be very difficult. Sometimes another nurse whose judgment you trust can help you in this assessment. Many institutions include peer evaluation in their evaluation systems.

Assessing your own decision-making skills should be part of your personal debriefing after any episode that required your decision-making skill. Debriefing is a technique of reviewing the entire situation, asking questions about what happened, and examining whether changes of some type might have improved your decision-making ability. For example, was other information needed that was not available? Is there a way to address the lack of needed information on a system-wide basis? If the problem was one of insufficient help to manage a crisis, what systems could the institution put in place for crisis management? By reviewing the situation, you can build your decision-making skill.

Technical skills are perhaps the easiest to self-evaluate. Do you perform skills quickly and efficiently? Do you follow the appropriate protocols or procedures? What are the outcomes for the patient when you are performing the technical skill demanded by that situation? In addressing your own technical skills, you may want to examine correct technique, organization, dexterity, and speed (Ellis et al., 1996). Correct technique means that the skill was done accurately, using the right equipment, and following the proper procedure. Organization has to do with your ability gather equipment and proceed through the skill from beginning to end without the wasted effort of finding some supplies that you need to obtain after starting, or forgetting to check the patient's record for information until you realize you do not have information you need. Dexterity has to do with the way you handle equipment. You handle sterile equipment without contaminating it. You move smoothly through procedures. Speed reflects on the amount of time you spent and whether that is a reasonable amount of time. Using correct technique is certainly the most important aspect, but the other aspects are essential to excellence.

Cultural competence requires that you examine your own values, beliefs, and background as well as become knowledgeable about others. Although you can never learn all about all the other cultures and backgrounds that exist in our pluralistic society, you can gain important knowledge that will help you in practice. The most important part of cultural competence is learning to ask questions and listen carefully to the individual to enhance your knowledge of that person at that time.

You will also need to assess your own attitudes and beliefs. What are your beliefs about other cultures? Other life patterns? Other races? Your own beliefs will affect your actions, whatever your knowledge base. A third aspect of cultural competence is your own actions. How do you behave toward others? What do you do with the knowledge you have? Do you strive to adjust care so that it is culturally and linguistically appropriate?

When we examine our own behaviors, we need to acknowledge the need to grow. It is not possible in nursing to remain stagnant and remain competent. With the changing nature of health care, the changes in responsibilities, and the changes in the patient population, if our practice as nurses does not change, we will soon be losing competence in relationship to our responsibilities.

Critical Thinking Exercise

For the next week, keep a personal journal reflecting on your own cultural competence. Examine your interactions with individuals from cultures different than your own. In your journal, describe the interaction and then reflect on the ways in which you did or did not demonstrate cultural competence in that interaction.

Enhancing Competence

What can the individual nurse do to enhance cultural competence? Campinha-Bacote (2003) suggests that before all else there must be what she terms **cultural desire.** This is defined as the "nurse's motivation to want to engage in the process of becoming culturally aware, culturally knowledgeable, and culturally skillful, and seeking cultural experiences." This motivation will determine whether the nurse seeks to become more culturally competent. One aspect of enhancing competence is learning from each new situation. It has been said that while some people are gaining 10 years of experience, others are gaining 1 year's experience 10 times. By that we mean that some people do not build on what they know. To build competence through experience demands a curious mind that is constantly asking questions and then seeking answers. One can learn from nursing colleagues, from patients, and from others on the interdisciplinary team. As you confront a new problem and solve it, you have added to your problem-solving repertoire. Even errors or difficulties can enhance your competence if the situation is used as a stepping stone to learning and improved function.

As we mentioned earlier in this chapter, CE is the standard by which many states measure ongoing competence. CE is now available by so many different avenues that it is accessible to everyone. Professional journals carry articles with testing to use for CE. There are online courses and online articles with tests. Conferences and workshops for nurses are held throughout the country. Most agencies that hire nurses provide CE in relationship to the needs of the institution. This might be the development of new technical skills, such as the use of a new intravenous pump or the ability to use decision support programs such as care pathways. Classes may be held to help staff improve documentation, manage pain more effectively, or address other commonly occurring problems.

Formal education is becoming increasingly accessible as online programs for registered nurses to continue formal education, the BSN for the associate degree graduate, the master's degree for the individual with a bachelor's degree, and the doctoral degree for the individual with a master's degree. Although traditional college programs are widely distributed, online programs now make formal degree programs ever more accessible.

■ KEY CONCEPTS

- ■ Regulatory authorities, accrediting bodies, and professional organizations all support the importance of assuring continued competence of health care professionals.
- ■ There are multiple approaches to assuring competence. Testing for entry-level competence, requiring CE for the professional in practice, requiring refresher courses for professionals wanting to return to practice, and competency testing by employers are used to assure continued competence of nurses.
- ■ The NCSBN identifies interpersonal competence, technical or psychomotor competence, and decision-making competence as aspects of competence for registered nurses.
- ■ Cultural competence encompasses both interpersonal and decision-making aspects of competence for nurses. Institutions also can set up systems to support culturally and linguistically appropriate standards (CLAS) for health care.
- ■ Self-assessment in relationship to personal competence requires that one examine one's own interpersonal skills, technical skills, decision-making skills, and cultural competence.
- ■ Each individual is accountable for establishing and carrying out actions to maintain personal competence in nursing.
- ■ A variety of CE programs are available to all nurses that help assure that competence in maintained.

REFERENCES

American Nurses Association. (2001). *Code of Ethics for Nurses With Interpretive Statements.* Washington, DC: American Nurses Publishing Co.

Bargagliotti, T., Luttrell, M., & Lenburg, C. (September 30, 1999). Reducing threats to the implementation of a competency-based performance assessment system. *Online Journal of Issues in Nursing.* Available at http://www.nursingworld.org/ojin/topic10/tpc10_5.htm. Accessed November 17, 2003.

Campinha-Bacote, J. (2003). Cultural desire: the key to unlocking cultural competence. *Journal of Nursing Education, 42*(6), 239-240.

Cross, T., Bazron, B., Dennis, K. et al. (1989). *Toward a Culturally Competent System,* Vol. I. Washington, DC: Georgetown University.

deVries, C. M. (October 1999). Continued competence: Assuring quality health care. *ANA Issues Update* [Online]. Available at http://nursingworld.org/ajn/1999/oct/issu109f.htm. Accessed November 18, 2003.

Ellis, J. R., Nowlis, E. A., & Bentz, P. M. (1996). *Modules for Basic Nursing Skills,* Vol. 1. Philadelphia: JB Lippincott Co.

Glazer, G. (November 3, 1999). *NursingWorld | OJIN:* Legislative Column: the policy and politics of continued competence. *Online Journal of Issues in Nursing.* Available at http://www.nursingworld.org/ojin/tpclg/leg_8.htm. Accessed November 23, 2003.

International Council of Nurses. (2000). Codes for Nurses: Ethical Concepts Applied to Nursing. Geneva, Switzerland: ICN.

Joint Commission for the Accreditation of Healthcare Organization (JCAHO). (2003). *Standards for Accreditation.* Chicago: JCHAO.

Lenburg, C. B. (September 30, 1999a). The framework, concepts and methods of the competency outcomes and performance assessment (COPA) model. *Online Journal of Issues in Nursing.* Available at http://www.nursingworld.org/ojin/topic10/tpc10_2.htm. Accessed May 16, 2004.

Lenburg, C. B. (September 30, 1999b). Redesigning expectations for initial and continuing competence for contemporary nursing practice. *Online Journal of Issues in Nursing* Available at http://nursingworld.org/ojin/topic10/tpc10_1.htm. Accessed May 16, 2004.

Meyer, C. R. (1996). Medicine's melting pot. *Minnesota Medicine 79*(5), 5, as quoted in *Transcultural Nursing: Cultural Competence* [Online]. Available at www.culturediversity.org/cultcomp.htm. Accessed May 16, 2004.

National Council of State Boards of Nursing (NCSBN). (1996). Assuring competence: a regulatory response. *National Council Position Paper* [Online]. Available at http://www.ncsbn.org/public/resources/ncsbn_competence.htm. Accessed May 16, 2004.

NCSBN. (2003a). Continuing competence summit to focus on action strategies. *Council Connector, 3*(5), 1 [Online]. Available at http://www.ncsbn.org/public/news/res/CC_Jun03.pdf. Accessed May 16, 2004.

NCSBN. (2003b). *Model Nursing Administrative Rules—Draft* [Online]. Available at http://www.ncsbn.org/public/regulation/res/Model_Rules_Web_Draft.pdf, accessed November 21, 2003.

National Standards for Culturally and Linguistically Appropriate Services in Health Care. (2000). Office of Minority Health, Public Health Service, U.S. Dept. of Health and Human Services [Online]. Available at www.omhrc.gov/CLAS/finalculturala.htm. Accessed November 22, 2003.

Pew Health Professions Commission. (1998). *Strengthening Consumer Protection: Priorities For Health Care Workforce Regulation.* San Francisco: University of California San Francisco Center for the Health Professions.

Rew, L., Becker, H., Cookston, J. et al. (2003). Measuring cultural awareness in nursing students. *Journal of Nursing Education, 42*(6), 249–257.

Trossman, S. (2000). Certified nurses report fewer adverse events: survey links certification with improved health care. *The American Nurse,* January/February, pp. 1, 9.

Whittaker, S., Smolenski, M., & Carson, W. (June 30, 2000). Assuring continued competence—policy questions and approaches: how should the profession respond? *Online Journal of Issues in Nursing.* Available at http://nursingworld.org/ojin/topic10/tpc10_4.htm. Accessed November 23, 2003.

12

The Challenging Workplace

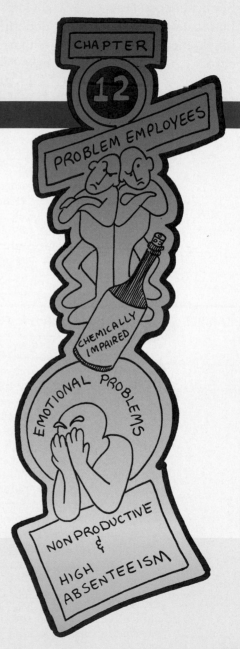

Learning Outcomes ■ ■ ■ ■

After completing this chapter, you should be able to:

1. Identify the common challenging interactions experienced by managers.
2. Discuss personnel problems commonly encountered when managing a nursing unit.
3. Outline the processes to be followed by a manager when working with a chemically impaired employee.
4. Describe what constitutes a boundary violation and describe the steps you would take if you encountered such behavior.
5. Explain the role of documentation in managing personnel problems and outline the content that should be included.
6. Discuss the issues to be considered when an employee demonstrates clinical incompetence.
7. Explain factors to be considered when working with an employee who exhibits high absenteeism.
8. Identify types of nonproductive employee behaviors and analyze strategies for working with each type.
9. Outline actions a manager can take that might improve performance of the marginal employee.
10. Discuss the role of the manager in working with employees experiencing emotional or personal problems.

Key Terms ■ ■ ■ ■ ■

absenteeism

anger

boundary violation

chemical dependence

chemically impaired

clinical incompetence

coerce

complaints

confidentiality

damage control

divided loyalties

documentation

embarrassment

employee assistance
    programs

humiliation

marginal employee

minimal disruption of the
    unit

nonproductive employee
    behaviors

problem employees

substance abuse

People who occupy management roles in health care facilities are faced with a wide variety of challenges. Concerns that the manager must handle include budgets, staffing, scarce resources, staff motivation, quality care, and maintaining positive interactions among the members of the interdisciplinary team. Perhaps the most challenging situation encountered by the manager relates to **problem employees:** those individuals who, for various reasons, are unable to perform as fully contributing team members.

EXAMPLE *Changing Work Performance*

Ten months ago you hired Julie James to work on the medical unit that you manage. When you checked references by telephone, her supervisor from another hospital in the community gave her excellent references. She graduated 2 years ago from the Associate Degree Nursing program at the local community college and has had three positions since then. For the past 2 months, she has been calling in ill frequently (five times in the last month) and has been late to work on several occasions. You have also noticed a dramatic change in Julie's behavior and work performance. Usually neat and well groomed, recently Julie's appearance is often disheveled with her make-up applied poorly. She frequently wears a long-sleeved polo shirt under her uniform top that covers her arms and she appears to have lost weight. On three occasions, patients have complained that she was unnecessarily abrupt with them. Other nurses on the unit have begun to complain that Julie "does not carry her load." You are aware that Julie is a single parent responsible for three children who are in elementary school.

Situations like the one described here are challenging to both the more seasoned clinical manager and the individual new to the management role. It is easy to gain satisfaction from working with people when operations run as expected. However, when faced with the responsibility of working with an employee whose performance is falling below expected standards, the personal rewards may not be as great. The manager must be able to distinguish between employees who need special assistance and support and those who have a problem that is so serious that progressive discipline is necessary. (Progressive discipline is discussed in Chapter 7.) Using management skills to assist employees who are having problems return to a productive status on the unit is not only cost-effective but also humanistic. This chapter explores the topic of the problem employee, including a discussion of the employee who is chemically impaired. We begin with a general overview of unpleasant behaviors that managers encounter in the work environment.

■ CHALLENGING INTERACTIONS

Fortunately, objectionable or distasteful confrontations are not everyday occurrences in nursing management. However, for the person experiencing them, they seem all too frequent and do present serious challenges. The offensiveness of these happenings can be reduced if one is prepared to deal with them. Next we discuss some of the more frequent incidences and offer some suggestions about how each might be managed.

Personal Embarrassment

Embarrassment occurs when one is caused to feel self-conscious or ill at ease. When this occurs, one often loses self-composure and may become flustered or confused. You can all remember some occasion on which you were embarrassed when you were called on in class and were expected to know something for which you failed to prepare. Can you remember how uncomfortable you felt at the time? How did you react? Because of the responsibility the nurse manager has and because of that person's visibility, it can be anticipated that he or she will be vulnerable to embarrassment. For example, the nurse manager or charge nurse is often expected to be the expert on all policies and when observed not following a particular policy may be embarrassed by having a lack of knowledge exposed.

If you find yourself in an embarrassing situation, put things into perspective. Remember that things are not as serious or as damaging as they may first appear to be. This is a good time to use some humor in your attitude and statements. The humor should be aimed at your own fallibility. Humor has the ability to lighten a situation and to take away the sting. Therefore, it is a powerful tool to keep in your professional repertoire.

However, a person might be embarrassed by deliberate action of someone trying to humiliate and cause distress. For example, a subordinate or a physician may launch a verbal attack and refer to you as incompetent in front of others about something he or she believes you should have controlled. In this situation, one may feel not only embarrassment but also humiliation. **Humiliation** reflects a loss of one's pride or dignity and feelings of shame. When experiencing a humiliating situation it is important to remain professional and detached. This is a good time to apply relaxation techniques (Kosmoski & Pollack, 2000). Take a long, deep breath, let it out slowly, relax your body, and think before you respond. The majority of observers will judge you not on the words intentionally designed to hurt you but on your response to those words. Respond without anger and emotion, but with assertive communication (see Chapter 5). Indicate that the comments or tone of voice are inappropriate in the situation and then immediately proceed to suggest a resolution to the current problem. Avoid being drawn into a verbal exchange of angry words that is unlikely to resolve anything.

Complaints

Complaints are a part of everyday life. A wise administrator once observed that one should not measure the organizational climate by the number of complaints but rather by the quality of the complaints. She meant that as an organization improved there would still be complaints, but they would be about minor rather than major issues. However, legitimate complaints, both major and minor, need to be addressed and dealt with promptly.

Kosmoski and Pollack (2000) advise that all complaints be taken seriously and considered valid until proven otherwise. This suggests that you will want to gather data about the complaint because you will want the important facts before you take action. If you already have the necessary knowledge, you can move quickly to rectify the situation. If others are involved, you will want to include these stakeholders in the decisions.

Use good interpersonal skills when relating to those lodging the complaints. Treat the individuals respectfully and thank them for bringing the issue to your attention. It may have taken a lot of courage on their part to approach you with their concern. Develop the view that complaints provide the opportunity for the organization and the people within it to grow and become more proficient at what they do. Looking at things from this perspective helps dissipate any threats that may seem to be present in the complaint. Avoid a defensive stand.

 ## Anger

Anger is an emotion frequently encountered in the health care environment. We mentioned in Chapter 9 that nurses often are the recipients of the anger expressed by members of the patient's family who are anxious about the medical outcomes of a loved one and displace this anxiety in the form of anger to nursing personnel. Occasionally, nurses experience the anger of physicians who find things not to their liking. Team members may become angry at one another in certain circumstances.

It is important to remember that anger is a normal human emotion that occurs in response to situations or circumstances that are unfair, unjust, or when someone's rights are not respected or his or her expectations are not met. It results when a person is frustrated, hurt, or afraid (Videback, 2001). When people become angry, they experience physiological changes. Anger causes one's heart to beat faster and the blood pressure to rise. The face may be flushed, the voice typically becomes louder, and speech may be more rapid. Anger is also culturally influenced. Asian and Native American communities may view the expression of anger as rude, disrespectful, and to be avoided at all costs. Other cultural groups freely express anger and expect others to do the same.

First, it is important to recognize that it is inevitable that you will encounter an angry person. What do you do when you encounter an angry person? Remember that the outburst you are hearing is not necessarily about you, and therefore try to depersonalize it. Focus on controlling your own voice and your choice of words so that neither provides additional threat or cause for frustration to the person who is already angry (Kosmoski & Pollack, 2000). Don't talk until you have thought about what to say. Practice techniques that will allow you to remain calm and in personal control. Be careful of your body language and gestures, and use those that convey genuine interest and concern. Develop active listening skills, and ask permission to ask questions or offer suggestions. As you work with and listen to the angry individual, try to determine what events prompted the anger. Be empathetic, and don't be afraid to agree with the content issues if it is appropriate to do so. Statements such as "I can understand why you are angry" will help defuse the situation. Make every effort to understand why the individual is complaining. What are the circumstances? What are the concerns? What does the individual want to have happen?

Because angry behavior can easily become physically aggressive behavior, it is important to take safety precautions for yourself and those around you. Stay calm but set limits such as "If we are to continue talking, you must lower your voice." If possible, move away from areas where others may be hurt. However, be careful that you do not position yourself so that you can be physically restrained or cannot leave if needed. If necessary, seek assistance.

Coercion

To **coerce** means to force or compel another to do something by threats or because of position or power. From an ethical standpoint, one would hope that this does not occur within the health care environment, but this is not the case.

EXAMPLE *Using Power to Gain Information*

> The clinical manager, to whom you report, calls you into her office. You have worked on the unit for only 6 months and are eager to receive a positive evaluation so that you can enjoy a raise in pay. The clinical manager states that she is very impressed with your work and your critical thinking skills and expresses the wish that others were more like you. She goes on to explain that she is particularly concerned about one of your colleagues but states that she has little time to observe that person. She asks if you would be willing to watch that person's performance and report back to her about behaviors that you notice, particularly those that might be questionable. You want to please the clinical manager, but your ethical standards are such that you do not want to find yourself in this type of relationship with a colleague.

Situations like the this one are stressful because they place us in intrapersonal conflict (see Chapter 9). We are eager to please those who supervise us but we are unwilling to compromise our own ethical standards to do so. To remain true to one's own convictions and values, it may be necessary to directly oppose one in a superior position.

The most straightforward manner in which to deal with such a situation would be to say, "I really cannot agree to doing that. If I observe substandard practice I believe I first need to discuss it with the individual whose behavior is questionable. Before I would report it to you, I would need to better understand why she chose those actions. If I felt they placed a patient in jeopardy and she was unwilling to change, I would need to let her know I planned to talk with you. I know this is what you would want me to do were you in her shoes."

In choosing this approach, it is wise to recognize the inherent dangers associated with it. The clinical manager could choose to make your professional life more unpleasant because of your unwillingness to cooperate. This could include anything from undesirable work hours to a poor employee evaluation. However, in most instances, if there is retaliation for actions that involve personal values, it is appropriate to ask for a transfer to another unit.

Another approach might involve asking for time to think about the request. This would give you time to think of alternative actions and to seriously review your own position. You might also hope that the request would be forgotten over time.

Divided Loyalties

Most nursing managers are in the role in middle management. That means that they are responsible for supervising the activities of others but they are accountable to higher administrative authority themselves. This can result in circumstances in which the nursing managers find themselves with **divided loyalties.** Are they to be honest and straightforward with their subordinates, or do they comply with the expectations of their supervisors? This becomes a real issue when it comes to maintaining **confidentiality** about organizational information or decisions, that is, the information cannot be shared.

EXAMPLE *Dealing With Confidential Administrative Information*

As a new unit manager you have been working diligently for the past 8 months to develop a sense of team spirit among the nurses and assistants on your unit. You have fostered this by role modeling collegiality and working on establishing a trusting and open environment. Following a meeting with your team, one of the licensed practical nurses (LPNs) walks back to your office with you and states, "There is a rumor that all employees are going to be asked to take three unpaid days off each month to reduce operating costs. Is this true?" At your last administrative meeting, you were told that this action would be taken and would be announced in 2 weeks. However, you were told to keep the information confidential until the announcement was made.

Circumstances such as this one are easy to fall into, especially for the novice in the management role. In an effort to develop an outstanding team, limits may not be established for the role of the manager. Although the trust that has been established with the LPN is such that she expects that an honest answer is forthcoming, it is better to state, "I'm sorry, but I have no information about such plans that I can share" or "I'm not at liberty to discuss this." Keeping your response short and succinct is desirable. Situations such as this can be avoided by planning in advance for them, starting with establishing guidelines regarding the manager's role with subordinates at the very beginning. As a member of the management team, when the original information and constraints on sharing it are discussed, you can request that the group develop a plan for how and when this information will be shared and how to respond to individuals who hear rumors. Both would help to avert such an uncomfortable situation.

Finally, it is important to recognize that there will be times when you will be unable to share information. In such cases, you must accept the professional responsibility for confidentiality.

■ THE CHEMICALLY IMPAIRED EMPLOYEE

We use the term **chemically impaired** to describe the individual whose practice has deteriorated because of drug dependence and **substance abuse,** specifically through the use of alcohol or drugs. Although it can be reasonably assumed that **chemical dependence** has been around as long as have been the substances that are abused, by the 1980s the nursing profession became seriously concerned about the impact on nursing. The American Nurses Association (ANA) publicly recognized the problem in 1984 (Dabney, 1995). As a result, most states and agencies have policies developed about the reporting of substance abuse and avenues for securing treatment instead of disciplinary action. These treatment programs are often referred to as diversion programs because they divert an individual from the disciplinary arena to the treatment arena. Diversion programs are used to assist those who acknowledge they have a problem. The state board of nursing and the Nurse Practice Act can be excellent resources regarding the legal aspects of chemical impairment and access to treatment. However, some states still respond to chemical dependence as a disciplinary issue rather than a treatment issue (Trossman, 2003). Therefore, you need to be aware of the policies of the licensing authority in your jurisdiction before deciding on the appropriate action. The state board of nursing and the Nurse Practice Act should be consulted as resources regarding the legal aspects of chemical impairment in your particular state.

Understanding the Problem

From September 1980 to August 1981 the National Council of State Boards of Nursing (NCSBN) collected data on disciplinary actions from its member boards. Of the cases reported during that period, it was determined that 67% of the disciplinary proceedings involving nurses were related to some form of chemical abuse (Sullivan et al., 1988). The statistics regarding substance abuse among nurses vary greatly. The ANA estimates that the prevalence of chemical dependency is 6% to 8% (Smith et al., 1998). Substance abuse is the number one reason listed by state boards of nursing for disciplinary action (Sullivan & Decker, 2001). Trinkoff and Storr (1998) report that emergency and critical care nurses are more than three times as likely to use marijuana or cocaine as nurses in other specialties and that oncology and administration nurses are twice as likely to engage in binge drinking. It is suggested that, in addition to the stress encountered by emergency and critical care nurses, having easy access to medication may contribute to the problem. Of the substances abused, meperidine (Demerol) and alcohol are by far the most commonly cited chemicals (Hughes & Smith, 1994), with drugs such as diazepam (Valium) and other narcotic drugs, such as morphine, frequently included (Landry, 1987). Recently, studies have been conducted to assess probable alcoholism among nursing students. The use of alcohol by nursing students was reported by Marion and colleagues (Marion, 1996), who found that the use of alcohol by nursing students paralleled the alcohol consumption of other college students. Sullivan et al. (1990) reported that the addiction process was starting earlier, sometimes even before nursing school, and that younger nurses were more likely to use narcotics, resulting in serious problems in job performance.

These studies, and others focusing on the problems of chemical dependency among nurses, reinforce that today's nursing manager will come face to face with this concern on the nursing unit. Institutions suffer a significant financial impact because of nurses with dependency problems in the forms of sickness, absenteeism, tardiness, accidents, errors, decreased productivity, and staff turnover. Early recognition and treatment are critical. The unit manager usually becomes responsible for the recognition of the problem and the confrontation of the employee.

The concerns about the chemically impaired nurse are twofold. The first concern is for the patients, whose care is jeopardized by the nurse whose judgment and skills are weakened. The second concern is a personal one for the nurse who is afflicted; the illness may go undetected and untreated for years.

Identification of the Problem

The behavior of the impaired nurse may vary tremendously, depending to a great extent on the degree of dependence on the substance. If used primarily for pleasure and in a recreational manner, the major problems seen in the work environment may relate to tardiness or absenteeism. As the abuse increases, the individual's defensiveness regarding substance abuse may also increase, with a great deal of denial occurring. Denial is a key aspect of both the nurse and of fellow coworkers (Hrobak, 2002). Leffler (1986) suggests that the "conspiracy of silence" established by nurses and managers, who have been slow to recognize the problem and are reluctant to help colleagues, has perpetuated this denial. An "out of sight, out of mind" attitude may prevail. Eventually, relationships break down among the manager, the impaired employee, and other staff members. As the problem becomes greater, the employee's personal and professional life becomes focused on his or her need for drugs, which has become so severe that abuse occurs during the working hours as well as at home. The employee may be obtaining the drugs by stealing the patients' medications and substituting other medications (Ashton & Bay, 1994). It is at this point that the behaviors identified in Display 12-1 can be most easily recognized.

Gathering and Analyzing the Data

An important step in working with the impaired employee involves gathering as much data to support your suspicions as possible. Another nurse may have confided to you his or her concerns. Patients may have registered complaints. You should note any changes in behavior or work performance and any unusual patterns of absenteeism or tardiness. All this information should be objectively recorded in writing with dates of when it was observed. If you are a charge nurse, you should report your concerns to the nurse manager who has the authority necessary to manage the process, including conducting a more thorough investigation.

If you are the nurse manager and suspect drug addiction, you will want to check narcotic records for inconsistencies. The procedure usually requires that you also consult with the pharmacy department regarding the steps you will need to take in checking all relevant records. Impairment related to alcohol abuse is more difficult to prove because it is more easily hidden than is drug abuse and most employees do not drink while on duty. The manager will need to look for more subtle clues. It is critical that you take the time to put this information into written format. (The importance of good documentation is discussed later.)

 ## Anticipating the Next Step

Unless you are already familiar with the hospital policies and protocols for dealing with poor work performance related to suspected chemical dependency, you also should review carefully the processes approved for use in the facility in which you are working. You will want to consider a number of factors. You will also want to know when it is appropriate to contact the board of nursing and which individual in your facility is expected to make that contact. Most hospitals have some written process for dealing with such issues, and it is important that you follow them. If you do not know where such policies are located, your immediate superior should be of assistance.

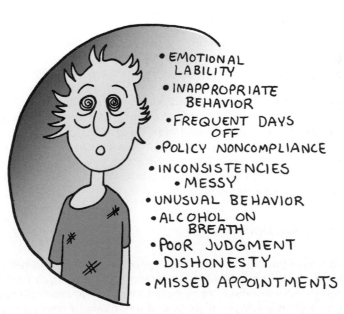

- EMOTIONAL LABILITY
- INAPPROPRIATE BEHAVIOR
- FREQUENT DAYS OFF
- POLICY NONCOMPLIANCE
- INCONSISTENCIES
- MESSY
- UNUSUAL BEHAVIOR
- ALCOHOL ON BREATH
- POOR JUDGMENT
- DISHONESTY
- MISSED APPOINTMENTS

The behavior of the impaired nurse may vary depending on the degree of dependence on the substance.

<table>
<tr><td>DISPLAY 12-1</td><td>Signs That a Professional May Be Experiencing Chemical Dependence Problems</td></tr>
</table>

- Emotional liability characterized by mood swings, irritability, and withdrawn behavior
- Inappropriate behavior
- Frequent days off for implausible reasons
- Noncompliance with acceptable policies and procedures
- Deteriorating appearance
- Inconsistent job performance
- Inadequate or "messy" documentation
- Unusual prescribing practices
- Alcohol on the breath
- Poor judgment and concentration
- Dishonesty
- Missed appointments
- Boundary violations

From Washington Health Professional Services. (1997). *A Confidential Program for Chemically Impaired Health Professionals* [Brochure], 6-25-97. Olympia, WA: Washington State Department of Health.

The Americans With Disabilities Act (ADA) of 1990 prohibits discrimination in hiring, job expectations, and promotion against the person with a qualifying disability. If an individual self-reports or is diagnosed with drug and alcohol dependency, then it becomes a qualifying disability prohibiting discrimination (Hrobak, 2002). However, protection under the ADA does not mean that the person does not bear responsibility for behavior in the workplace. The person is protected while under treatment and while maintaining that treatment program, which in the case of chemical dependence includes remaining drug or alcohol free. The person is subject to the same expectations of appropriate behavior as all other employees. Because of the various interpretations and applications of the ADA, such as maintaining confidentiality of records, provision of sick leave, and treatment opportunities, it is wise for the manager to consult with the human resources department to assure accurate information before proceeding with actions if an individual is believed to have a chemical dependence problem.

Meeting With the Employee

Once sufficient data have been gathered to assure that there is a genuine concern, a meeting will need to be arranged with the employee to discuss the situation. If you are in this position, do not expect such a meeting to go smoothly. The employee who has a problem with substance abuse typically uses many defense mechanisms, especially denial. The employee also may be angry at having been confronted. With this in mind, it is important that you do not preach, moralize, rebuke, or blame the individual. The focus of the conversation must be on the employee's unacceptable performance and the absenteeism, poor patient care, irritability, or other behaviors that have been noted. Your observations should be supported by the documentation you have gathered. In a kind and concerned manner, you need to help the employee see what aspects of behavior did not meet professional standards. Expectations for improved performance must be set forth and a second meeting scheduled. It is very common for the employee to deny any problems with substance abuse, perhaps because he or she has not acknowledged personally that a problem exists. Using the example presented at the introduction of this chapter, let's review how such a meeting might proceed.

EXAMPLE *Meeting With an Employee*

You schedule a meeting with Julie toward the end of the shift. It is your intention to discuss her increasing pattern of calling in ill and the complaints that have been registered by patients in her care. You also decide to discuss with her the changes you have noticed in her appearance. You hope that as you discuss these concerns, Julie will provide you with a clearer insight into bases for these behaviors. Inwardly, you are concerned that she may be involved in some type of substance abuse. Julie appears 10 minutes late for your meeting, explaining that at the last minute one of her patients required pain medication. You tell her that you are concerned about the number of sick days she has taken in the last month, reminding her about the additional stress her absences place on other staff members when the unit is understaffed. She states that two of the ill days were because one of her children had a communicable disease and was unable to go to school. She was not able to arrange childcare until the third day. On the third absence, she was unable to obtain transportation because her car would not start, and on the fourth occasion she had a migraine headache. When you mention the complaints from patients, citing specifics, she seems surprised but does acknowledge that she had been unusually tired lately and perhaps had been "a bit short" on occasion. In response to your concerns that her appearance has been disheveled lately, she indicates that getting three children ready for school before leaving in the morning does not leave her with much time for herself; however, you are left with the impression that she does not really recognize this as a concern. Despite opportunities that you provide for her to share other information that might impact the situation, she does not do so. In response to questions about her health, she states she is fine, just a little tired. You state your expectations regarding her performance and make suggestions for improvement. She promises to improve her appearance and be careful about her response to patients. She says she does not anticipate any more ill days. The two of you agree to meet in another month to review how things are going with her. Following the conference, you are a little disillusioned because you feel you accomplished very little. Two weeks later, Julie again calls in ill.

As a manager, you must realize your own role in assisting the impaired individual. Some managers find themselves wanting to care for the impaired person as they would for others who are ill. Such behavior on the part of the manager may be enabling (Navarra, 1995). The manager should not assume the role of confidant, counselor, or treatment provider. The impaired employee should be referred to others who have expertise in the area and who can view the situation objectively.

 ## Documentation

One of the most important aspects of working with any employee problem is **documentation.** This includes documenting the date, the time, and the behavior you observe, reports made to you by other employees, complaints made by patients, or any other factual information related to your concern. The statement of the incident that has occurred should be objective and relate only the facts surrounding the situation. Any actions taken by the manager when the problem occurred should also be noted. Notes should not draw conclusions or express opinions. Documentation must also be kept on any meetings that take place as a result of the incident. The documentation should include the date, time, and general content and decisions reached at any meetings that take place. Although thorough documentation is time consuming, it cannot be left to memory. Important details cannot be remembered unless immediately recorded before times and responses become clouded. Many managers state that taking time to adequately document such incidents and meetings is one of the management responsibilities most difficult to consistently implement.

Referral and Follow-up

Many institutions have implemented **employee assistance programs** that are available to employees at no charge or at a minimum fee. In facilities in which this is an option, the manager can refer any troubled employee to this program for professional help and move away from the counseling role. If the employee does not wish to take advantage of this benefit, documentation and meetings on the unit will need to continue until sufficient data have been gathered for the unit manager to implement policies developed by the institution for working with employees with problems. However, data related to drug dependence indicate that job-related pressure is often effective in getting someone into treatment.

In some instances, there may be clear evidence of chemical impairment or substance abuse. In these instances, the employee assistance program may arrange for an intervention. An intervention is a meeting planned by a trained chemical dependency counselor to which colleagues, supervisors, and even family may be invited. The purpose of the meeting is to clearly tell the person that the behavior has been identified and that it is harming the individual and those around him or her. The counselor plans ahead for access to treatment and guides the meeting. The purpose of the meeting is to overcome denial and push the person into treatment. Treatment entered into through the force of an intervention in the workplace may be very effective. The intervention overcomes the denial and the importance of the job in an individual's life provides motivation to enter treatment.

Many states now have programs in place at the state level to provide support for treatment of health care professionals with chemical dependency. These programs usually provide a specific contractual agreement in regard to professional practice during the treatment and monitoring period. This is often done without formal disciplinary proceedings. These programs work best when the nurse involved voluntarily seeks assistance. The actions that follow will depend on the seriousness of the problem, but in all instances the goal is to rehabilitate the impaired nurse. In some states, the licensing boards may institute formal disciplinary proceedings to suspend a license or issue a license with limitations on practice and to provide monitoring and supervision while the individual seeks treatment. When treatment is completed, the board may reinstate the license with temporary limitations and continued monitoring support. The determination that treatment is complete will vary among individuals, depending on the nature of the problem and the person's willingness to comply with expected steps of rehabilitation. Trossman (2003) reports that some nondisciplinary assistance programs for nurses with chemical dependence report 80% recovery rates whereas some report up to 95% recovery.

Some institutions have developed guidelines for reentry into the workplace. Typically, such guidelines spell out expectations of the returning employee, such as assignment to the day shift, willingness to consent to random urine samples, and continued work with support groups. The goal is the eventual full rehabilitation of the health care professional and return to the service of the community.

The NCSBN (www.ncsbn.org) has produced a video and facilitation package, *Breaking the Habit: When Your Colleague is Chemically Dependent*. This package was developed to assist boards of nursing to deal proactively with chemical dependency in licensed nurses through education, prevention, and early detection. The program, which won the 2002 Nursing Electronic Award of Sigma Theta Tau International (STTI), is appropriate for nurses in every practice setting or level of practice, including students.

Critical Thinking Exercise

You are concerned that one of the nurses on your unit is diverting drugs. What steps should you take before you deal with this problem? Which of those activities must be accomplished first? Are there other individuals within the institution with whom you should talk before taking any action? Are there legal ramifications to consider? If you are the charge nurse, what are your primary responsibilities? If you have never dealt with a problem such as this before, with whom should you consult?

■ BOUNDARY VIOLATIONS

Boundary violations are currently receiving much attention in nursing and health care. **Boundary violation** refers to a situation in which nurses move beyond a professional relationship and become personally involved with their patients and the patients' lives. All boundary violations have in common the recognition that any health professional in a relationship with a patient has a position of power. The patient is more vulnerable in the relationship and is often unable to set limits with the professional. When the professional crosses out of a professional relationship into another type of relationship, it is an abuse of the power of the position.

Professional sexual misconduct is one of the most serious types of boundary violation. Professional sexual misconduct has been defined as "any expression by a nurse or other health care provider of erotic or romantic thoughts, feelings, or gestures that are sexual or may be reasonably construed by the patient as sexual"

(Smith et al., 1997). This consists of any behavior in which a provider initiates sexual interaction with a patient or responds to a patient in a sexual manner. According to the Florida Nurse Practice Act, this would include sexually suggestive or explicit comments, off-color jokes, nontherapeutic hugs, or other overt sexual acts. Keep in mind the importance of the perception of the patient or client as to whether an action is sexual in nature.

Although most of the attention regarding boundary violation has been focused on sexual misconduct, other types of boundary issues can emerge. Overinvolvement and inappropriately moving from a professional relationship to a personal relationship also constitutes a boundary violation. For example, nurses sometimes find themselves overidentifying with a particular family member, such as the wife of a patient dying from cancer or the mother of the pediatric client. On occasion, nurses have become involved to the point that they moved into a pseudofamily relationship, that is, beginning to act like the daughter, sister, or other family member. When this happens, the family may question the nurse's motives, wondering if she is looking for a bequest in a will or other tangible benefit. The patient may begin to be dependent on that one professional and be very hurt if the professional sets limits or changes the relationship.

Although this type of overinvolvement with patients does not create the degree of concern we see focused on sexual misconduct, it does have serious implications. The nurse's work and personal life may suffer. Families may bring suit against the nurse and/or the health care facility. Because of the serious ramifications of letting relationships move beyond that which is professional, nurses should be alert to situations in which they are becoming too involved with the client or the client's family and take action to bring that relationship back into professional bounds.

At the present time, there is no official reporting of the violation of sexual boundaries; thus, statistics regarding its frequency are lacking. However, the NCSBN formed a focus group to study sexual misconduct among nurses. Although the number was relatively small, video tapes and instructional materials have been developed by the group to assist with recognition of the problem. It is of particular concern because it represents a violation of the trust relationship that exists between the patient and nurse. Because of the highly personal nature of the routine assistance that nurses provide to patients, they have access to privileged and confidential information. In a nurse–patient relationship, the nurse necessarily holds the power, creating a vulnerable situation for the patient. Boundaries allow the patient and the nurse to connect safely in a therapeutic relationship that is based on the patient's needs. Misconduct occurs when the boundaries begin to erode. The opportunity for occurrence of such behavior is greater in some settings than in others. For example, misconduct tends to occur more frequently in long-term settings in which supervision may be minimal.

Early indications that boundaries are beginning to break down include spending extended time with a patient beyond assigned duties, visiting the patient when not on duty, showing favoritism or possessiveness of a patient, meeting patients in isolated areas not required in direct patient care, or personal disclosure by the care provider.

It is important that you, as a professional, be able to recognize situations in which a colleague may have crossed sexual boundaries. As a manager, you have an even greater responsibility to respond to the situation. Like many nurses, you may be initially shocked that such behavior is occurring. This emphasizes the nursing profession's responsibility to educate nurses about the problem of sexual misconduct—teaching them how to identify indicators of sexual misconduct in colleagues and the

DISPLAY 12-2	**Preventing Sexual Misconduct**

- Be aware of any sexual attraction you feel toward a patient. Discuss those feelings with a trusted friend or colleague.
- Transfer the care of a patient to another nurse when sexual attraction threatens the therapeutic relationship.
- Learn to recognize indications that the patient may be interested in forming a sexual relationship. The enforcement of professional boundaries is in your hands.
- Respect patient privacy and dignity at all times.
- Provide a professional explanation for all aspects of patient care. This is particularly important when examination or treatments involve sexual or private parts of the body.
- Maintain clear, appropriate, and professional communication with patients. Do not engage in the sharing of sexual jokes or comments.
- Do not discuss your personal life or problems with the patient.

Adapted from guidelines provided by Smith, L. L., Taylor, B. B., Keys, A. T. et al. (1997). Nurse–patient boundaries: crossing the line. *American Journal of Nursing, 97*(12), 26–31.

steps that should be followed when it occurs. Staff education is extremely important in preventing and identifying the problem.

If you believe sexual misconduct is occurring on your unit, the steps you would follow are similar to those you have learned to use in dealing with chemical abuse. Carefully document the behavior you have noted. Identify dates, times, and names of individuals involved. Document only factual information and objective data. This information should then be shared with your immediate supervisor. Allegations may need to be reported to outside agencies, such as the board of nursing or another state regulatory agency. Most facilities have policies that guide action in relationship to sexual misconduct. Most boards of nursing, in addition to possible discipline, evaluate the nurse for possible treatment. Display 12-2 outlines guidelines for preventing sexual misconduct.

The NCSBN has also produced a facilitation package on professional boundary violation. The package, which was honored with the STTI Nursing Electronic Award in 1999, is titled *Crossing the Line: When Professional Boundaries Are Violated.*

■ THE INCOMPETENT EMPLOYEE

Dealing with an employee's **clinical incompetence** may be one of the most challenging problems faced by charge nurses and unit managers. First, professionally we would like to believe that all nurses would be ethically responsible and not undertake tasks for which they were not adequately prepared. Complicating the problem of clinical incompetence is the fact that peers will often help cover for the inept employee, thereby delaying recognition of the problem. Frequently, employees who lack the necessary skills can be very clever in persuading a colleague to do the procedures they are incapable of performing themselves.

To prevent the occurrence of clinical incompetence among employees, health care facilities now have checklists and skills tests to determine competency that must be administered to new employees at the time they are hired, a process required by the Joint Commission on Accreditation of Healthcare Organizations (JCAHO). These checklists tend to cover the nursing skills and procedures essential for safe functioning on the unit to which the employee will be assigned. Thus, the skills required in an obstetrical unit would be different from those administered on a medical unit. Identifying deficits in underlying knowledge and the application of this knowledge to problem solving is much more challenging. This type of deficit may be identified when an error in judgment occurs and the problem is investigated.

If deficits exist in the performance of an employee, plans for remediation can be established. Although initially time consuming, assessment of clinical competence can have very beneficial outcomes. Again, the steps discussed earlier (problem identification, data gathering, meeting with employee, documentation, and follow-up) are critical to resolution of the concerns. The role of the manager as coach and counselor takes on new proportions in such situations. (See discussions of the role of coach and counselor in Chapters 5 and 7.) If there is a staff member who is willing to serve as a mentor to the employee who is performing poorly, such a relationship is often valuable with the three individuals (manager, employee, and mentor) working as a team to improve the deficient clinical skills of the employee.

■ THE EMPLOYEE EXHIBITING HIGH ABSENTEEISM

Absenteeism represents another major challenge to a manager, especially when it exceeds what is normal or expected. The right to be absent from work with pay due to illness for a certain number of days each year has long been accepted as one of the prerogatives of employees guaranteed through collective bargaining agreements or through official personnel policies when no collective bargaining agreement exists. Even in facilities that have no formal contractual agreements, the right to take a certain number of paid sick days each year may exist as a common understanding between management and employees. Such benefits result in significant costs to the institution.

In addition to the salary and benefits of the nonproductive employee, there are the additional costs of a replacement or perhaps overtime hours for others if a replacement is not available. The level of functioning and the quality of patient care on the nursing unit also can suffer from employee absences. Other members of the nursing team often feel stress even when a replacement, who may not be familiar with the unit, can be found. On some occasions, the nurse manager may feel compelled to take a partial patient care assignment, thus neglecting important management activities that day. Although the legitimate need for time off when ill is not to be questioned, when the privilege is misused it can have deleterious effects on the unit. In addition to loss of productivity, the demoralization of unit staff can become a critical factor. Unit staff may see the abuse of sick time as ethically improper and also may resent the extra time and effort required of them because a colleague is unable or unwilling to fulfill working responsibilities.

In addition to sick days, which are typically accumulative to a certain number, some organizations now have provisions for personal necessity leave or personal leave days, which were established to allow employees to carry out personal responsibilities that cannot be accomplished if they are at work. The usual activities considered would include such things as appearing in court, signing papers to purchase or sell a house, or meeting with a professional on some personal matter. Personal leave days may be deducted from allocated sick leave days, but when the sick days have accumulated to a fairly high number this is not a concern.

Increased rates of absenteeism are also noted when an individual is experiencing role stress. Absenteeism becomes a way to withdraw from an undesirable situation and is frequently seen prior to resignation (Lee & Eriksen, 1990). When this occurs, the manager may also note that the interpersonal interactions of the individual have decreased. An interview with the employee may reveal that this individual is receiving far less satisfaction from the job.

Most employees use all leaves in the manner in which they were intended. In fact, there are those employees who need to be encouraged to stay home when they are ill so that they do not infect others with the cold or flu virus that is incapacitating them. However, there are a few employees who take advantage of all leaves. The tendency among these individuals is to view the leave days as something they have coming to them and, with this thinking, very religiously take the maximum time allowed each year. When sick leave, personal leave, family leave, bereavement leave, and any other leave provided in the contract are all taken into consideration, the amount of lost work time can be significant.

When the right is abused, dealing with it is as frustrating to the experienced manager as to the individual new in the role. The frustration the manager feels can stem from a number of causes. First is the time required to find a replacement and the time taken from other duties to assure that the substitute is able to function adequately in patient care. If a replacement is not available, care assignments will need to be adjusted. The morale of other members of the nursing team is also important. If allowed to continue for too long without some action on the part of the manager, unit employees may turn their criticism to the manager, seeing it as the manager's responsibility to do something about all the absences. Another consideration that affects the situation and often makes it difficult for the manager to positively address the issue is the discrepancy that may exist between the employee's value system and that of the manager. When an employee honestly believes he or she is entitled to the days off and the managers see this as a benefit to be used only as needed, a built-in conflict exists in the situation. The provisions created by the ADA, which allows that emotional stress may be a legitimate basis for illness, only adds to the complexity of the issue.

The difference between the value system of the employee and the manager may be the most difficult for a person new to management responsibilities to accept and understand. New to a management role, anxious to do a good job, eager to establish a reputation for managing a unit noted for quality patient care, and willing to put in extra time to see all this occur—there is little room in this manager's set of values and beliefs for the individual who views his or her obligations as simply a job and who is willing to meet minimum work standards. At this point, not only are values at odds, but so are commitment and professionalism. However, in the real world, such situations exist, although hopefully not often. Before any positive discussion can occur between the manager and the employee, the manager must recognize that this difference exists and minimally accept the right of the employee to have his or her own views.

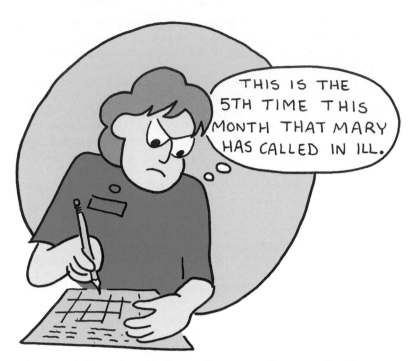

A manager's frustration with absenteeism can stem from a number of causes.

Recognizing that differing values and standards exist in this situation will assist the manager in the discussions that must follow with the employee. Discussing problems of absenteeism from a factual perspective rather than an emotional one is important. It is possible that personal problems are interfering with an employee's ability to meet expectations. However, if a contract is in effect between the institution and employees and if the employee has not taken more leave than is allowed within that contract, there may be little to discuss. Although the manager may not be convinced that the employee was ill when "sick" days were taken, there is little that can be done about the situation. The manager will then be challenged to do appropriate record keeping and reporting and make a distribution of assignments so that there is minimal disruption of the unit.

What is implied by the words **minimal disruption of the unit?** Is that an acceptable management strategy? How is it accomplished? These and other questions are reasonable to ask. When it is apparent that the manager is dealing with a situation which existing policies and protocols will not allow to be changed, altered, improved, or otherwise influenced, often the best solution is to manage assignments so that the actions of the person in question can have as little effect on the operation of the unit as possible. For example, it would be undesirable to have this individual serving as a mentor for a new employee or filling the role of unit representative to a critical hospital committee. These assignments are best given to employees exhibiting greater stability. More seasoned managers label this **damage control,** referring to the limitation that can be placed on harm that can occur to the day-to-day operation of the unit. It is a management technique used in any situation in which it appears there is no other positive resolution to the existing problem.

When working with absenteeism, we need to remember that when it occurs as a change in the behavior of an employee, it may be one of the more obvious symptoms of a more serious problem. Often this problem can be corrected with help and understanding.

Critical Thinking Exercise

Elizabeth Jones, LPN (LVN), has worked on your unit for 5½ months. In that time, she has been late on at least six occasions. She tends to take 45 minutes for her lunch breaks instead of the expected 30 minutes. On occasion, her uniform has been wrinkled and stained and her shoes usually need polishing. Her patients make positive comments about the care they receive and she is willing to make adjustments in her own schedule to work around the needs of others on the staff. How much documentation do you believe you should have before talking with her? How would you approach Elizabeth regarding her tardy behavior and long lunch breaks? What information would you share with her? What notes would you make following your meeting with her?

■ NONPRODUCTIVE EMPLOYEE BEHAVIORS

The problems discussed in this section, which we have grouped as **nonproductive employee behaviors,** may provide the manager with frustration more than anything else does. The situations cited usually are not serious enough for any formal actions to be instituted. Some of the behaviors tend to be a reflection of basic personality types, which can be challenged but seldom changed.

The Employee Motivated by Self-Interest

In the best of institutions, there will always be some employees who declare themselves "only in it for the money," who are interested solely in the necessities or the conveniences wages can buy. Although all of us recognize the importance of adequate and appropriate wages for nurses, there is much more to a professional commitment than working for a wage. (See Chapter 10 for more discussion of professional commitment.)

Individuals who see their responsibilities only in terms of hours and paychecks are less likely to be fully functioning members of the profession with a view of the larger picture. Critical to professional practice and an expectation of nurses at all levels is the obligation to be involved in maintaining current practice. Participation in professional organizations, self-governance, and serving as advocates for the profession are additional aspects of professionalism. Nurses who see their responsibilities ending at the completion of the shift are missing opportunities to make a contribution to the profession.

A wise manager needs to realize that some individuals have such time constraints on their lives that it makes extra activities hard to fit in after a full shift.

Young mothers who are busy with the activities of school-aged children that involve Girl Scout or Boy Scout activities, soccer games, and music lessons provide good examples of this situation. This individual might be offered other opportunities, such as assignment to a hospital committee that meets during the work hours.

The Employee Who Is a Doomsayer

The incurable pessimist has a vested interest in portraying any problem as one without an acceptable solution. If there is no solution to any given situation, then the individual cannot be held accountable for failures. Doomsayers typically bemoan the lack of supplies, the shortness of staff, the insensitivity of management, the inadequacy of secretarial assistance, or other inconveniences without attempting to make realistic suggestions for change. It is wearisome to work with these individuals, because each effort made by others to improve the situation merely meets with a different explanation for why the suggested innovation will be inadequate. Doomsayers need to be helped to see that their input is valued and can result in productive change. They may respond well to team-building activities. Each nurse must realize the responsibility for contributing to finding solutions to problems.

An astute manager realizes that a well-managed unit still experiences complaints. As mentioned previously, rather than consider the number of complaints, it is wise to look at the nature of the subordinate's complaints. Objections that focus on the lack of time available to review and analyze patient questionnaires or to reevaluate discharge plans are of an entirely different nature and seriousness than complaints about the need to always work overtime to complete the day's assignment or the lack of enough bath towels to assure all unit needs. Yet the number of complaints may be rather constant.

The Employee Who Demonstrates Insubordinate Behavior

Insubordinate behavior is that which, whether done consciously or unconsciously, undermines the leadership of the manager or the group. Frequently dissident employees feel disappointed with their own situation and seek to exert some measure of control by subverting the goals of the manager or the group. Other times, this behavior is manifest by individuals who have an antipathy toward authority figures, whom they suspect of some organizational bias that must be guarded against. For example, the facility may have decided to adopt a different charting form. Some nurses are enthusiastic about the new form; others are not. A subversive employee would plot to defeat the new forms without a trial by encouraging others to fill them out improperly or not to fill them out at all, substituting the original forms instead. Many times the behaviors displayed by the subversive employee are passive–aggressive in nature, making them all the more difficult to deal with.

Persistent concern about the welfare of the individual may assist in turning the situation around. Frank discussion of the behavior may help bring to light issues that would otherwise be overlooked. In such instances the manager should not make any comments that might reflect anger or disdain. The focus should be on helping the employee recognize and change unproductive behaviors.

Working with the insubordinate employee is difficult because all managers may be viewed by this individual as unreliable or as the voice of the administration. Encounters with such individuals tend to be taxing. If you find yourself having difficulty maintaining a positive attitude, seeking the assistance of a mentor may be helpful. A mentor will provide a safe environment for "letting off steam" and will help keep things in perspective. The mentor also may suggest approaches to working with the individual that you had not considered.

EXAMPLE *A Dissident Employee*

> Susan Amour worked part-time as a charge nurse on the day shift in a small rural nursing home. She had experienced a particularly busy day, and she and her staff had managed to complete all the various aspects of care with the exception of catheterizing one resident who had a suspected urinary tract infection for a specimen to be sent to the laboratory. Performing the catheterization would require that she work overtime and the evening shift had already arrived. The evening staff for the 45-bed unit, which was divided into east and the west, included two LPNs, each of whom took one end of the unit and did all treatments and medications, and a registered nurse, who was the evening charge nurse and was expected to help out when and where assistance was needed. Susan gave report, mentioning that the catheterization was not done. She asked the evening charge nurse if she would please do it. The charge nurse, who was looking forward to taking vacation time within the next 30 days replied, "I'm not going to do anything tonight. I'm just going to sit here."

The Employee Who Is an Accommodator

Just as there are those who try to undermine the activities of the manager, there are those who always accommodate or uncritically agree with all ideas that are proposed. Although this may outwardly seem to be a positive situation, it robs others of information that may be critical to the implementation of changes. For example, the nursing assistant who consistently smiles, agrees to everything that is asked of her, and provides no comment with regard to assignments given to her is not providing input regarding the organization of activities on the unit. All employees have the responsibility for providing feedback in a consistent and positive manner, because it is not possible for a single individual to have all the information that is needed to make the best decisions. When an employee just agrees to, or accommodates, a suggested plan rather than voicing any concerns he or she may have prior to its implementation, a poorer decision-making process results, and the manager does not function as effectively because of the lack of input.

Productive managers develop skill in soliciting and reinforcing input from team members. Recognizing good ideas and giving or sharing credit for endeavors that produce good outcomes help create a climate in which people are more willing to trust and take chances. Accepting all ideas or suggestions as worthy of consideration also encourages such behavior. Perhaps most important of all is taking time to celebrate successes. This need not be as elaborate as a formal party or gathering. Simply bringing doughnuts or special refreshment to the unit for all to enjoy can provide recognition of a job well done.

The Employee Who Is a Superachiever

The employee who is a superachiever represents a special challenge to a manager. Because this individual frequently has the greatest work output and outstanding technical know-how, the manager is inclined to overlook or tolerate the undesirable behaviors that may be present. Superachievers tend to believe that their ideas and ways of doing things are superior to those of all others. Those who see themselves in this light may treat colleagues in a patronizing or demeaning and arrogant manner. The behavior of the superachiever often is viewed as aggressive and uncompromising. The interactions with others may be intimidating and often critical, causing others to acquiesce to this person's judgment or decisions, thus reinforcing the dominant actions. Individuals who lack self-confidence and assertiveness are easy prey for the superachiever.

In working with this employee, the manager must move in a calm, assertive manner, pointing out the behaviors that are not acceptable. The goal is to help the employee recognize and change the undesirable behaviors. It is important that the manager maintain a quiet, assured manner when talking with this individual and not allow challenge to the manager's role or position on the issue to take place. Discussions should not be allowed to evolve into arguments.

Critical Thinking Exercise

Alice Johnson has been working on your unit for 9 months. A recent graduate, she has quickly learned the routine on the unit, is clinically very skillful, highly motivated, always well groomed, and finishes her assignments in time to assist others. You believe she has the potential for advancement with the exception that as she has become more comfortable in her role she has become more critical of others. Recently, she has been demonstrating impatience with newcomers or those who learn more slowly than she, is sometimes abrupt, and often communicates that she knows best. Do you think you should do anything about this behavior? If so, how will you approach it? What cautions should you consider? What outcomes would you want? What would be the best time to discuss your concerns with Alice?

The Marginal Employee

Unlike the superachiever, the **marginal employee** is one whose work meets only the minimum standards considered acceptable. Usually, the performance is not serious enough to consider terminating the individual but is poor enough to frustrate all with whom this individual works. The general feeling is that such individuals are not carrying their share of the responsibility for organizational efficiency. Unlike the incompetent employee who does not meet established standards, the marginal employee just barely meets them on a consistent basis.

There are many reasons for marginal behavior. First, it may be due to insufficient knowledge. It may be the result of burn out. There may be personal problems that are affecting the work performance. Health problems, including emotional difficulties, may be a cause.

In working with this individual, the manager will once again begin by gathering as much information as possible. In this instance, a good beginning point is to look at previous work records of marginal employees. Has there been a change in their ability to perform or is this a pattern that has been present for a long time? If it is a change when did it change? How long has it persisted?

Then the next step would be to try to discover what factors have led to this change and what actions can be taken to turn the situation around. On the other hand, if the behavior has always been marginal, other solutions will have to be implemented. This is a good time to employ some of the coaching behaviors mentioned in Chapters 5 and 7. As you work with the individual, you will gain a better understanding of factors that motivate him or her. If additional training or education will help remedy the problem, it can be arranged. If personal problems are the cause of the poor performance, referrals can be made to individuals within your institution who are skilled in that area. You do not want to try to become the counselor in this type of situation. If personal health problems are a problem, again a referral is appropriate. Perhaps you can help arrange a work schedule that would allow for needed appointments.

As you work with the individual, you will be able to establish goals and timelines for improvement. Perhaps in the process, the marginal employee will discover that there is another area in which he or she would be happier working. At the very least, the marginal employee's self-esteem may be raised by your professional investment and you may be able to identify skills at which that individual will be most productive. In the worst-case scenario, the employee may need to be terminated. If this is the case, all the guidelines discussed in Chapter 7 should be followed.

■ THE EMPLOYEE EXPERIENCING EMOTIONAL OR PERSONAL PROBLEMS

The astute nursing manager recognizes that certain changes in the performance of an employee may be manifestations of emotional problems. Illness of a parent, problems with adolescent children, separation from a partner, and concerns about finances are but a few examples of personal concerns that can take on significant proportions, and, at times, interfere with work performance. It is important that the manager recognize and discuss these with the employee. It is equally important that the manager, after identifying the concerns, assist the employee to get professional help. The manager's role is not to attempt to provide the required counseling or other assistance needed to cope with the problem but rather to make the necessary referrals or connections. The manager needs to be supportive, understanding, and helpful. This is another instance in which an established employee assistance program or the employee health services area may be of help. If available, the problems can be referred to these areas. Let's once again review the example presented at the beginning of this chapter.

EXAMPLE *Resolving a Concern With an Employee*

You have met with Julie regarding her absences, dress, and patient complaints. A second meeting was scheduled as a follow-up. Since the first meeting, which occurred 1 month ago, three more absences have occurred. Julie appears at your office at the scheduled time. She looks more tired than a month ago and her dress is little improved. You review with her your previous conversation about concerns and tell her that the problem with absences is not improving. You indicate that she has only two more sick days left for the year and that you are concerned that her many absences are affecting staff morale and patient care. You advise her that if the behavior continues, more serious steps will need to be taken. Julie suddenly bursts into tears, and when she has regained some composure, tells you she is in a terrible situation. She started dating a man who moved in with her 3 months ago. Two months ago, he lost his job and seems not interested in really searching for another. He has become very jealous of the time Julie spends with her children or other friends and this has resulted in serious arguments. She states that on several occasions he has become so angry that he has physically attacked her, leaving bruises on her arms and body but not on her face. Julie states that is why she has taken the sick days and has started wearing the long-sleeved polo shirts. She states she is too frightened for herself and her children to kick him out, but she realizes the situation cannot continue as it is. You state that both she and her children deserve to be safe and that there is help in the community for her problem. You suggest that she immediately seek assistance through the local domestic violence project. You offer to dial the call and then step out of the room while she talks with the counselor. She accepts your offer, you dial, tell the person who answers that you have a colleague who needs their help and advice. You hand the phone to her and step out of the room.

Clearly, in situations such as the one detailed here, the problems of the employee are beyond anything for which the manager can provide adequate assistance. However, the manager does have an ethical obligation to direct the person toward appropriate resources.

In working with employees exhibiting symptoms of emotional illness, there are some similar constraints. Although a manager may suspect that an employee has a mental health problem, the manager's role is not to diagnose. The manager should focus on the behavior and the standards. If the employee indicates a mental health problem, the manager would then provide an appropriate referral and then consult with someone in the human resources department who is knowledgeable about how this fits into the employer obligations under the ADA.

■ THE IMPORTANCE OF THE COACHING ROLE

We discussed the importance of the coaching role in Chapters 5 and 7. We reemphasize it here because it has such significance in the management role. It is important that coaching be a part of a management style. That means that it is used in everyday activities, not just when there are problems. Coaching involves providing support and encouragement to employees. The manager acting as a coach should set a good example and recognize good work with praise that is provided in public. This role involves listening attentively and providing feedback. It involves letting people know what is going on and what you expect as a manager.

When working in a situation in which a problem exists, it is especially important that you are seen as trying to be helpful. Keep reminding yourself that you are trying to help someone improve. Although there may be some punitive steps to be followed at some point in the future, a caring attitude is important throughout. Show that you care. Be certain that the employee understands what you expect in terms of performance. Express your sincere concern about ways the individual must change in order to be successful and to meet those expectations.

Select the right time and place to discuss your concerns with the employee. There is an old adage that states, "Timing is everything," and this is certainly true in these situations also. Although nursing units have little downtime these days, typically, some of the best times to discuss concerns with employees on a nursing unit are during the late morning hours, right after lunch, or just before the end of the shift. If you believe that your comments are going to disturb and upset the employee, planning your meeting just before that employee would leave the unit for a break or for the end of the day might be desirable. Such meetings always must be held in a private place, such as an office, where interruptions can be avoided and privacy can be assured.

Avoid using language that is preachy or carries a judgmental impression. It is preferable to discuss the employee's behavior in relation to the standards that prevail, avoiding the use of such language as "You should have done. . . ." "Should" language often creates the impression that you are rigid or pedantic. Be sure that you communicate the message that your primary concern is helping the individual improve. Deal with the performance rather than with personalities or personal characteristics.

Give specific suggestions for change. If you are vague, the employee may not understand exactly what it is that you expect to change. You also leave yourself open to such comments as "She wants me to change, but she can't tell me what she really wants." Identify ways in which the employee will benefit from making the changes that you are expecting will occur. Your goal should be to motivate the employee to improve performance rather than threatening or challenging the individual. It is important to involve the employee in setting timelines and goals for change.

When the changes that you desire take place, it is also critical that you recognize this change and commend the employee for what has been accomplished. This recognition helps build self-reliance and self-esteem in the employee and results in the employee feeling more empowered and willing to seek others ways in which performance can be improved. All these result in more positive feelings about work and the work environment.

When the manager first realizes that a serious problem may exist requiring significant change, it is wise to contact the human relations department and the manager's immediate supervisor. Most contracts or policy manuals have sections that spell out the steps for dealing with disciplinary problems. By knowing and following the established protocols, the manager would be using correct evaluation procedures in order to avoid infringing on the employee's right to due process.

In addition, the people to whom the manager reports will wish to be aware of the problem if it is going to involve disciplinary procedures. The situation should be discussed with them and approval obtained before moving ahead. The administration will want to be certain that the disciplinary steps are carried out fairly and are legally defensible.

In summary, it is not easy to work with problem employees. Sometimes, little progress can be made. Other times, you will be limited in what you may do because of rules or regulations. You may experience frustration. It is helpful to remember that no one is perfect, and that includes you. If you find that you have mismanaged a situation, do not hesitate to apologize. Saying "I'm sorry" or "I'm sorry you feel this way" tends to express comfort and empathy when said sincerely. If you find yourself in an uncomfortable confrontation, heed your body messages. Little is accomplished when people are upset. It is best to defer taking any action until the situation has cooled and the involved individuals are calmer. As you continue to work with tough situations, you will find that the skills you will learn to use as a manager have some commonalities with the skills you learned to become a competent clinical nurse. For example, you will remember that the more you used the skills, the easier it became to perform the expected behaviors. Your self-evaluation of the manner in which you functioned was critical to improving your performance the next time. When you were in doubt about a particular way you should complete a task, you asked a more experienced person or researched the topic in a textbook. You gave yourself credit for things that went well and made a mental note to continue to use that approach in the future. These same approaches will serve you well in the interpersonal aspects of the management role just as they have as you worked to improve your clinical performance.

■ KEY CONCEPTS

- Some of the more challenging responsibilities a manager must deal with involve personnel problems. As with other skills, managing personnel concerns comes easier with experience.
- Managers must learn to deal with unpleasant confrontations. These take many forms and include dealing with anger, complaints, coercion, divided loyalties, and situations in which the manager is embarrassed or humiliated.
- Chemical dependency among nurses is growing. It is critical that managers are able to identify the problem, gather and analyze data related to it, meet with the employee, document all behavior and meetings, and complete a referral and follow-up. Many states now have programs to assist the chemically impaired employee.
- Clinical incompetence is a problem requiring that the manager exercise skill in the role of coach and counselor. In the interest of quality patient care, problems must not be brushed aside but must be dealt with openly and effectively.
- Employees who exhibit a high absentee record can significantly impact productivity of the unit. In working with the employee who has many absent days, the manager may have to come to terms with a difference in value systems. There are times when the best management of the situation is one involving damage control.
- A number of nonproductive employee behaviors can also create concerns for the manager. Some of the more common behaviors include the employee motivated by self-interest, the employee who is a doomsayer, the employee who demonstrates subversive behavior, the employee who is an accommodator, and the employee who is a superachiever.

■ The marginal employee is one whose work performance meets only the minimum established standards. There can be many causes for marginal performance and remediation begins with looking for the cause. The situation may be improved if the manager assumes a coaching role. Termination is the final alternative.

■ Managers must also be able to work with employees who have personal or emotional problems. Once the problems are identified, the manager should help the employee seek professional help with the concerns. Employee assistance programs can be of great help in these instances.

REFERENCES

Ashton, J. T., & Bay, J. (1994). Investigating narcotic diversion. *Nursing Management, 25*(3), 35–37.

Dabney, D. (1995). Workplace deviance among nurses. *Journal of Nursing Administration, 25*(3), 48–55.

Hughes, T. L., & Smith, L. L. (1994). Is your colleague chemically dependent? *American Journal of Nursing, 94*(9), 31–35.

Hrobak, M. L. (2002). *Narcotic Use and Diversion in Nursing* [Online]. Available at http://juns. nursing.arizona.edu/articles/Fall%202002/hrobak.htm.

Kosmoski, G. J., & Pollack, D. R. (2000). *Managing Difficult, Frustrating, and Hostile Conversations: Strategies for Savvy Administrators.* Thousand Oaks, CA: Corwin Press.

Landry, D. (1987). The impaired nurse. *California Nursing Review, 9*(6), 14–18.

Lee, J. B., & Eriksen, L. R. (1990). The effects of a policy change on three types of absence. *Journal of Nursing Administration, 20*(7/8), 37–40.

Leffler, D. (1986). Addicted nurses: how you can lend them a helping hand. *Nursing Life, 6*(3), 41–43.

Marion, L. N., Fuller, S. G., Johnson, N. P. et al. (1996). Drinking problems of nursing students. *Journal of Nursing Education,* 35(5), 196–203.

Navarra, T. (1995). Enabling behavior: the tender trap. *American Journal of Nursing, 95*(1), 50–52.

Smith, L. L., Taylor, B. B., & Hughes, T. (1998). Effective peer responses to impaired nursing practice. *Nursing Clinics of North America, 33*(1), 105–118.

Smith, L. L., Taylor, B. B., Keys, A. T. et al. (1997). Nurse–patient boundaries: crossing the line. *American Journal of Nursing, 97*(12), 26–31.

Sullivan, E., Bissell, L., & Leffler, D. (1990). Drug use and disciplinary actions among 300 nurses. *International Journal of the Addictions, 25*(4), 375–391.

Sullivan, E., Bissell, L., & Williams, E. (1988). *Chemical Dependency in Nursing: The Deadly Diversion.* Menlo Part, CA: Addison-Wesley.

Sullivan, E., & Decker, P. (2001). *Effective Leadership and Management in Nursing.* Upper Saddle River, NJ: Prentice Hall.

Trinkoff, A.M., & Storr, C. L. (1998). Substance abuse among nurses: differences between specialties. *American Journal of Public Health, 88,* 581–585.

Trossman, S. (2003). Nurses' addictions. *American Journal of Nursing, 103*(9), 27–28.

Videbeck, S. L. (2001). *Psychiatric Mental Health Nursing.* Philadelphia: Lippincott Williams & Wilkins.

Washington Health Professional Services. (1997). *A Confidential Program for Chemically Impaired Health Professionals* [Brochure], 6-25-97. Olympia, WA: Washington State Department of Health.

13

Nursing Informatics and Evidence-based Practice

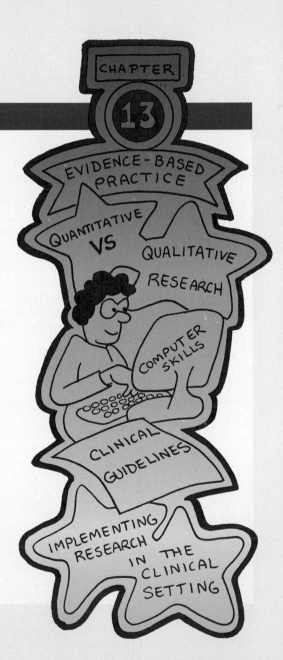

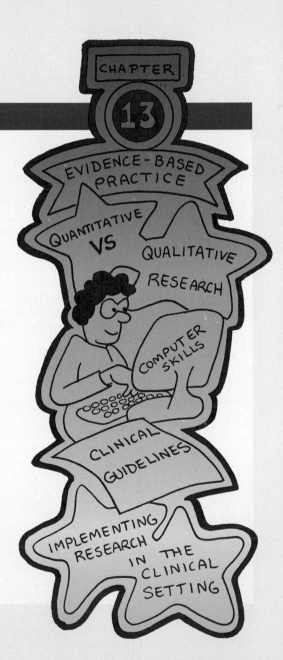

Learning Outcomes

After completing this chapter, you should be able to:

1. Discuss how nursing informatics affects today's nursing practice.
2. Evaluate yourself in relationship to competency in the core computer skills needed by nurses in the workplace: word processing, e-mail, spreadsheets, databases, bibliographic retrieval, the Internet, and the World Wide Web.
3. Explain the various types of information resources useful to nurses, the purpose of each resource, and strategies to access appropriate resources.
4. Describe a systematic analysis of information accessed for use in nursing practice.
5. Discuss what is meant by the term *evidence-based practice (EBP)*.
6. Explain the types of evidence used to support EBP in nursing.
7. Demonstrate a beginning understanding of research terminology.
8. Describe the characteristics of quantitative and qualitative nursing research.
9. Describe the legal ethical standards for safeguarding research subjects.
10. Apply a framework for understanding research reports that includes analysis of the steps of the research process.
11. Identify how research findings can be implemented in the clinical setting.

Key Terms ■ ■ ■ ■

abstract	Internet service provider	population
control group	(ISP)	probability
convenience sample	journal	qualitative
dependent variable	level of significance	quantitative
descriptive research	listserv	random sample
ethnography	maturation	reliability
evidence-based practice	MeSH	research
(EBP)	meta-analysis	research design
experimental group	mortality	samples
experimental research	newsgroup	selection
extraneous variables	null hypothesis	subject
findings	nursing informatics	subject headings
history	particpant	testing
hypothesis	peer reviewed	thesaurus
independent variable	phenomenology	validity

In many modern businesses there is an emphasis on creating more effective systems for many functions. Health care is no exception to this need for more effective systems. One major aspect of this is the emphasis on evidence as a basis for health care practice. This has become more possible as computer technology has enhanced communication, enabled information to be recorded in methods that allow for study and aggregation, and created mechanisms for all types of health information to be more broadly accessible. At present, nurses are expected to possess the skills that will allow them to use computers effectively and are challenged to consider the evidence on which they based their practice.

■ NURSING INFORMATICS

Nursing informatics is an emerging field related to the use of technology to retrieve and manage information relevant to nursing practice. Nursing informatics is part of a larger field of health care and medical informatics and is growing in importance as a mechanism to collect and analyze data from care that is occurring. Within the field of informatics, some individuals and groups are working on systems of terminology to help collect and compare data from different settings. Some groups are setting standards for the use of computer information systems in various health care set-

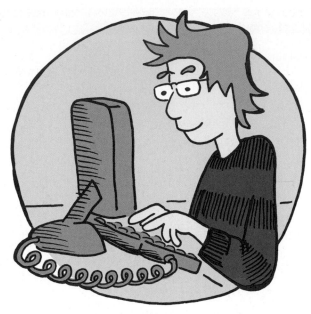

Nurses are being prepared to design and implement systems for nursing informatics.

tings. Individuals in informatics are working with health care agencies and systems as they establish and maintain computerized documentation systems.

Employers Expectations Regarding Information Technology Skills

As information technology becomes more widespread, nurses will need basic skills and an understanding of informatics to assure that they provide patients with the most up-to-date and appropriate care. Many hospital systems have developed integrated information systems that allow information from all sources—nursing, admissions, pharmacy, laboratory, therapy, billing, and so forth—to be combined into one computer system. This type of integrated system facilitates interdisciplinary cooperation and planning. Although long-term care facilities originally were slower to develop these systems, the prospective payment system that relies on comprehensive assessment data that must be submitted electronically for Medicare and Medicaid payment spurred a rapid move into computerization for long-term care.

To gain a greater understanding of the computer skills considered critical for nurses entering the nursing profession currently, two surveys were conducted that provided background on the information technology needs. Both the surveys revealed increasing expectations for nurses. Members of the American Association of Nurse Executives were asked about the software skills that are critical for new nurses as well as about the need for using a Windows operating system, searching the Internet, and using e-mail. All these skills were reported as critical for nurses entering today's workforce. Specific software that was seen as important included nursing-specific software such as bedside charting and computer activated medication systems. One area not seen as critical was the use of handheld computers for managing calendars and organizing time (McCannon & O'Neal, 2003).

As part of an information technology survey sent to nursing education programs, responders were asked to identify the information technology tools that were used by practicing nurses in their areas. They identified that the tools currently used most frequently are remote monitoring devices, online consumer health tools, and handheld computers (McNeil et al., 2003).

Strategic Directions for Nursing

In 1998, the National Advisory Council on Nurse Education and Practice of the Department of Health and Human Services, Division of Nursing recommended five strategic directions to enhance nurses' preparation to use and develop information technology (Gassert, 1998).

The first strategic direction was the inclusion informatics content in nursing curricula, one of the goals of this chapter. Nurses are being challenged to use effectively the technology currently available. Only with this type of use will nurses be able to function within the health care system of the future. Core computing skills have been identified, which include word processing, e-mail, spreadsheets, databases, bibliographic retrieval, the Internet, and the World Wide Web. Although some students enter with these skills, many do not, and therefore find it necessary to develop computer abilities. Most basic nursing programs include requirements for students to acquire many of these skills. Fifty percent or more of the nursing programs responding to a survey indicated that information technology skills are currently being taught (McNeil et al., 2003). However, many nurses in practice have not had opportunities to learn computer skills. Health care institutions are beginning to recognize the need to support the education of nurses in core computing skills.

The second strategy identified was the preparation of nurses with specialized skills in informatics. Nurses are being prepared at the master's degree level to design and implement systems for nursing informatics. With an interdisciplinary focus, the specialist in nursing informatics will help to systematize the nursing language, making data more retrievable and enhancing the ability to use the data to build aggregated information upon which practice decisions can be based. At present, there are many master's degree programs in nursing informatics, and specialists are available in major health care systems. Smaller agencies often rely upon self-taught individuals with an interest in the field.

The third strategy was the enhancement of nursing practice and education through informatics projects. The goal of the nursing informatics agenda is to fund innovative and collaborative projects that can be used as models for others. Projects may be of direct benefit to patients or may support decision making by health care professionals. Some informatics projects are being supported through grants.

The fourth strategy was increasing nursing faculty preparation in informatics. Faculty must first learn to use this technology before effectively teaching students to use it. A variety of approaches to this strategy have been proposed, such as independent study modules and the use of online technologies. Faculty with recent education have been required to develop these skills. Individuals whose formal education occurred before the advent of information technologies may have learned the skills on the job, but some still need to have support for upgrading their technological abilities. In the survey of nursing programs conducted by McNeil et al. (2003), 18% rated their faculty as novices, and 39% rated their faculty as advanced beginners; and in the area of information technology only 29% rated their faculty as competent, and 2% rated their faculty as experts. Clearly, progress is still needed in this strategic direction.

The fifth strategy was advancing nursing informatics by encouraging collaboration among individuals and organizations, both public and private. Collaboration can serve to stretch limited funds and advance the profession more rapidly.

■ USING COMPUTERIZED SYSTEMS WITHIN THE CARE SETTING

As almost all care settings are moving toward the use of computers for all health care information, nurses are challenged to explore new ways of working and documenting their practice. Computers are making it possible to audit records on an ongoing basis and provide feedback to care providers on the completeness of their documentation. Information retrieval may become easier and individual segments of data may be pooled to enable statistical analysis of the effectiveness of various practices in achieving desired patient outcomes. As nurses participate in these changes, it is imperative that there be thoughtful evaluation of how computer systems can contribute to quality of care rather than the computer system being the controlling force for practice.

Common Features of Computerized Documentation Systems

There are many companies creating computerized documentation systems, and some institutions create their own systems. An individual system may not incorporate documentation of all aspects of patient care; some aspects continue to be documented on paper forms. Although each computer documentation system is unique in the screens and entry expectations, all systems have some elements in common.

SECURITY SYSTEMS

To safeguard patient/client information as required under the Health Information Portability and Privacy Act (HIPPA), every computerized patient record system must have in place a wide variety of strategies for security. One of the most basic requirements is a computer server that is protected from outside access. Although nurses are not responsible for any aspect of this important patient protection, they should know that the institution has put safeguards in place in order to be able to assure patients who express concerns.

Passwords are assigned to each person who has a legitimate need to access information. Passwords usually restrict individuals to the information pertinent to their own role in the institution. For example, a nurse's password would not usually provide access to hospital billing records. Computer systems have in place tracking systems that identify when a particular password has been used and what information was accessed. The institution will track this information to identify when individuals are accessing information inappropriately. The inappropriate use of your computer password either by giving it to someone else or by using it to access information for which you do not have a legitimate need can result in disciplinary action and even termination from employment.

Automatic date and time records for all documentation are an important legal safeguard. This eliminates the forgotten date or time on a note in the patient record.

From a legal standpoint, it assures that time and date information is reliable. This feature also facilitates tracking computer entry and makes it possible to identify unauthorized entry.

BILLING SYSTEMS

Management of the financial and billing aspects of any health care institution has been computerized for many years. The federal programs of Medicare and Medicaid require that billing be done through computerized systems that communicate with the appropriate governmental agency. Both hospital and long-term care charges must be billed in this way. Once the federal government required this type of billing, most health plans also began requiring this. Using computerized systems for this large amount of data has brought both advantages and complexity to health care.

Several major systems (such as Pyxis) are available to health care institutions that require entering both patient information and a provider password into a computer in order to access supplies or medications. This means that no items can be taken without proper authorization and expenses can be attributed to the appropriate patient. In addition, these systems often make it possible to track expenses related to particular medical diagnoses or surgeries. This contributes to the overall financial planning of the institution.

PATIENT INFORMATION RETRIEVAL

Results of laboratory and diagnostic tests have been posted to computer records in many agencies. These results are then made rapidly available to those who need the information. Accessing this information may be critical to caring for some patients. A security concern arises when staff print out data to carry with them and do not recognize that this is protected health information under the federal HIPPA regulations. Data found on computers should not be routinely printed out unless the protocol in the facility is to print the data and place it in a written patient record.

ORDER ENTRY

Entry of physician's orders for medications, laboratory tests, diagnostic tests, and therapies is often one of the earliest aspects of nursing responsibilities to be put on the computer. The system may allow a unit secretary or clerk to do the initial data entry and then the nurse rechecks the information and submits it.

An increasing emphasis has been moving to provider entry of all orders. Although this has been slow to expand across systems, this may eliminate many sources of error, such as illegible handwriting, mistakes regarding abbreviations, and confusion over spelling of similar drug names. Some order entry systems can be used to create a more standardized order format, double-check available dosages forms, and remind physicians of parameters needed (such as laboratory tests to accompany certain drugs). Some physician now use handheld computers to create orders and download them to the hospital computer.

NURSING DATA ENTRY

Establishing data entry systems for nursing departments has often come near the end of a planned computerization of health care services. Nursing data is complex and with the large numbers of care providers providing access points is costly.

Many long-term care facilities have nurses complete assessment forms such as the minimum data set (MDS) and then have a data entry person in medical records enter the data in order to facilitate the computerized billing process. Because residents remain for a longer period of time and only periodic assessment must be entered, this has proven successful, especially for small facilities.

In an acute care facility, the large quantity of data that must be up-to-date means that for computerized data entry to be useful, it must be done by the care providers. Some facilities have provided multiple terminals at the nurses' station. These terminals may have both keyboard entry and entry with light pens or touch screens for information that appears on tables, charts, and items from which a person might choose from a list. In some systems the primary information appears on one screen; on others multiple screens are used to focus the nursing documentation. Narrative notes are entered on the keyboard. Some systems include an array of possible narrative notes that the nurse can copy and paste into a specific note. This is a time saver and tends to systematize the language used. An increasing number of hospitals are placing terminals at each bedside so that some information may be entered immediately. This also saves nursing time, because the nurse does not need to make separate notations on a piece of paper that must be rewritten on the actual patient record.

COMPUTERIZED MEDICATION ADMINISTRATION SYSTEMS

The Institute of Medicine has been encouraging all health care institutions to create safer systems for the administration of medications. One rapidly increasing approach to this is the computerization of all medication records along with bar coding of the medications and patient identification bands. When a medication is accessed for the patient, the barcode is used to read the label and verify that it is the medication on the medication administration record (MAR). In the patient room, the patient's identification band has a barcode that is read and must match the barcode reading on the medication itself. The medication administration is then automatically charted. If the MAR, medication label, and the patient identification do not match, an alarm is provided to alert the nurse to a potential error.

Other Computer Resources

Many agencies are adding to their computer systems resources that support staff decision-making. A computerized drug reference provides easy access to information on medications, actions, side effects, and administration. Computers may also make available similar references regarding diagnostic tests, including patient preparation and care after the test. Having the policy and procedure manual on the computer facilitates frequent updates without the need to reprint many copies. In this way a hospital can assure that each unit has access to the most current policies and procedures.

Some systems may allow access to the medical center library reference page. This creates easy access to searching the literature and requesting copies of articles needed. Some systems have access to digital copies of many journals that can be easily accessed from the unit.

■ ACCESSING INFORMATION RESOURCES

Skill in finding the information resources needed to support nursing care is critical to improving practice. Although computerized searches are especially useful, traditional means of accessing information through print indexes remain available in many places. Many different types of information resources are available to help you.

Texts and Reference Books

For students, the most familiar information resource may be textbooks and reference books in the field of nursing. As you progress in your career, you may use primarily books from a library, but you may want to purchase books that will be a major reference source in your area of clinical practice. You may encourage your agency to purchase reference books that are of particular relevance to your nursing unit, such as a reference on traction for an orthopedic unit. Medical dictionaries and drug references are essential for ongoing practice and many hospitals are making these available on the computer. Some nurses purchase electronic references that can be loaded onto a personal digital assistant (PDA). See the information given in the following regarding evaluating texts and references used in your practice.

Libraries as Resources

Libraries are a familiar source of information resources in which you may find additional books for reference as well as professional journals that will provide more up-to-date information. The availability of adequate library resources is a key support for excellence in nursing practice. Part of the challenge of using a library is finding the information you need from a wide array of sources. A library may have personnel who can help with your search for information, making it more time efficient.

Books not available on a nursing unit may be obtained from a library. To determine what books are available on the topic of interest to you requires that you understand the way books are catalogued or indexed. Although the card catalog may still exist in smaller libraries, larger libraries have been converting rapidly to computerized catalogs. Even bookstores are beginning to provide computerized book lists to facilitate customers to find the books they wish to purchase. A computerized catalog may allow you to search for books by **subject,** by title, or by author.

The most up-to-date information is usually found in journal articles. A **journal** is a professional periodical as opposed to a magazine, which is a general-interest periodical. This distinction is important when you are seeking professional-level references. Medical libraries at universities or large medical centers may be very extensive, with hundreds of journals available. Hospitals have medical libraries with a collection focused on the various aspects of care they provide. College libraries that are not part of research institutions may have a much more limited selection of health-related journals and books. The community library may carry a small selection of health and medical related periodicals. Small libraries may be able to obtain specific articles you need through an interlibrary loan. There may be a charge for this service. If you are fortunate enough to live near a university or medical center, you may be able to use their resources even if not employed or enrolled there.

Some journals have articles available online through Internet resources. Unfortunately, this is a small percentage of the available health care journals. However, **abstracts** of articles are frequently available online, which will allow you to screen potential resources to find the most appropriate ones before ordering them through interlibrary loan.

Some libraries subscribe to CD-ROM systems that distribute on a set of CD-ROMs the citation information, the abstract, and sometimes the full text of many journals along with a system for searching the information. CD-ROMs are updated periodically and are accessed from a library computer that has a multiple CD-ROM drive. Using a variety of subject, author, and title indexes, CD-ROMs can be searched. The article abstract or full-text article can be read when it is part of the service. When the full text is not available, the abstract can be used to determine whether the article is appropriate.

Policies and Standards as Resources

Individual agencies have policy manuals and procedure books as a quick reference for commonly used information. These documents are valuable for their purpose, but must be evaluated on an ongoing basis in relationship to current best practice because of the changing nature of health care. Some agencies are now making their policies available on the computer to assure that the latest information is always available.

Many organizations publish standards that are an excellent reference for care. Some of these are legal standards, such as those established for Medicare and Medicaid certification. Others are voluntary standards, such as the *Accreditation Manual* of the Joint Commission for the Accreditation of Health Care Organizations (JCAHO). When you are part of an organization that is seeking certification or accreditation, the *Accreditation Manual* is the most accurate reference in regard to those standards.

The Internet as a Resource

The *Internet* is a worldwide network of computers that provides rapid communication between distant sites. The origin of the Internet was the linking of major universities and defense installations so that messages could travel by many different routes between sites; therefore, disruption in one site or on one link is unlikely to disrupt the communication among all other sites.

Internet resources are often referred to as *online* resources because you must be connected to other computers by some kind of communication line. Access to the Internet may be provided at a work location, through an educational institution, at a library, or you may set up your own access by subscribing to a commercial **Internet service provider (ISP).**

Individuals commonly access their ISP through dial-up access. This requires having a device in their computer called a modem, which is capable of transmitting signals from the computer through a telephone line. The computer is then plugged into the telephone line. The computer is programmed to dial and connect into the ISP that links into the Internet. Access to an ISP also can be attained through hook-up to a cable system or through a DSL (digital subscriber line) telephone system connection. These systems provide much more rapid communication and are "on" all the time, eliminating the need to dial a number and wait for a computer to answer. There are many Internet service providers from which to choose. Educational institutions and research health care centers may be connected to the Internet by direct fiberoptic cable, which is much faster and more reliable than the connections available to individuals. The Internet offers access to information through e-mail, group discussions, and the World Wide Web. Each of these provides different opportunities for gaining information.

E-MAIL ACCESS

E-mail is shorthand for electronic mail. E-mail allows you to send and receive messages rapidly around the world. To send and receive e-mail, you must have a specific e-mail account with a provider and an e-mail address. Each provider of e-mail services has a designated name. Names that end with *.gov* are governmental agencies. Those ending with *.edu* are educational institutions. Names ending with *.com* are commercial companies. Names ending with *.org* are nonprofit organizations. Some clinical agencies provide all employees with e-mail access for professional purposes. In these agencies, general communication with employees occurs through the e-mail account rather than through paper memos.

Through e-mail you may contact experts in the field, ask specific questions of manufacturers regarding the use of their products, seek answers to questions from governmental agencies, and simply share information with other health care professionals. These same communications can be completed in regular, written correspondence sent by the post office (sometimes referred to humorously as "snail mail") or by telephoning. The advantage of e-mail is the rapidity of the message exchange and the ease with which you may ask the same question of many different people simultaneously. Directions for using e-mail are specific to the various software programs that may be used. E-mail is necessary to participate in group discussions on the computer. It is possible to have e-mail access without having access to the World Wide Web.

GROUP DISCUSSIONS ONLINE Blogs

Group discussions online are a means for many individuals to send and receive messages from a large number of people with a similar interest. In an editorial on the value of online communities of professional practice, Billings (2003) discussed how these environments can enhance communication and the dissemination of the best in nursing practice. She suggests that all who participate become learners, whatever their formal roles. These communities may be formed in a variety of ways.

A **listserv** is a type of group discussion conducted by e-mail messages. To join a listserv, the individual subscribes to the computerized distribution list. A subscription fee may be charged to join the list, but many online listservs are free. The membership in the listserv may be limited to a specific group of people who need to share information. A computer is programmed to manage the list, adding new subscribers and deleting those who unsubscribe. All individuals send their discussion topics, questions, and comments to the address of the listserv by e-mail. The listserv computer then sends the e-mail message to everyone subscribed to the list. In a moderated list, a designated moderator reviews each message to determine whether it is appropriate for posting to the list. Many lists are unmoderated, which means that all messages received are forwarded to all subscribers.

The person who controls the listserv site is called the owner. This person oversees the e-mail address list of subscribers and usually keeps an archived copy of the messages. An archived copy is a permanent copy kept in a specific computer location. Often, the archived messages can be searched for topics of interest. The owner may also compile a list of frequently asked questions (FAQs) with their answers that a newcomer to the list may review so as not to burden others with questions that have already been answered on the listserv. The general topic of the listserv may be as broad as "nursing" or as narrow as one for the nurse legal consultant.

A **newsgroup** is another type of group discussion. Each newsgroup is focused on a specific topic. In a newsgroup, you need not subscribe to the service. Your Internet access provider may make a variety of newsgroups available to you. Individuals may send messages to the newsgroup where the messages are posted. You can review any of the groups at any time to determine whether there is information pertinent to your needs, but you will not receive individual messages.

If you participate in group discussions, you should take time to familiarize yourself with what is called "netiquette" (Internet etiquette). Netiquette is simply trying to be respectful of the time, effort, computer space, and feelings of others. Some key points are listed in Display 13-1.

Critical Thinking Exercise

Identify a listserv or newsgroup that would be of value to a practicing nurse. Subscribe to that service for at least 1 month. Analyze the messages over this month. Report to your class on the types of questions discussed on this forum. Evaluate the responses to questions that have been posed.

WORLD WIDE WEB

The *World Wide Web* (often referred to simply as "the Web") is a use of the Internet for the connection of computers that all use a common protocol for information exchange. A *Web site* is a computer file that resides on a computer connected into the Internet. A Web site may house multiple Web pages. A special software program called a Web browser, such as Netscape, Windows Explorer, or Mosaic, is necessary to view the graphics on a Web site. Any individual with access to the Web may create and operate a Web site that anyone else can access as long as the Web site computer is turned on and connected. Web sites have become popular because of the ease with which they may be accessed from a home computer. Most Web sites have free access, but some charge a fee and then require a special password for subscribers to access the site.

A search engine is a World Wide Web site that offers a computerized search of the Web. See Display 13-2 for a list of search engines. All have directions that assist you in entering your search terms. A site that is deemed to match your search terms is called a hit. One problem you may encounter after entering your search terms is that you may get hundreds of hits. Some search engines make it easier for you to use several terms in combination in order to make the hits more relevant and to limit the number. Different search engines use differing techniques for seeking relevant Web sites. Therefore, you may find that one search engine meets your professional needs better than another.

DISPLAY 13-1	**Suggestions for Internet Communication**

- Remember that all e-mail is potentially public, and therefore you need to take care with the content of your messages.
- Excessive e-mail becomes burdensome; therefore, be careful when your purpose is to reply to an individual that you do not reply to an entire group.
- The brief nature of e-mail may make communication seem more brusque or even rude than you intend; therefore, consider your wording carefully. The use of emoticons (typing symbols used to represent feelings) such as :) for a smile or ;) for a wink may clarify your intent.
- Do not routinely copy messages back to the originator when you reply unless the original message is needed to make your response clear. Especially avoid recopying other messages to groups simply to say "Me too." This takes space on computer servers and clutters the screen for readers.
- Most group discussions online frown on using them for commercial advertising of any sort.
- If the group has posted a resource of frequently asked questions (FAQs) be sure to review those before asking questions of the group.

See Display 13-3 for a list of specific Web sites of interest to health care providers. Many of these sites provide *links* to other sites. A link is an embedded computer command that moves you to another Web site by simply clicking on a designated word or graphic on the screen. A link is a simple way to move from one site of interest to another that has a related topic. When you have found a site of value, you can usually save the Web address of that site in your program making it easy to return. Journal articles may also provide a list of Web sites relevant to the journal's area of focus.

DISPLAY 13-2	**Selected Search Engines for Use on the Internet**

TITLE	ADDRESS
Altavista	http://www.altavista.digital.com
Excite	http://www.excite.com
Google	http://www.google.com
InfoSeek	http://www.infoseek.com
Lycos	http://www.lycos.com
Webcrawler	http://www.webcrawler.com
Yahoo	http://search.yahoo.com

DISPLAY 13-3	**Selected Internet Sites for Nursing Resources**

TOPIC	ADDRESS
Federal Sites	
Agency for Health Care Policy and Research— clinical guidelines	http://www.ahcpr.gov
Centers for Disease Control and Prevention	http://www.cdc.gov
National Institute of Neurological Disorders and Stroke	http://www.ninds.nih.gov
National Institutes of Health	http://www.nih.gov
National Library of Medicine	http://www.nlm.nih.gov
Occupational Safety and Health Administration	http://www.osha.gov
Cancer	
Association of Cancer Online Resources	http://www.acor.org
National Cancer Institute	http://cancernet.nci.nih.gov
Directories of Health-Related Internet Sites	
AIDS Info Bulletin Board Database	http://aidsinfobbs.org
CINAHL Sources	http://cinahl.com/csources.index.htm
Hardin Meta Directory	http://www.lib.uiowa.edu/hardin/md/ idx.html
Healthfinder	http://healthfinder.gov
Healthweb	http://healthweb.org
Medical Matrix	http://www.medmatrix.org/index.asp
Human anatomy	http://www.InnerBody.com
Nursing Organizations	
American Nursing Informatics Association	http://www.ania.org
National Health Information Center (referrals to organizations and sites)	http://nhic-nt.health.org
National Council of State Boards of Nursing	http://www.ncsbn.org
National League for Nursing	http://www.nln.org
NursingNet	http://www.nursingnet.org
Nursing World (ANA)	http://www.nursingworld.org
Sigma Theta Tau	http://stti-web.iupui.edu
Publishers	
Elsevier (Mosby and Saunders)	http://www.us.elsevier.com
Lippincott Nursing Center	http://www.nursingcenter.com
Medical articles and columns Medscape	http://www.medscape.com
Prentice Hall Publishers	http://vig.prenhall.com/catalog/academic/ discipline/0,4094,2341,00.html
Slack Publishers	http://www.slackinc.com/idirectories/ nursenet-w.htm

Critical Thinking Exercise

Choose a health problem and search on the World Wide Web for sites that would be useful for clients to learn more about that health problem. Make a list of the sites, including the address, the sponsor, a summary of what is available at the site, and an evaluation of the site. Use the criteria in the chapter for your evaluation.

■ HEALTH CARE INDEXES FOR FINDING INFORMATION RESOURCES

Finding the specific information that you need requires library reference skills. Indexes to the health care literature are the primary means to find resources. Each has developed a set of **subject headings** under which articles are indexed. These subject headings reflect the terminology in use by the discipline and are gathered together in the subject heading list or **thesaurus** for the index. Some indexes also have articles indexed by author. Most computerized indexes index articles by a wide variety of categories in addition to specifically identified subjects. Each health care index has specific instructions available to facilitate your effective search.

Indexes Available

Two of the most common indexes used by nurses are MEDLINE, produced by the National Library of Medicine (NLM), and CINAHL (Cumulative Index for Nursing and Allied Health Literature) produced by the CINAHL corporation. Both of these are available in print and computerized forms. The International Nursing Index, RNdex, Hospital Literature Index, Psych Index, and Social Sciences Index are other commonly used indexes that would reference articles and books pertinent to nursing practice. Many libraries subscribe to computerized databases such as *Ebsco* and *Proquest*, which provide citations, abstracts, and some whole articles.

Many journals publish annually their own indexes to the articles that have appeared in their journals. For example, *RN* and *Nursing Education Perspectives* each provides a useful list of its articles annually, although the indexes are more limited in scope. Some publishers provide a Web site that contains indexes, tables of contents, and some full-text articles of journals they publish. Lippincott Nursing Center Online at http://www.nursingcenter.com is one such source. Some indexes are available in print forms only, but increasing numbers are available either online by subscription or on CD-ROM.

MEDLINE is a government-sponsored service of the NLM that indexes a wide variety of biomedical journals, videos, and other resources from throughout the world. In addition, selected articles from general-purpose journals such as *Science* are indexed. As a print index, MEDLINE is published as *Index Medicus*, which is generally found in the reference section of a medical library. Because the complete *Index Medicus* involves many volumes and includes non-English resources as well as English resources, many libraries choose to subscribe to the *Abbreviated Index Medicus*, which is a smaller index to more commonly available resources.

MEDLINE is also available as a computerized online data source in many libraries and to anyone who has access to the World Wide Web. There is no charge for accessing MEDLINE at the NLM. Direct MEDLINE access is available at the Web site http://www.nlm.nih.gov. Each article in the various journals indexed by the NLM is reviewed by experts for the subject matter of the article. The *subject headings* used for this indexing are **MeSH** (medical subject heading) terms. In addition, each article is indexed by author, title, date, name of journal, language, type of article (**research,** editorial, other), and other bibliographic data.

CINAHL focuses on nursing and allied health journals, all publications of the American Nurses Association (ANA) and National League for Nursing (NLN), conference proceedings, standards of nursing practice, nurse practice acts, state nursing journals, and consumer health materials, as well as nursing dissertations and research projects. CINAHL also indexes media resources for nursing, such as videos, computer-assisted learning programs, and films. CINAHL uses MeSH terms for disease-related topics, but also includes nursing-related terms for subject headings. Nursing diagnoses, nursing interventions, and nursing outcomes are included as subject headings in CINAHL. CINAHL designates both major and minor subjects included in the publication as well as other categories, such as author or date, that are used by MEDLINE. CINAHL is also available online through the World Wide Web by subscription at http://www.cinahl.com.

Critical Thinking Exercise

Choose a specific disease entity, an age group, and a gender. By using a computerized literature search database (such as MEDLINE or CINAHL), find a list of references of articles published within the last 5 years. Identify how many articles you originally found. Print a list (or copy a list from the computer screen if you cannot print) of the article citations you believe would be the most relevant to nursing care.

Techniques for Effective Searching of Indexes

Both *Index Medicus* and CINAHL in print have two indexing systems in each volume. You may look up information by subject or by author. To search for the same subject in multiple years, you would need to search in each volume of the index. Articles are listed under more than one subject heading when that is appropriate to the content. The *thesaurus* for the index is a list of the subject headings used for indexing purposes. Consulting the thesaurus will help you determine what terminology might be used for indexing a subject that is of interest to you.

Searching any print index allows you to look for only one subject heading or author in the index for 1 year at a time. By using a computerized or CD-ROM search, you can combine subject terms and author names, designate specific time frames, specify journals or languages to be searched, and use a variety of other techniques to make your search more exactly fit your needs. Some computerized searches allow you to use *connectors* to make your search more precise, such as the words *and, or,* and *not.* For example, you might search for diabetes *and* children *and* nursing. This would indicate that you wanted articles that pertained to all these in one article and that you were neither interested in articles that did not discuss children with diabetes nor in articles about research into insulin, because that would not be indexed as nursing.

In addition, computerized searches can search for key words that might be found in the title or abstract of the article instead of through indexed subject headings. Searching for key words instead of subject headings is easy but will produce many more hits, of which many may not relate to your needs. For example, a key word search will not differentiate between a word that occurs as an incidental part of an abstract and the same word when it is a major subject of the article.

Part of the skill needed to use indexes effectively lies in understanding the ways in which publications are indexed. Some programs used for searching have easy-to-use menus to construct searches. In others, more knowledge of the basic structure of the index is needed to make the most effective search. A health sciences librarian can be of great assistance in helping you learn to search for information resources.

Critical Thinking Exercise

Identify a nursing diagnosis in which you are interested. Use at least two computerized literature search systems to gather a list of citations for articles that provide information on this nursing diagnosis. Were different articles found on the two systems? Compare the two systems in relationship to the ease of finding relevant articles. Analyze your results and identify which system you would recommend for this purpose.

■ EVIDENCE-BASED PRACTICE

Many definitions of **evidence-based practice (EBP)** for nursing have been suggested. The definition by Goode and Piedalue (1999, p.15) encompasses the broad view most commonly used: "Evidence-based clinical practice involves the synthesis of knowledge from research, retrospective or concurrent chart review, quality improvement and risk data, international, national, and local standards, infection control data, pathophysiology, cost effectiveness analysis, benchmarking data, patient preferences, and clinical expertise."

Background

Evidence-based medicine (EBM) was the original approach to the use of evidence in health care. It originated during the 1980s, when the McMaster Medical School coined the term and began emphasizing the importance of data-based studies and research over authority opinions to guide decisions about medical therapy (Rosenberg & Donald, 1995). Evidence-based medicine is defined as "the conscientious, explicit, and judicious use of current best evidence in making decisions about the care of an individual patient. The practice of evidence-based medicine means integrating individual clinical expertise with the best available external clinical evidence from systematic research" (Sackett et al., 1996, p. 71). Sorting through the myriad of detail available regarding diagnosis and treatment of disease has always been complex; advances in medical science make it even more challenging. EBM is focused on identifying the specific therapy to be used for a specific medical diagnosis. After the evidence has been evaluated and the best practice determined, the next step is to disseminate the information and affect medical practice in a broad way.

In the United States, one of the earliest groups that attempted to support systematic use of the best available practices was the Agency for Health Care Policy and Research (AHCPR), now the Agency for Healthcare Quality and Research (AHQR). This federal agency formed expert panels to systematically review the literature and make recommendations for overall health care practice in relationship to broad problem areas that were of particular concern in the health care system. These problems included pressure ulcers, surgical pain, incontinence, and others. The work of these panels resulted in a series of guidelines that were published and distributed free of charge and made available on the Internet at www.ahpr.gov. Each of these guidelines identifies the type of evidence used in decision making by the expert panel. Many of these guidelines also provided direction for nursing practice.

The Centers for Disease Control and Prevention also make recommendations regarding infection control. The agency bases its recommendations on a variety of evidence that is weighted for use in decision making.

As nurses consider evidence-based nursing practice they must understand some basic premises. Much of the data that EBM has relied on involve multiple randomized controlled trials of therapies. These types of studies are rare in nursing, in which the phenomena of interest are often much more global and related to quality of life. The quality-of-life aspects of health are less amenable to a traditional research study. For this reason, nursing scholars have supported the view that the scientific, experimental way of knowing is only one of the ways of studying and understanding nursing practice. Therefore, nursing experts encourage the use of a variety of types of evidence, as is indicated in the definition of EBP given previously.

Types of Evidence Used

Many different types of evidence are used to support health care practice, which are presented in the following, moving from the type considered the most reliable to the type that is less reliable. Remember that for any given health care action there may be limited evidence (see Display 13-4).

DISPLAY 13-4	**Sources of Evidence for Evidence-based Practice**

Research
Retrospective or concurrent chart review
Quality improvement and risk data and benchmarking
International, national, and local standards
Infection control data
Pathophysiology
Cost-effectiveness analysis
Patient preferences
Clinical expertise

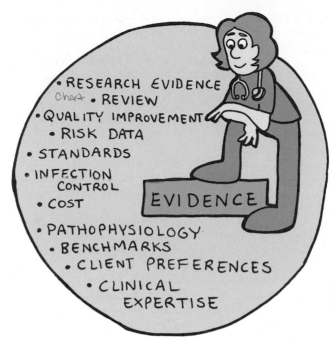

Many types of evidence are used to support health care practices.

Most experts consider the well-designed double-blind experiment (often referred to as the randomized control trial) the best type of evidence. Although this type of study is appropriate for medications and major medical treatments, it is not feasible for many aspects of care; therefore, there are few studies in nursing of this nature. Another type of evidence is found in research studies that have fewer controls. Some of these types of studies are included in the discussion of reading research. The Centers for Disease Control and Prevention identify these types of research evidence as the most important in devising their guidelines for disease and injury prevention and control (Centers for Disease Control, 1992).

Retrospective or concurrent chart reviews, quality improvement and risk data, and benchmarking data were discussed in Chapter 4. Aggregating data across an institution or several institutions provides an opportunity to assess how well current practices are working. Determining patient outcomes for large groups provides a firm foundation of data that, although not part of a research study, can guide practice. Individual health care institutions and health plans are compiling information for statistical analysis and making decisions about health care based on these statistical measures. For example, when a health maintenance organization analyzes its data on compliance with preventive care by those with a chronic illness, the data may reveal that depression has been a major barrier to effective participation in self-care. Based on this evidence, the plan then institutes training of health care professionals in assessing for depression in people with chronic illness and setting up protocols for treatment.

International, national, and local standards bring together the opinions and expertise of many health care providers. The standards are based on the collective experience and goals of individuals who are intimately involved with health care practice. Individuals who have worked with many patients, seen the results of multiple trials, and identified at first hand the complexity of the care have a special insight into effective practice. Because of this involvement and knowledge, the standards provide guidance and support for practice.

Because infection remains a major complicating factor in health care, infection control data assume major importance as guide for practice. The incidence of infection is of critical importance to both the patient and the entire system in terms of its impact on overall health outcomes. Practices that decrease the potential for infection have high priority.

Modern understanding of pathophysiology at even the cellular level has changed thinking about many health care practices. As this knowledge grows, it is used as a basis for deductive reasoning regarding the initiation of health care practices and the evaluation of proposals.

Information regarding cost-effectiveness analysis helps an institution weigh possible benefits against costs. It compares how much improvement a certain practice makes versus how much that practice costs. Sometimes changes are so slight that they are not reasonable to institute.

Patient preferences are gaining in importance. As we recognize the importance of self-care in managing health and illness, practices to which patients will adhere and ones that make their lives simpler are more likely to be incorporated. For example, one of the factors that often interferes with the willingness of patients with diabetes to check their blood glucose level frequently during the day is the discomfort and inconvenience associated with this process. New devices that allow smaller samples to be used and that can be taken from the forearm rather than from the fingertip may be more expensive, but if they result in greater adherence to treatment and thus fewer complications, the devices may be worth the cost. Failure to take into consideration patient preferences may make the best-designed therapy ineffective.

Opinions of clinical experts remain an important aspect of evidence. Individuals who have worked with many patients, seen the results of multiple trials, and identified at first hand the complexity of the care have a special insight into effective practice. Their collective wisdom creates an opportunity for improved practice.

■ READING RESEARCH

"Nursing research is a form of systematic search for knowledge about issues of importance to nurses" (Polit & Hungler, 1997, p. 5). Like management, research is an area that beginning nurses sometimes feel is not directly related to their patient care practice. In reality, all nurses need to appreciate and read research if they are to practice safely and effectively. The importance of research is emphasized in the Standards of Clinical Nursing Practice of the ANA.

By becoming more knowledgeable about research, learning to identify clinical problems that can be addressed by research, and applying research **findings** to practice, nurses can gain the benefits of this process, and, in addition, can contribute to the development of nursing knowledge.

Understanding Research Terminology

Nurses sometimes fail to use research findings, because the findings are difficult to interpret unless the nurse has a basic understanding of research language. A nurse need not be a statistician or a doctorally prepared nurse researcher in order to use research information. All nurses should have a basic understanding of research terminology.

Just as you initially learned health care terminology and now find it easy to read patient records, learning research terminology will facilitate your reading of research reports. Although in-depth knowledge and advanced education are needed to design and conduct research, reading research can become comfortable and useful for any nurse.

ABSTRACT

An **abstract** is a brief synopsis of the contents of the article. A well-written abstract tells you about the purpose of the study, gives a brief description of the population of interest, mentions the methodology used, and indicates the overall results. Reading an abstract carefully will enable you to determine whether the research is relevant to your needs. Those familiar with research publications often read many abstracts but focus their in-depth reading on a few well-chosen articles that address their specific practice area.

RESEARCH QUESTION AND PURPOSE

The research question or problem is the concern that researchers are attempting to answer through the research study. This question might be as simple as "Where do parents learn of the immunization recommendations for their children?" The clarity of the question helps the reader to have a clear picture of the purpose of the research. Sometimes a question is not provided, but instead a statement of purpose is given. This might be stated as "The purpose of this study is to learn the various sources of immunization information that parents report using." Some studies provide both a broad statement of purpose and one or more specific research questions.

HYPOTHESIS

The **hypothesis** is a statement of a relationship between variables that the research study is designed to test. There are two different types of hypotheses. The first, more traditional one is called the **null hypothesis.** In this statement, the researcher suggests that there is not a relationship, and the purpose of the study is to falsify (find false) that statement of no relationship. An example of a null hypothesis would be "There will be no relationship between parents' knowledge about immunization and the immunization status of their children."

Although meaningful in terms of planning for statistics, many readers find the null hypothesis quite confusing. Therefore, many articles are written using a research hypothesis. This is a statement of the relationship that researchers expect to find based on their study of previous research. In the research hypothesis, the author states explicitly the kind of relationship expected, based on the research of the literature. An example of a research hypothesis would be "The immunization knowledge level of the parents will be positively related to the immunization status of their children."

POPULATION VERSUS SAMPLE

The entire group of people who have the problem or would be affected by the question of concern is termed **population.** A study of the treatment of pressure ulcers might be trying to find answers for every person who has a pressure ulcer—this is the population.

Because it is not possible to obtain information about an entire population, researchers select a representative group, called a **sample,** to study. The researchers make inferences about the population based on this sample. The degree to which the sample, or selected group, can provide information about the population from which it is drawn depends on how similar to, or how representative of, the population the sample is. To study immunization status of children in relationship to their parent's immunization knowledge, you might study parents of children coming to a particular day care center.

Each member of the sample is called a **participant** or a **subject.** Although the term *subject* has been used for many years, there is increasing emphasis on acknowledging the autonomy and value of those who are in the study by using the term *participant*. Specific criteria are established regarding who will be asked to be a participant in the study.

Obviously, the way in which each participant is chosen is very important. Researchers generally like to choose participants randomly (totally by chance) from the population and then assign participants to comparison groups by the process of randomization (without definite aim or intent). A **random sample** is considered the most representative, because each member of the population has a potential for being included in the sample and each participant in the sample has an equal chance of being in any group. This means that any differences between the groups are due to chance. Obtaining random samples and assigning individuals to groups on a random basis may be very difficult or even impossible in health care settings. Therefore, a variety of other approaches to selecting and sorting participants may be used.

A **convenience sample** is composed of those whose participation may be "conveniently" obtained. This is often through volunteers. When volunteers are requested, the sample may be biased by the traits that make individuals interested in volunteering. In a study of immunization, parents who are interested in participating in a study might be the parents who felt they would appear in a good light because their children were immunized. Parents declining to participate might be those who had not carried through on immunization recommendations.

A particular concern is the lack of minority groups in many samples. Minority individuals often have less trust in the system because of past unethical treatment and are reluctant to trust researchers. Another aspect is that convenience samples are often sought in places where there are fewer minority individuals, such as the campuses of research universities. When minority groups are not included in samples, then the information obtained may not apply to the health problems of minorities. There is increasing evidence that genetic factors contribute to response to drugs and other therapies. Members of minority groups share many genetic factors within the group that may differ from genetic factors in majority groups.

When a particular population at the location at which the research is being conducted is too small to effectively sort on a random basis, a sample that includes all the clients admitted for the particular problem may be used. This is still a sample if they are being used to represent all the individuals with that problem regardless of the institution to which they are admitted. This same group is the entire population if you intend that results will be used in the one institution only.

GROUPS

Members of the sample are often divided into two or more groups that will be treated differently. Having more than one group allows the researcher to make comparisons and to evaluate the effect of the **independent variable** (e.g., a treatment or intervention) on the **dependent variable** (the phenomenon of interest). One group, the **experimental group,** can be exposed to the intervention, whereas the other, the **control group,** is not. The function of the control group is to help the researcher determine that the change in the experimental group is due to the intervention. For example, if our immunization study was being designed to include a teaching component and then check on the children's immunization levels 1 year later, those volunteering to participate might be randomly assigned to one of two groups: one group would receive the teaching intervention and one group would not. Many nursing studies cannot be carried out in the classical experimental way, because people cannot be subjected to harmful interventions and helpful interventions cannot be withheld.

VARIABLE

The term *variable* is used to describe something in the environment that varies or changes. Independent variables are those variables that vary by themselves or that can be caused to vary. The dependent variable is that which changes as a result of the independent variable. In our immunization study, teaching would be an independent variable.

Other variables are known as **extraneous variables.** These are variables that might also affect the dependent variable and could confuse the relationship between the independent and dependent variables. Extraneous variables might include such things as previous life experience or family relationships. For our parents, personal experience with having a preventable communicable disease might be an extraneous variable that would affect their response.

VALIDITY AND RELIABILITY

Validity is defined as the degree to which an assessment tool actually measures what it is supposed to measure. When a physical measure is used, such as temperature, validity refers to whether the device being used accurately measures temperature. This validity is easy to determine. When questionnaires are used, determining validity is more problematic. A set of questions measuring perceived stress might have responses from 0 to 6 for each item. A total score is obtained by adding the scores for each question. Validity refers to whether the person with a higher score actually has more stress than the person with the lower score. Is this questionnaire really measuring stress? Much work goes into determining whether any given instrument is valid. For some types of measuring, a group of experts is asked to examine the tool and give its opinion as to whether it is measuring what it says it measures. A new tool can be used along with an older, established tool as a basis for validity. In our immunization study, we would have to measure knowledge level about immunizations. This would require some type of test. We would also need to have a way to measure immunization status of the children. Would we use a verbal report by the parents? This might not be valid (a true measure), because some parents might be forgetful and some might not be truthful. Would we require copies of medical records? These might be accurate, but what if the child received an immunization in a school program and this does not appear in the medical record? These are the types of questions that must be considered to determine validity.

Reliability is defined as the degree of consistency or dependability with which an assessment tool measures something. If an assessment tool is reliable, it will produce the same results when used again or in different circumstances. A glass thermometer is very reliable. Time after time it will measure temperature accurately. However, if untrained people are reading the thermometer, the reliability of the reported temperature goes down. Reading a glass thermometer is a learned skill. A questionnaire that provides accurate information when used with a person reading and explaining the questions may not provide accurate information if people are asked to complete it independently.

PROBABILITY AND STATISTICAL TESTS

Probability refers to the likelihood that something will happen. In research reports, we are interested in the likelihood that a result is due to chance variation rather than to the interaction of the dependent and independent variables. Through the use of statistical techniques, the researcher can identify the probability that the observed result is due to chance variation. This is generally stated in the form of a mathematical expression. For example, $p > 0.10$ means that there is less than a 10 in 100, or 10%, probability that this result could be explained by chance. A 10% level of chance is quite high and would not be considered very good evidence for the results of the study being useful.

Another term associated with probability is the **level of significance.** This is a level of probability chosen by the researcher that identifies what will be judged to be meaningful in the context of the study. Frequently used levels of significance are 0.05 and 0.01. The first means that the probability is less than 5 out of 100 that the result was due to chance. The second means that only one time in 100 events of this type could the result be expected to be due to chance rather than to the interaction of the dependent and independent variables. This latter is considered more significant. When researchers speak of "significant" findings, they are referring to results with statistical evidence of a low probability that the result was due to chance.

Readers of research reports will also find references to statistical tests. Statistical tests are used to determine the probability of the results. Each statistical test has a different purpose and can be used only when specific criteria are met. In the research report, the researcher generally gives both a figure for the test result itself and a figure for the level of probability. This allows the researcher and the reader to make judgments about the hypotheses.

In addition to statistical tests for probability, additional figures are reported in most research reports. These figures are easier for the beginning reader of research to understand. They include the following:

■ The mean or average score of subjects on the variables examined
■ The range of scores from the highest to the lowest
■ The standard deviation (SD)

The mean and range are measures with which most individuals are familiar. The SD is a mathematical statement that provides information on how much those in the sample tend to vary from the mean. A high SD would mean that a large number of participants were considerably below or above the mean. A low SD would mean that more participants were close to the mean. This is important information for readers of research reports. If the group to whom you wish to apply the research findings is not similar to the group studied, the results may be quite different. Information on the mean, range, and SD helps readers make judgments about the applicability of the results to their own settings.

Beginning readers of research reports who have not yet had course work in statistics can still understand the implications of the research findings by reading the researchers' interpretation of findings. In the following sections, the various statistical tests are interpreted.

CLINICAL SIGNIFICANCE

Clinical significance refers to whether a result produces clinically important change in the participants. There is a difference between statistical level of significance and clinical significance. A result can be statistically significant without producing clinically important changes. In a study of bladder decompression, nurses found that there were statistically significant changes in blood pressure and heart rate in patients whose bladders were emptied at one time as compared with patients whose bladders were emptied by stages. However, these changes had little clinical significance. Both blood pressure and pulse normally go up and down based on such things as exercise and excitement. These changes are not a problem. In the same way, the changes in blood pressure and pulse that occurred when the bladder was rapidly emptied were not a problem.

The Research Process

Like the nursing process and the scientific method, the research process itself has discrete steps that may vary according to the type of research done. Understanding what the steps entail and why they are important will facilitate your understanding of research reports. A typical research study might have the following steps.

STATEMENT OF THE PROBLEM/QUESTION

The first step in the process is the identification of or statement of the problem. This is often stated as a question to be answered. This might seem to you to be self-evident: What you want to know is the statement of the problem. Frequently, however, what we want to know is too general to be properly researched, and the first task of the researcher is to define and state the problem carefully.

REVIEW OF LITERATURE

This is a step that beginning researchers often feel is less important than getting to the task at hand. However, becoming familiar with what is already known about the problem, including what other investigations have been done and what populations have been studied, can save the researcher much time and effort. Previous studies can also help the researcher identify an appropriate way to carry out the study and reveal useful measurement instruments. Another important reason for reviewing what has been done is so that the planned research can be constructed in an orderly way to add to the development of nursing knowledge. It is the responsibility of all nurse researchers to relate their investigations to the established body of nursing knowledge and to the work being done by other researchers.

THEORETICAL FRAMEWORK

The third step assists the researcher further to relate this specific study to established knowledge. Development of the theoretical framework requires the researcher to set the stage for the particular project. It defines the way in which the researcher views nursing and the particular problem to be investigated. In research reports, the reader will often find a discussion of a particular nursing theory and how it relates to the planned research. Such linking of research to theory helps connect the various investigations into a fabric that can help nurses understand better not only the problem currently studied but the larger realm of nursing as well.

REFINING THE PLAN

The fourth, fifth, and sixth steps in the research process are identification of variables, formation of hypotheses, and selection of **research design,** respectively. It is at this stage that the methods of the study are identified. The fourth step involves clearly identifying the specific dependent variable to be studied. Often, it is hard to identify the specific elements that might be causing the change in the dependent variable. Nursing is a complex activity, and it is challenging to identify the most important variables without eliminating others that might significantly influence the variable of interest. Once the variables have been ascertained, the researcher must identify what he or she believes is the nature of the association between or among them and state a hypothesis.

The research design is determined by the nature of the variables and the type of relationship thought to exist between them. The design must be appropriate to the study planned; otherwise, the conclusions drawn will be invalid. A valid and reliable research tool must be found to measure the desired variables. The researcher must plan how the participants will be found and the method for selecting participants. In addition, the details of actually dividing people into groups will be decided. How the tests will be conducted and who will do all the tasks of collecting the data must be planned. The types of statistical tests to be used must be determined in advance. Many nurse researchers work collaboratively with statisticians at this point to ensure that the planned research design and analysis of data will provide the type of information the researcher is seeking.

IMPLEMENTING THE STUDY

Actually conducting the study is the moment most researchers have been waiting for. Once data collection has begun, the possibility of gaining new knowledge is growing closer. In some instances, additional people are hired to serve as data collectors. In some nursing studies, nurses who are caring for patients collect the data needed for the study. If multiple people are collecting data, it will be important to assure that all are carrying out the study tasks in the same way. If different data collectors function differently, the results of the study may not be accurate.

ANALYZING THE DATA

The eighth step in the process is the analysis of data. During this process, specific statistical tests appropriate to the study are performed. Researchers summarize information about the subjects and compute the results of their statistical tests. For some studies, researchers must try to organize narrative interviews and other types of data.

PRESENTING AND INTERPRETING FINDINGS

The last two steps in the research process are, respectively, the presentation and interpretation of findings. Often they are discussed together in the research report. The presentation of findings involves reporting the data gathered. This step generally includes giving information on the sociodemographic variables as well as the dependent and other independent variables. Usually, the data are reported in terms of mean score, range, and SD. Following this, the results of the analysis are presented and the hypothesis is either rejected or not rejected.

In a section titled "Discussion," the importance of the findings is discussed, including the implications of the results for nursing practice. This is an important section for readers of research reports. Although it may be difficult to understand the intricacies of the statistical analysis completely, it is generally very clear what the researchers feel are the implications for nursing practice. They will make recommendations to practicing nurses and to other nurse researchers who may want to repeat the study or to investigate other questions suggested by the research.

LIMITATIONS OF THE STUDY

The discussion will usually include factors that might have made the results of the study unreliable or invalid. These are referred to as threats to reliability and validity. Many different things might occur to threaten the usefulness of research results.

One problem that might arise is measurement error. Measurement errors can occur for a number of reasons. If the nurses investigating the question are measuring blood pressure, each person must use the same accurate procedure. If the person taking the reading fails to follow the protocols established for the study, results may vary. The environment itself, such as the temperature or humidity level, may affect the variables measured. The reagent strips used to test for presence of blood in one type of study may be difficult to read. All these factors can affect the results obtained. If interviews were part of the data collection, the individual approaches of the interviewers may alter the results. Nurses involved in caring for patients who are involved in research studies can help identify threats to measurement accuracy that might result in misleading or inaccurate data. If the nurse draws such factors to the attention of the researcher, it may be possible to correct or control for them and to safeguard the integrity of the research.

In addition to measurement error, a number of other factors can limit the usefulness of the research study. Some of these limitations are subject variables, which include history, maturation, testing, selection, and mortality.

History refers to the fact that events other than the experimental variable can affect outcome. Suppose, for example, that researchers were studying a technique to reduce anxiety in preoperative patients and that during the time of the study there was a fire drill in the hospital. The noise and commotion of the fire drill might strongly affect the patients' level of anxiety, making it difficult for the researchers to evaluate the effect of a treatment designed to reduce anxiety.

Maturation refers to the fact that subjects are growing and changing and that differences measured from one point in time to another may be due to these changes. This factor is especially important in research studies that deal with populations undergoing rapid changes, such as patients in a pediatric unit.

Testing refers to the fact that a testing procedure can itself pose a threat to research integrity, because it can produce changes in a patient. This is particularly true if the research design uses a time-series format. If the experience of being tested makes it easier for a patient to respond to the question a second, third, or fourth time, the changes may be due to experience with the test instrument rather than to the nursing intervention the test is designed to measure.

Selection refers to choosing subjects and sorting them into control and experimental groups. If the choice of subjects and the assignment to groups are not random, there may be significant undetected differences between the two groups. Volunteers for a research study may represent only one segment of the population of interest, or a researcher may choose only those subjects who can conveniently be studied. Thus, basic, undetected differences between groups could produce misleading results.

Mortality refers to the loss of subjects from a study for any reason. Another term for this phenomenon is *attrition.* Even when the two groups being compared are basically similar, the differential loss of group members may change the composition of the groups. This is an even greater problem when the groups are not basically equivalent.

DISSEMINATING RESEARCH RESULTS

An important part of the research process is the dissemination of findings to other nurses. Researchers frequently disseminate findings by publishing research reports or by presenting research at nursing conferences. The beginning reader of research reports will increase his or her understanding of reported research by becoming involved in research conferences and nursing research discussion groups and by regularly reading nursing research journals.

■ TYPES OF RESEARCH

As mentioned earlier, not all research problems can be addressed in the same way, and the design of the research must fit the type of problem being studied. The two major types of research are called **quantitative** and **qualitative.**

Quantitative Research

Quantitative research emphasizes experimentation and statistical analysis. It is generally what is thought of when research is mentioned. Generally, quantitative research focuses on measurable observations (those that can be reported as numbers). It is very objective and tries to be value-free. The three principal types of quantitative research are experimental, quasi-experimental, and nonexperimental designs.

The **experimental research** design has three characteristics:

1. The subjects are randomly assigned to groups.
2. The researcher manipulates (gives a treatment to) one group.
3. The other group, called the control group, does not receive the treatment and is used for comparison purposes.

This structure allows the researcher to observe differences between the two groups and to make conclusions about the effect of the treatment from empirical observations.

Quasi-experimental and nonexperimental designs have less control; for example, a quasi-experimental study may lack a control group. One type of quasi-experimental design is called the time-series design. It uses the experimental group itself as a kind of control, by taking a series of measurements prior to the treatment and then following it. Changes can be reliably linked to the treatment if the multiple readings before and afterward show the change to be connected in time with the treatment.

Nonexperimental designs are the least controlled and therefore are the hardest to interpret and the hardest from which to generalize results. One kind of nonexperimental research is called *ex post facto* research. It deals with an event in the past, such as the death of a child, and another variable of interest, such as the subsequent development of maternal depression. Obviously, a researcher cannot manipulate the independent variable, but he or she can assess naturally occurring groups to see what relationship there might be between the death of a child and development of maternal depression. These studies are also referred to as cross-sectional, because they study all the participants at one time in their lives.

Longitudinal studies are those that follow selected research questions over time. Longitudinal studies are very expensive and are especially subject to problems with maturation and loss of the participants (attrition). An example of a major longitudinal research has been the study of residents of Framingham, MA, over many years to investigate the effects of various aspects of their life patterns on subsequent health issues.

Descriptive research is a type of nonexperimental research that has as its purpose a more accurate and more precise description of the population. No attempt is made to alter or manipulate variables. For example, a descriptive research study might be used by a hospital to identify the ages, gender, marital status, and other details of their patient population. This might enable them to more effectively target a new wellness program. Surveys are one subtype of descriptive research. The survey asks people to answer specific questions of fact or opinion and the aggregate results are reported. Hospitals commonly use surveys of former patients as one method of evaluating their services.

Methodological research is aimed at developing tools to be used in future research studies. Methodological research may be used to develop technical measuring instruments or to develop questionnaires and rating scales that are both valid and reliable. A high degree of sophistication in statistical methods is usually important to critiquing methodological studies.

Qualitative Research

Qualitative research aims at a different sort of information. The goal of qualitative research is a more comprehensive, contextual understanding of the topic in question; that is, it looks at phenomena in their environment instead of attempting to isolate them, as is frequently done in quantitative research. Qualitative research is reported with descriptions, quotations, and models. Unlike quantitative research, qualitative research is not reported with statistical tests. Examples of qualitative research methodologies are **phenomenology** and **ethnography.**

The aim of phenomenology is "to describe experience as it is lived by people" (Munhall & Boyd, 1993, p. 70). The information sought draws on the patient's subjective interpretation of an experience, which itself reflects previous experiences as well as current factors, and involves small groups of people who are studied in depth. A phenomenological approach has been used to examine whether patients perceived their nurses as caring or noncaring. Other examples of research that might use a phenomenological approach are the examination of what it means to experience pain, the approach of death, or recovery from disease.

Ethnography is probably best known as a tool of anthropologists who seek to describe the characteristics of a particular culture. The subject of the study can be very large and inclusive, such as the health culture of the Hmong refugees, or very small, such as the health practices of a single family. The ethnographic researcher becomes involved in the culture being studied and tries to describe it as completely as possible. Rather than try to isolate variables, as the quantitative researcher would do, the ethnographer tries to include as many as possible. As the ethnographer gathers information, themes and patterns become evident, and the researcher gains an understanding of "norms, values, belief systems, language, rituals, economics and role behaviors" in the group studied (Munhall & Boyd, 1993).

Other qualitative research designs include the life story and case history approaches and action research strategies. Action research strategies emphasize the importance of viewing nursing as a practice discipline and research as having ethical and moral implications. Action researchers are particularly interested in research that produces change in clinical nursing practice.

Combined Research Strategies

Both quantitative and qualitative research are important for nursing. Sometimes a quantitative research design is the most effective, and at other times qualitative approaches are most appropriate. Many researchers are now combining both approaches in a method called triangulation or multimodal research. This type of research allows researchers to look at phenomena from two different perspectives, which can add depth and validity to the study.

To compare the two approaches, consider the following situation. Suppose the staff nurses on a surgical unit are considering a variety of brochures designed to help prepare patients and their families for surgery. The brochures vary in the amount of detail provided, the variety of illustrations, and the degree to which they involve nurses in the teaching process. The staff members identify two brochures that look promising and attempt to compare them.

A quantitative research design would allow the nurses to compare the effectiveness of the two brochures in a number of ways. They could identify two surgical units on which patients were basically similar and have the patients on one unit read one of the brochures and those on the other unit read the other brochure. The nurses could assess individuals for physiological signs and symptoms of nervousness, such as respiratory and heart rate before and after reading the brochures. They could assess understanding by giving each subject an objective pretest and posttest. These quantitative measures would allow the nurses to decide which of the two brochures better reduced physiological signs of anxiety and produced increased understanding. Statistics would be used to analyze the quantitative measures (the pretest–posttest results).

A qualitative research design might approach the question of which brochure was better by asking the patients about the feelings they had before they read the brochures and how their feelings were different afterward. The nurse researchers might ask such questions as, "What concerns did you have about the surgery before reading the brochure?" "Did you feel more at ease about the surgery after reading it?" or "Do you still have questions or concerns that we can answer?" The answers from patients from one unit who had read one brochure could be compared with those from the other unit who had read the other brochure, and judgments could be made about which one was more effective, although no statistical test could be used to compare the feelings of the subjects.

The advantages of a quantitative design are that it is easy to measure differences and to understand their significance. In the first example, the staff nurses could actually measure the difference in their patients' physiological responses and the difference in their scores on pretests and posttests. Using one brochure with one group of patients and the second brochure with another, similar group of patients, they could compare the numerical differences by using a statistical measure to determine whether the differences were actually significant. The disadvantage is that this approach might not tell them much about how the patients actually felt about their impending surgeries and how the brochures influenced those feelings.

The advantage of a qualitative measure is that it allows the researchers to address the question more broadly, using as a primary source of information the patient's subjective response. The disadvantage is that it is harder to compare the responses of the different patients. The use of a combined strategy that includes a qualitative as well as a quantitative approach is often most informative.

Meta-analysis

Meta-analysis is a process of examining multiple research studies about the same topic and combining the findings of all for analysis as a group. By combining research studies, samples are larger, a broader representation of populations may be present, differing interventions may be compared, and application to practice is facilitated. Meta-analyses can be problematic because of wide variations in the different research studies being combined. Therefore, a meta-analysis is not considered as strong a support for any result as is a single study with the same number of participants. Conducting meta-analysis requires complex statistical skills and an understanding of a variety of research methodologies.

■ LEGAL AND ETHICAL CONSIDERATIONS IN RESEARCH

Regardless of the type of research, the researcher must be concerned with certain legal and ethical considerations, especially in relationship to those who are participants or subjects in the study. The most fundamental consideration has to do with consent. Before any research project can be initiated, the individuals who will be the subjects in the study must be informed about the study and give their consent to participate. It is important to recognize that just as nurses have a duty to serve as patient advocates in the daily delivery of nursing care, they also have an obligation to see that patients are safeguarded during any research study. Certain types of patients, such as the very young and the mentally incompetent, require particular protection.

The first internationally recognized code of conduct for research was developed after World War II. This code, called the Nuremberg Code, provides a set of principles to govern research on human subjects. The code was a response to the appalling experimentation conducted by German researchers on prisoners during World War II.

In 1975, the ANA developed a code of ethics for research that is found in a document titled *Human Rights Guidelines for Nurses in Clinical and Other Research* (ANA, 1975). In 1978, the United States Congress enacted the National Research Act. The act established a National Commission for the Protection of Human Subjects of Biomedical and Behavioral Research, which then developed regulations for the protection of human subjects in any research that is supported in whole or in part through federal funds. The most recent revision of this code was in 1983 (Code for Federal Regulations, 1983). Three principles guide these regulations. First, the research should do no harm. Second, the participants should be free from exploitation. Third, there should be careful attention to the risk:benefit ratio of the research. To safeguard patients' ethical and legal rights, the following rules for ethical research are used (Code for Federal Regulations, 1983):

1. Voluntary consent of the human subject is essential.
2. Experiments should be based on the results of animal experimentation and knowledge of the natural history of the disease or other problems and should be so designed that the anticipated results will justify the experiment.
3. The degree of risk to be taken by the subject should never exceed the potential humanitarian importance of the problem to be studied.
4. Through all stages of the experiment, the highest degree of skill and care should be required of those who conduct or engage in it, and the experiment should be conducted only by scientifically qualified persons.
5. At any time during the course of the experiment, the human subject should be at liberty to end participation in the experiment.
6. The scientist in charge must be prepared to terminate the experiment at any stage if there is probable cause to believe that continuation of the experiment is likely to result in injury, disability, or the death of the subject.

Just as patients must give informed consent for any medical procedure, they must be fully informed about any proposed research before they can legally give their consent. The formal consent form generally describes the researcher's credentials; how the participant was chosen; purposes of the research; procedures that will be followed; and risks, discomforts, and benefits expected. The subject is generally guaranteed anonymity or at least confidentiality. If alternative treatments are available, they must also be described. Finally, the subject must be assured that participation is voluntary and can be terminated at any time. Similarly, just as it is appropriate for a staff nurse to inform a physician of patient questions that indicate a lack of understanding of a planned procedure, it is also appropriate for the staff nurse to communicate to the nurse researcher any misgivings or misunderstandings a subject may voice concerning proposed research participation.

Research that is undertaken in a health care setting requires approval by one or more review boards. There may be an institutional review board that evaluates and approves all proposals before they can be implemented. If the research is being conducted in conjunction with a school of nursing, medicine, or other academic discipline, that institution will also have a review committee that will evaluate and approve the research proposal. Funding agencies may have yet another approval process. The aim of these multiple reviews is to ensure that the legal and ethical rights of patients as research subjects are protected.

■ PERSONAL INVOLVEMENT IN RESEARCH

We have already mentioned one important way in which staff nurses can assist the research process: by helping ensure that patient rights, both ethical and legal, are safeguarded. Other ways include helping identify nursing problems that need research, assisting with ongoing research, and implementing the results of nursing research in the practice setting.

Identifying Problems for Research

Staff nurses are in an ideal position to identify important research needs. First, nurses generally are excellent observers because they have been carefully trained in the assessment skills that are so important to the research process. Second, nurses are responsible for putting the whole complex of patient care together. As a consequence, it is they who notice when the overall plan of care is ineffective.

You may find situations in which research might help answer nursing questions, and you might want to suggest them as possible topics to your head nurse or clinical specialist. As mentioned previously, you may be searching for new strategies that would be effective in improving care for the clients in your setting. When no information is available, you might recognize that a carefully performed study would benefit not only your own clients but also others with similar problems.

Assisting With Ongoing Research

Although you may not be actively involved in research, patients you are assigned to care for may be involved as participants in a research study. This may be through taking an investigational drug, completing a written survey, or having an experimental procedure done. You must be knowledgeable about the study and the research process so that you can plan your care so as not to compromise the research results. As a nurse providing care to individuals in a study, you should consider yourself a participant in the process and do your best to make it successful.

Staff nurses need to understand the factors that can affect research results and to help ensure that the data collected will be as accurate as possible. The staff nurse is in a good position to help observe for threats to the research study. By helping ensure that other variables do not affect the outcome, the results obtained and the interpretations made will be as reliable and valid as possible. If you are asked to be the actual data collector, you will need to follow procedures and protocols exactly so that the data collected are both reliable and valid.

■ IMPLEMENTING NEW PRACTICES BASED ON EVIDENCE

Staff nurses who read research reports and search for other evidence of best practices and who look for opportunities to apply these findings to clinical practice can make an important contribution not only to patient care but also to the expansion of nursing knowledge. Implementing new practices based on evidence requires that you identify sources of evidence that can be helpful in an individual nursing environment, evaluate that evidence in relationship to your setting, work collaboratively to introduce changes based on the evidence, and evaluate the effectiveness of the changes. This should sound to you like the nursing process taken one step further, and in fact it is.

As you participate in continuing education and in-service presentations and as you read nursing journals, you may identify evidence that will allow you to make positive changes in your nursing practice. This may be a proactive process, which means that you change your practice before a problem is identified. You focus on continuous improvement.

Barriers to utilizing research in practice include insufficient time on the job to read research and attempt to implement new ideas (Omery & Williams, 1999). Barnsteiner and Prevost (2002) identified several strategies for nurses seeking to implement EBP. These include changing one's viewpoint about the importance of reading research, increasing one's knowledge about the entire EBP process, harnessing new knowledge through accessing resources, instituting system changes and collaborating both locally and globally.

Critical Thinking Exercise

Identify an area of nursing that is of interest to you. Use the MEDLINE, CINAHL, or other indexes to help you find appropriate resources. Your reference librarian can help you locate the various indexes and provide information and assistance with computer searches. Retrieve and read the *abstract* of the article. Repeat this until you find an abstract that describes a study of interest to you. Retrieve the full article.

As you read the article, you might first skim the whole article to get an overview. Is this a quantitative study or a qualitative study? What specifically were the research questions? Skim the authors' discussion to have a perspective on the results. Then go back and read the article and use the information you have learned about research as a basis for using the study guide in Display 13-5 to assess the usefulness of the research report for your own practice.

■ SYSTEMATIC ANALYSIS OF INFORMATION AND EVIDENCE

Analysis always includes the careful evaluation of information you obtain from any resource and provides an essential foundation for practice. Whether the information comes to you verbally, is found in print, or is accessed through a computer, critical thinking must be applied in your evaluation process. After the information is obtained, analysis includes a systematic process of weighing the various pieces of evidence, determining their importance, and coming to a conclusion as to the appropriate approach for practice in an individual setting.

Analysis may include the use of meta-reviews: studies that aggregate across many different research studies that attempt to use statistical measures to aggregate the results. These are useful when multiple research studies are identified. When

DISPLAY 13-5	**Reading Research Reports: A Guide**

Author:
Title:
Journal Name and Issue:

Statement of the Problem: What were the researchers attempting to learn about? Is it clear to you what they were investigating? What questions would you like to ask them if you could?

Review of the Literature: What do the researchers tell you about the level of our knowledge regarding this problem? Are there research reports that you might want to review? Does this research seem to address the questions earlier research has raised?

Theoretical Framework: Do the researchers indicate how their study fits into nursing knowledge as a whole? Do they relate their study to theories from other fields, such as education, psychology, or sociology?

Identification of Variables: Do the researchers clearly point out dependent and independent variables? Do the researchers explain how the variables will be measured? If variables are not identified, what is being studied?

Formation of Hypotheses: Do the researchers clearly indicate how the dependent and independent variables are linked? Is it clear what their research is designed to test or to examine? (Qualitative research does not usually contain hypotheses.)

Research Design: Do the researchers say what type of design they have chosen? Can you see things that might interfere with their data collection? Have the researchers taken these threats into account and attempted to control for them?

Collection of Data: How did the researchers go about obtaining their information? Did they provide for voluntary consent and withdrawal of subjects at any point desired?

Analysis of Data: Do the researchers tell you how they analyzed the data? If this is a quantitative study, do they identify the statistical tests used and the level of significance they have chosen? If a qualitative approach is used, do the researchers describe what techniques have been used to draw their conclusions?

Presentation and Interpretation of Findings: Based upon their analysis, what do the researchers say about the hypotheses? Do they present their findings objectively? Do they relate their findings to earlier research and their theoretical framework? Do they indicate how their findings can be used in practice? How will this information help you in your clinical practice? What additional questions does it raise?

Your Contribution: With the information from this research report, what changes might you want to make in your own practice? What implications does this have for you as a student? With whom would you need to share this information? What are the implications of not using the knowledge you have gained from this research report?

data are from other sources, the decisions about the appropriate use of the evidence to guide practice are usually made by groups of experts. In the case of nursing practice, this may be a specially constituted nursing committee comprised of expert nurses with skills in evaluating data.

Some of the aspects that must be included in their deliberations are the reliability of the source of the data, bias in the data, the timeliness of the data, the purpose for which the evidence will be used, and the setting in which it will be used. Each of these is discussed in the following. Pearson (2002) suggests that in addition to all other criteria for analysis, evidence for establishing practice should include a look at what he termed the *FAME scale*. Nursing practices are examined for feasibility, which relates to the practicality of implementing the action on a widespread basis. Appropriateness refers to whether it is acceptable and justifiable within ethical guidelines. Meaningfulness provides the rationale for the practice being adopted. Effectiveness relates to how much evidence supports the practice and what evidence provides divergent viewpoints.

Reliability of the Source of the Information

What is the *source of the information* you have found? You need to examine the credentials and affiliation of the person or organization speaking, writing, or posting the information. In addition, what is the affiliation or organization that sponsors an individual writer or Web site? Sites that do not identify the author or responsible organization should be considered unreliable.

Professional and scientific sources may provide you with actual research-supported information or may provide information based on the judgment of experts in the field. References to the research or source of factual data may be a part of an excellent site. When a site alludes to research but does not provide a reference, it is not considered as reliable.

Many nonprofessional resources, such as magazines for the lay person or Web sites operated by non-health care personnel, are subject to the interpretation of editors and writers of general literature rather than of health care experts. Thus, even when trying to present very accurate information, they may omit essential details, make unwarranted assumptions, and apply data to inappropriate individuals. In other cases, the author or editor does not attempt to be scientific and factual but rather has a goal of creating interest and controversy.

How was the information found at this source screened or verified before being made available? Sources from federal government agencies such as the Food and Drug Administration, the National Institutes of Health, the Agency for Health Care Policy and Research, and the Occupational Health and Safety Administration are reviewed for content by expert scientific panels before being published in any form. Government-sponsored sites can be recognized by the *.gov* at the end of the site address.

Many professional journals assist you in the evaluation process by printing only **peer-reviewed** (sometimes called *refereed*) articles. This means that any article submitted for publication is sent to one or more reviewers who are experts in the field. The reviewers read carefully to assure that research was conducted appropriately and that the article meets professional standards. This does not mean that you do not need to read critically, but it does give you a baseline of trust in the material. You can usually learn whether a journal is peer reviewed by reading the information for authors that is printed within the journal. This information may also appear where the editorial staff is listed.

Some journals, although not peer reviewed, have knowledgeable staff who review articles. If the journal is not peer reviewed, you will need to examine carefully the credentials of the authors and look at the references to help you determine whether this is material that you wish to use as a basis for practice.

Major universities with medical centers often offer access to many Internet resources that are based on the research and practice of that center. There may be some sites that are designed for the client and others that are resources for professionals. University sites also may have many links to other related sites. The Hardin Meta Directory at the University of Iowa is a source for health care related Web site links that have been verified by the Hardin Medical Library staff. Sites sponsored by educational institutions can be recognized by the *.edu* at the end of the site address.

Be sure, however, to distinguish between official sites sponsored by the university medical center or library and individual sites of students at that university, which may also have the *.edu* suffix. For example, a nursing student who posts tips for overcoming test anxiety may have useful ideas for other nursing students. However, these ideas may not be tested nor appropriately generalized to a wide population of nursing students. If you have a problem with test anxiety and the suggestions are not difficult or costly, the tips might be useful for you to try. If they fail to work for you, you will just discard them. On the other hand, these tips are inappropriate as widespread recommendations from a professional, because people receiving professional recommendations are expecting that the suggested strategies have a degree of reliability for success.

Any individual or organization is free to post personal opinions and experiences through various Internet forums and sites. These may or may not be verifiable or applicable to your setting and needs. Anyone with the appropriate computer technology can develop a World Wide Web site. Many sites are not clearly identified as to their origin or the name of the person appears without any credentials. Individual nurses may post information by using their medical center site or a personal computer. Be sure to differentiate one nurse's viewpoint from the official policy or protocol of an institution. For practicing nurses, it is sometimes useful to learn about procedures and protocols in use at other health care facilities. Be cautious in accepting these protocols for adoption without further research. The protocols in use at one facility may not be based on the latest research data.

Just as you evaluate information from print sources, you will need to develop skill in evaluating sources found on the Internet. You can use the criteria discussed next to evaluate all types of information accessed.

Bias of the Source

Bias refers to presenting one viewpoint of an issue about which there are multiple viewpoints or presenting a preferred viewpoint as the best one without evidence. You will want to ask "Is the particular source I have found biased in some way?" Often, bias is difficult to discern even when it is present. For example, an alternative health care resource may be so biased against conventional health care that individual problems are presented as general situations or half-truths may be presented.

Conversely, some conventional health care resources are so biased against alternative health care that reliable information is ignored or discounted. Even within the conventional health care field there are sometimes strong differences of opinion with regard to appropriate treatment plans. Different individuals may give differing weight to supporting data. Sometimes the background and affiliation of the author are clues to bias that might be present. Often bias can be detected by seeking a variety of resources and comparing them. The use of a variety of resources is an effective way to minimize bias in your information.

Critical Thinking Exercise

Identify a health-related topic that is of common interest to the public. Use the World Wide Web to identify sites designed for consumers in regard to the topic. From the sites found, identify one that you believes shows bias in its presentation of information. Provide the rationale for your judgment regarding the presence of bias.

Timeliness of the Information

The timeliness of information is another aspect to be evaluated. How current is the information you are obtaining? Although dates on journals and other publications are usually clear, dates of Internet sites may be hard to find or even absent. You may be unable to ascertain when the information was posted. Old information may remain on sites long after newer information has replaced the information. Again, good information is clearly identified with a date.

Another aspect of timeliness is to consider how current the information should be for your purposes and compare it with how current the newly found information is. Sometimes arbitrary limits, such as 5 years, are set for whether something is timely. Although this is a simple approach to use, it may not be appropriate. Information on the treatment of HIV infection could be within this 5-year framework and yet omit some of the most promising new approaches to treatment. Valuable information on the physiologic effects of bed rest that was discovered through research many years ago would be omitted from consideration if anything older than 5 years was discounted. Individual critical thinking is the key when determining whether information is timely for the purposes you have in mind.

Purpose for the New Information

Consider your purpose in seeking the new information. When you are seeking another option to solve a difficult individual patient problem, you might accept evidence that a particular approach was successful for a small group of clients. If the approach did not have adverse effects of concern, you might then try this approach. However, data from a very small group would be inadequate to support a generalized policy or protocol to be used on many patients.

DISPLAY 13-6 | **Key Questions for Evaluating Information**

1. Is the source identified?
2. Is the source reliable?
3. Is the source biased?
4. How timely is the information relative to the need?
5. How does the information fit with the purpose for which it will be used?
6. How does the setting that originated the information compare with your setting?

Research evidence should always be sought for instituting new practices; however, it is not always available. In those instances, accustomed practice or deduction from physiologic or pathophysiologic information may be the only option. If this is true, one of your obligations would be to continue to have an open mind about the subject and therefore to continue to seek more evidence. In some settings, you might be able to support the development of a research study to provide more definitive answers.

Comparing Settings/Situations

How does the source setting or situation in the research report or article compare to the one you are considering? When you are looking for new ideas for protocols, procedures, or approaches to problems, consider whether the possible solutions have been used in a setting or situation comparable to your own. For example, a protocol that works well in a large medical center with 24-hour physician availability may not be appropriate to a small rural facility in which the private physicians are in their homes a 30-minute drive away. Approaches that have worked well with elderly patients may not be effective when used with adolescents. The assessment instrument that is effective in long-term care, in which the residents will reside for months, may be inappropriate to use in an acute care hospital, in which patients will be hospitalized only a few days.

Although patient problems may appear on the surface to be similar, they may have important differences. A leg ulcer found in an elderly diabetic individual will respond differently to treatment than one in a young person who developed the ulcer under a cast. Thus, you must look at the individual patient situation and ask whether the participants in the study have characteristics that are similar to or different from the clients that you are considering.

Economic resources differ among different settings also. Cost-effectiveness is a critical concern in most health care environments. A very costly approach may have a high rate of success but not be feasible in a setting in which the clients rely on public assistance for health care support. Sometimes, decisions must take into account the cost/benefit data. See Display 13-6 for a summary of key questions to consider when evaluating information.

■ KEY CONCEPTS

- ■ Nursing informatics is the use of technology to retrieve and manage information relevant to nursing practice.
- ■ Five strategic directions have been developed to enhance nurses' preparation to use and develop information technology; among these is the inclusion of core informatics content in nursing curricula.
- ■ Computerized systems are increasingly essential components of the health care delivery environment and require that nurses participate in the use and evaluation of these technologies for improving quality of care.
- ■ Nurses use computer documentation systems for scheduling, ordering, retrieving patient information, and for entering patient data.
- ■ Individual agencies have differing computer documentation systems, but all include the use of security systems and may include billing systems, order entry, patient data, and nursing data entry.
- ■ Other resources available on agency computer systems may include drug and diagnostic test references, policy and procedure manuals, access to the Internet, and access to library resources.
- ■ To maintain and improve practice, nurses must access the latest in information resources to seek evidence for best practices.
- ■ Information resources to support EBP include materials found in libraries, such as texts and journals, indexes to literature, and CD-ROM systems for literature searching. Policies and standards also serve as resources to support nursing practice.
- ■ The Internet is a growing resource for health care information and includes the use of e-mail, group discussions online, and the World Wide Web.
- ■ Health care indexes are an essential resource for accessing specific, relevant literature. *Index Medicus* (print version) and MEDLINE (online computer version) are indexes developed by the NLM and provide references to biomedical journals, videos, and resources from throughout the world. CINAHL, an index available in print, CD-ROM, and online computer forms, focuses on nursing and allied health journals, publications of the NLN and ANA, standards of nursing practice, nursing practice acts, state nursing journals, consumer health materials, as well as nursing dissertations and research projects.
- ■ Other indexes found in libraries provide citations, abstracts, and sometimes full-text journal articles.
- ■ Effective searching of indexes requires that you understand the particular system, but all computerized systems allow you to construct searches with multiple terms that more precisely describe your aims.
- ■ EBP requires that nurses base their approaches on those strategies that are based in strong evidence of effectiveness.
- ■ Evidence from research; retrospective or concurrent chart review; quality improvement and risk data; international, national, and local standards; infection control data; pathophysiology; cost-effectiveness analysis; benchmarking data; patient preferences; and clinical expertise may all be used for evidence-based nursing practice.
- ■ The research process is designed to provide a structure for examining questions in a systematic manner.

■ Research terminology that is necessary for beginning users of research data to understand includes the concepts of population, sample, participant/subject, control group, experimental group, randomization, statistical significance, and clinical significance.

■ The steps of the research process provide an orderly framework for designing and carrying out a research project. They include statement of the problem, review of literature, development of a theoretical framework, identification of variables, formation of hypotheses, selection of the research design, collection of data, analysis of the data, presentation of the findings, and interpretation of the findings.

■ Nurses working with research need to be aware of threats to the integrity of the study, such as measurement errors and the subject variables referred to as history, maturation, testing, selection, and mortality.

■ There are two basic types of research, quantitative and qualitative, which provide different types of information and a different perspective on problems. Meta-analysis involves the integration of multiple studies into a useful pattern for possible application.

■ Nurses involved in caring for patients who are subjects in a research study have responsibility for protection of the legal and ethical rights of subjects through informed consent and adherence to specific protocols.

■ To read research reports, you need to review the report in light of each of the steps of the research process to evaluate whether the research has relevance for your practice situation.

■ Nurses providing direct care can assist in validating research findings and in suggesting other areas for investigation and they can help ensure that ongoing research is conducted under optimal circumstances.

■ Evidence retrieved to support nursing care must be systematically analyzed and subjected to expert scrutiny to determine what will used to guide practice.

■ Evaluation criteria include the reliability of the source, bias of the source, timeliness of the information, your purpose for using the information, and comparability of the settings in which it is to be used.

REFERENCES

American Nurses Association (ANA). (1975). *Human Rights Guidelines for Nurses in Clinical and Other Research.* Kansas City, MO: Author.

Barnsteiner, J., & Prevost, S. (2002). How to implement evidence-based practice: some tried and true pointers. *Reflections on Nursing Leadership, 28*(2), 18–21

Billings, D. M. (2003). Online communities of professional practice. *Nursing Education, 42*(8), 335–336.

Centers for Disease Control. (1992). A framework for assessing the effectiveness of disease and injury prevention. *MMWR,* 41(RR-3).

Code of Federal Regulations. (1983). *Protection of Human Subjects: 45CFR46* (revised March 8, 1983). Washington, DC: Department of Health and Human Services.

Gassert, C. (1998). The challenge of meeting patients' needs with a national nursing informatics agenda. *Journal of the American Medical Informatics Association, 5*(3), 263–268.

Goode, C. J., & Piedalue, F. (1999). Evidence-based clinical practice. *Journal of Nursing Administration, 29*(6), 15–21.

McCannon, M., & O'Neal, P. V. (2003). Results of a national survey indicating information technology skills needed by nurses at the time of entry into the work force. *Journal of Nursing Education, 42*(8), 337–340.

McNeil, B. J., Elfrink, V. L., Bickford, C. J. et al. (2003). Nursing information technology knowledge, skills, and preparation of student nurses, nursing faculty, and clinicians: a U.S. survey. *Journal of Nursing Education, 42*(8), 341–349.

Munhall, P., & Boyd, C. (Eds.) (1993). *Nursing Research: A Qualitative Perspective* (2nd ed.). New York: National League for Nursing.

Omery, A., & William, R. P. (1999). An appraisal of research utilization across the United States. *Journal of Nursing Administration, 29*(12), 50–56.

Pearson, A. (2002). Nursing takes the lead: redefining what counts as evidence in Australian health care. *Reflections on Nursing Leadership, 28*(4), 18–21.

Polit, D., & Hungler, B. (1997). *Essentials of Nursing Research: Methods, Appraisal, and Utilization.* Philadelphia: Lippincott-Raven.

Rosenberg, W., & Donald, A. (1995). Evidence based medicine: an approach to clinical problem-solving. *British Medical Journal, 310*(6987), 1122–1126.

Sackett, D. L., Rosenberg, W. M. C., Gray, J. A. M. et al. (1996). Evidence-based medicine: what it is and what it isn't. *British Medical Journal, 312*(7023), 71–72.

14

Anticipating the Future

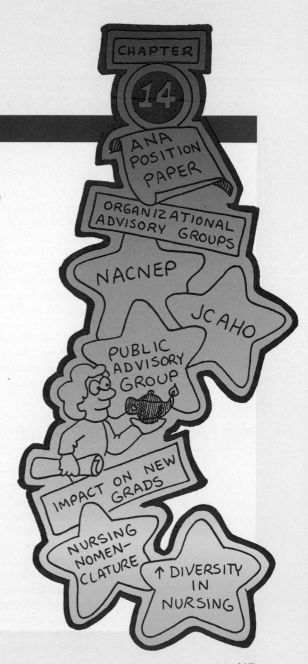

Learning Outcomes ■ ■ ■ ■ ■

After completing this chapter, you should be able to:

1. Briefly sketch the history of nursing education from its beginnings as apprenticeship-type training to a college or university-based professional education.

2. Discuss the various aspects of the American Nurses Association's position on nursing education, its impact on the profession of nursing, and the effects the position might have on you as you move into the role of registered nurse.

3. Describe two approaches to differentiated nursing practice and the efforts to implement it.

4. Identify how differentiated practice might affect your own practice as a registered nurse.

5. Explain how a nursing practice model may be used to improve the delivery of nursing care.

6. Identify how working in an agency with a nursing practice model would affect your role.

7. Identify ways in which advisory groups impact the nursing profession.

8. Discuss the development of systematic language for classifying and describing nursing phenomena.

9. Identify the characteristics of four major systems of nursing nomenclature: North American Nursing Diagnosis Association (NANDA), Nursing Interventions Classification (NIC), Nursing Outcomes Classification (NOC), and the Omaha System, and relate these to their use in the care environment.

10. Analyze the factors that have resulted in increased efforts to recruit and retain minorities in nursing.

Key Terms ■ ■ ■ ■

accreditation
advisory groups
apprenticeship
certification
classification systems
competencies

differentiated nursing
    practice
entry into practice
malpractice
NANDA
NIC

NOC
nursing nomenclatures
Omaha System
scope of practice
taxonomy

When we are able to anticipate activities or events before they occur, we place ourselves in a better position to deal with the outcomes. In some instances, anticipation of the events to come can lead to prevention of undesirable conclusions. You are already familiar with this concept from clinical nursing courses in which you were expected to provide anticipatory guidance to your clients. As you move into a professional role, being able to anticipate some of the issues and concerns with which the professional will be dealing will put you in a better position to have an effect on decisions that will be made. You will be able to study issues and make personal decisions about them. How will you know what activities or events to anticipate? Are some more critical than others? Do these events affect all nurses? Although we do not profess to predict or to possess unique insight into the future, certain issues will continue to seek resolution. Activities that have been initiated will continue to grow, take on new dimensions, and impact the profession. Many of these involve nursing education and, as a result, nursing practice.

■ A BRIEF LOOK AT THE HISTORY OF NURSING EDUCATION

Nursing education found its roots embedded in an **apprenticeship** type preparation of its practitioners. In an apprenticeship, the student works for a given period of time with a master craftsman to learn the skills of that trade. Thus, if you were living in the 1800s and wanted to be a nurse, you would work closely with someone in your community who would teach you the necessary skills. In reality, this likely would have occurred in a facility operated by a religious order, and you would have made a commitment to a religious group, because the first schools of nursing were not founded until the last quarter of the nineteenth century. In 1877, the Training School of the New York Hospital offered an 18-month course to prepare graduates for nursing; other schools opened soon thereafter. Even the early schools had an apprentice-type approach to teaching. Students worked with more experienced nurses until they had learned the skills necessary to care for the sick and ailing. There were few actual classes. When there were lectures they were often delivered by physicians.

EXAMPLE *Miss Peabody's Schooling During the Late 1870s*

Sadie Peabody had completed her 1-month probationary period in nurses' training. She was happy to have moved beyond the responsibilities for arranging the linen closet and folding clothes (which had to be completed in a particular order), sweeping and cleaning, polishing the floors, and washing and ironing. Her board, lodging, and laundry were furnished and she now received a monthly stipend of $7 for clothes, textbooks, and incidental expenses. Considered a junior nurse, 6 months of the remaining 2 years of Sadie's clinical time was spent on 14-hour night shifts. Her training was divided into several "service" rotations among medical, surgical, maternity, pediatric, and other areas of the hospital—that is, that was how it was to have occurred. However, the rotation was often overlooked if a particular area of the hospital was short of staff; students were required to fill that need. Days started early (before 6:00 a.m.) and ended at 8:00 p.m. When there were lectures by the physicians, they occurred after she completed her ward work, and it was difficult to remain alert during the lectures. Instruction was also provided by the superintendent, assistant superintendent, and head nurses, who were students themselves. Sadie looked forward to next year when she would be a senior and there would be no more lectures or quizzes, and the stipend would increase to $12. She would dispense medications and be given charge of an entire ward. She also cherished her half-day off each week, which she often spent sleeping.

The period from 1900 until 1950 saw tremendous changes in society. The world experienced two world wars; the United States moved from a predominately agricultural nation to an industrialized one, hospitals were built to house the ill and infirm, and women were granted the right to vote as they also realized economic and intellectual emancipation. Women moved into many roles in society; however, teaching and nursing were often favored as professions for females.

The development of hospitals and the advance of medicine created a need for nurses who would staff the hospitals. Many hospitals found that this was most easily accomplished by opening a school of nursing. Thus, during the early 1900s, many nursing schools were started in hospitals. These schools operated without the benefit of guidelines or accreditation, and there was no accountability for quality of education as measured by licensing examinations. It was not until 1923 that all states had enacted nursing licensure laws; however, the licensure was not mandatory.

By the mid 1900s, concern was being voiced regarding the quality and standards of the many nursing programs. Fueled by a study conducted by Esther Lucille Brown, nursing education began to move away from the system of apprenticeship that predominated at the time toward a planned program of education similar to that offered by other professions. A program for accreditation of schools was developed, and the first mandatory licensure law took effect in New York in 1947. Nursing organizations were established and became active in issues surrounding nursing education and practice.

Starting in 1909, 4-year baccalaureate nursing programs continued to grow in colleges and universities, although slowly. Then in 1952, as a result of a research study, associate degree nursing programs that could be completed in 2 years were initiated in community colleges. Thus, nursing found itself with three educational routes to preparation for registered nursing: the traditional hospital-based diploma program, the college or university-based baccalaureate degree program, and the college-based associate degree program. Any differences in abilities and skills of the graduates, regardless of length or depth of study, were undetermined. The commonality was that all nursing education programs within a state had a similar required core curriculum and the graduates of all types of programs were required to pass the same state licensing examination. The law provided the same **scope of practice** (the activities a person with a particular license may legally perform) for all registered nurses.

■ THE AMERICAN NURSES ASSOCIATION POSITION PAPER ON NURSING EDUCATION

By the early 1960s the educational preparation of nurses became a major concern of nursing leaders who were members of the American Nurses Association (ANA). Believing that the improvement of nursing practice and the profession as a whole depended on the advancement of nursing education, this organization published its first position on nursing education in December 1965 (ANA, 1965). This paper took the position that the minimum preparation for beginning professional nursing practice (sometimes referred to as **entry into practice**) should be baccalaureate degree education in nursing. It also stipulated that the minimum preparation for beginning technical nursing practice should be associate degree education in nursing.

Thus began what many believe to be the most contentious issue in nursing. After almost 50 years, the issue is still debated among those concerned. At their Spring 2000 meeting, the ANA Board of Directors reaffirmed the long-standing position that baccalaureate education should be the standard for entry into professional nursing practice.

Although the ANA has continued to hold its position regarding entry into professional nursing practice, the various states have continued to require the same competencies of all those preparing for registered nurse (RN) licensure. Thus, in all states, those graduating from associate degree programs, diploma programs, and baccalaureate programs continue to take the same licensing examination. Employers hire graduates of all types of programs into entry-level positions in hospitals, nursing homes, clinics, and home care.

Public health nursing, with the community as the client, continues to be taught exclusively in baccalaureate programs. Thus, public health departments usually require employees to have a baccalaureate degree. Some public health departments operate ambulatory clinics, for which they do hire nurses with other credentials. Baccalaureate degree programs usually require content related to reading and understanding nursing research along with the statistics needed for that process. They traditionally include a larger leadership component. These added components are not part of the licensure examination.

Specialization in nursing occurs at the master's degree level and a baccalaureate degree is required for entry into master's education. Many master's degree programs admit nurses with an associate degree in nursing and a baccalaureate degree in another field.

Critical Thinking Exercise

Gather as much information on the ANA position paper as possible. Review the various aspects of the issue. Do you support the requirement of a baccalaureate degree for entry into professional nursing? Why or why not? What would be the issues that must be settled if this were to occur? How would individual nurses be affected? Do you have a creative approach to this nursing concern?

The debate over this issue continues. As a new graduate, it is one with which you will grapple. A part of this concern is how the competencies of graduates of various programs differ. Thus, closely akin to the concern regarding entry into practice is that of differentiated practice.

■ DIFFERENTIATED NURSING PRACTICE

Differentiated nursing practice can be defined as "the practice of structuring nursing roles on the basis of education, experience, and competence" (Boston, 1990, p. 2). Differentiating nursing practice has gained increasing attention and importance as the reform that has occurred in health care has placed greater emphasis on cost containment, downsizing of acute care hospitals, the shift of care to ambulatory and community settings, and the increased focus on outcomes of care. Efforts to place the right nurse with the right competencies with the right patient at the right cost became the goal of health care professionals. Nursing organizations pushed for recognizing that different nursing competencies were needed in different settings and for different roles within the health care system and that the variety of educational programs should direct their resources to preparing graduates with differentiated skills.

Throughout the country, various projects began to emerge to address the issue of differentiated practice. In 1984, facilitation of differentiated practice was a goal of the National Commission on Nursing Implementation Project (NCNIP), which was funded by the W. K. Kellogg Foundation. It defined two types of differentiated practice: education-based and assessment-based. The education-based differentiated practice rested in the differing educational credentials of the nurse. Thus, nurses with different educational preparation would be both prepared for and expected to work in different roles within nursing. Both education and experiential learning that the nurse brought to the situation formed the base of the assessment-based differentiated practice model and was the most commonly used form. In this model, nurses were assessed for different competencies that might have been obtained through a variety of educational opportunities as well as experience in nursing and their roles would be assigned based on those competencies.

The Midwest Alliance in Nursing (MAIN) carried out two projects as part of the NCNIP activities. The first of these, a 3-year project funded by the W. K. Kellogg Foundation, was entitled "Defining and Differentiating ADN and BSN Competencies and Facilitating ADN Competency Development." The second, entitled "Continuing Education for Consensus on Entry Skills," was funded by a grant from the Division of Nursing of the Department of Health and Human Services. Both resulted in the development of general statements on roles and the delineation of

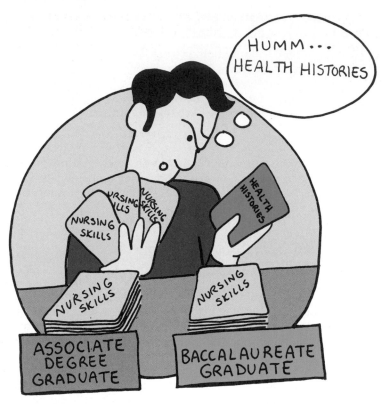

Education-based differentiated practice rests in the differing educational credentials of the nurse.

specific competencies in the area of direct care that would be based on educational preparation.

In 1988, Colorado developed a statewide plan that facilitated articulation of nursing education programs of various types and developed a differentiated model for nursing practice based on educational credentials and degrees of experience. A differentiated pay scale was recommended in this model. This plan included a detailed set of competency statements and job descriptions, and moving from one role to another required the acquisition of the appropriate degree. However, this model has never been widely implemented.

The Healing Web Project involved six midwestern and western states in which representatives of nursing education and practice came together to design, implement, and evaluate a variety of educational and practice differentiation activities. Associate degree and baccalaureate students are educated in concurrent laboratory experiences to differentiated roles. One of the sites for this project was Sioux Valley Hospital in Sioux Falls, South Dakota, where differentiated roles for nursing staff were implemented. Shared governance and case management accompanied this.

Another approach exists in the development of competency models. These models were often an outgrowth of the work of one of the twenty Colleagues in Caring projects throughout the United States that were funded by the Robert Wood Johnson Foundation. These projects frequently incorporated the ANA's standards of care or other standards along with the Benner (1984) levels of practice—novice, advanced beginner, competent, proficient, and expert—or in some cases most of them. One such model, developed in New Jersey, aimed to "bridge the disconnect between nursing education and practice and develop a patient care delivery model that was designed to utilize the RN role effectively across settings" (Cadmus, Dickson, and Tuella, et al., 2004, p. 2). The New Jersey model planned for two levels of practice and licensure in their differentiated practice models. Other states, including California, Mississippi, New Mexico, Alaska, South Dakota, Arizona, and South Carolina, became involved in developing pilot projects for differentiated practice.

In 1995, working with the American Organization of Nurse Executives (AONE) and the National Organization for Degree Nursing (NOADN), the American Association of Colleges of Nursing (AACN) published *A Model for Differentiated Nursing Practice.* This document outlined current efforts and presented a model for differentiated learning and practice (AACN, 1995).

Defining Competencies

The key to these models lies in identifying the competencies of nurses. The term **competencies** refers to what an individual is capable of performing and includes cognitive skills such as decision making and interpersonal skills as well as the psychomotor or technical skills associated with nursing procedures. Competency may be achieved through formal education. It is also acquired by work experience and practice (see Chapter 11). Nurses with differing competencies are assigned to different practice roles.

The term *competency* has become very popular in nursing and health care over the past decade. Thus, you will find it used in a number of references, but always with regard to what an individual is capable of doing. For example, in 2000, the Pew Health Professions Commission's Final Report addressed skills needed to function in health care in the twenty-first century. Twenty-one competencies were identified as critical to practice (Bellack & O'Neil, 2000). Display 14-1 lists the competencies identified by the Pew Commission. In 2003, a report released by the Institute of Medicine (IOM), titled "Health Professions Education: A Bridge to Quality," called for all programs that educate health professionals and adopt five core competencies: the abilities to deliver patient-centered care, work as a member of an interdisciplinary team, engage in evidence-based practice, apply quality improvement approaches, and use information technology (*IOM*, 2003).

EXAMPLE *Application of IOM Competencies*

Sally Jones was completing the last year of her nursing program. Her clinical instructor had asked the students to complete a client care plan that would incorporate all the IOM competencies in the care they delivered. One of the clients assigned to Sally's care was Jim Carding, who was diagnosed with chronic obstructive pulmonary disease (COPD). Sally was secure in the fact that her care was patient centered and therefore focused her efforts on the remaining competencies. She joined the pulmonologist and members of the nursing and respiratory therapy team as they met to discuss the client's care. At the conference she expressed concern regarding the increased mucus production she had noted and reported that Jim's cough appeared ineffective, that he tired easily, and experienced shortness of breath. Following the conference, Sally reread all the information in her textbook and accessed information regarding COPD on the Web site maintained by the publisher of the book that had been selected for her class. She also researched data on COPD in other nursing literature via the Internet. She found three recent studies related to caring for patients with this diagnosis. She was alerted to potential complications of atelectasis, pneumothorax, respiratory failure, pulmonary hypertension, and status asthmaticus. Based on her findings, she incorporated into her plan of care the monitoring of respiratory status and pulse oximetry, patient instruction and encouragement in diaphragmatic breathing and effective coughing techniques, and the administration of oxygen therapy as prescribed. She established outcomes focused on establishing a normal respiratory rate and pattern, normal pulse oximetry values, and improvement in respiratory function. When the patient was discharged several days later, he rated the nursing care he had received as excellent on the patient evaluation form provided by the hospital.

DISPLAY 14-1	**Twenty-one Competencies Defined by the Pew Health Professions Commission**

1. Embrace a personal ethic of social responsibility and service.
2. Exhibit ethical behavior in all professional activities.
3. Provide evidence-based clinically competent care.
4. Incorporate the multiple determinants of health in clinical care.
5. Apply knowledge of the new sciences.
6. Demonstrate critical thinking, reflection, and problem-solving skills.
7. Understand the role of primary care.
8. Rigorously practice preventive health care.
9. Integrate population-based care and services into practice.
10. Improve access to health care for those with unmet health needs.
11. Contribute to continuous improvement of the health care system.
12. Advocate for public policy that promotes and protects the health of the public.
13. Continue to learn and help others learn.
14. Practice relationship-centered care with individuals and families.
15. Provide culturally sensitive care to a diverse society.
16. Partner with communities in health care decisions.
17. Use communication and information technology effectively and appropriately.
18. Work in interdisciplinary teams.
19. Ensure care that balances individual, professional, system, and society needs.
20. Practice leadership.
21. Take responsibility for quality of care and health outcomes at all levels.

Implementing Differentiated Practice

The nursing profession has debated the issue of differentiated practice for years. Who should do what? What education should be required for the task? How much prior experience is required? At present, the growing demands for accountability and the pressure of the nursing shortage that expects the most efficient use of each nurse push the profession to renew its efforts and sharpen its focus on efficient delivery of care. Rick (2003, p. 11) states, "In the future high quality, state-of-the-art patient care that will require a spectrum of differentiated nursing roles to optimally configure nursing practice."

To this end, almost every state has initiated some type of program aimed at implementing differentiated practice. To encourage this breakthrough, several philanthropic organizations, such as the Robert Wood Johnson Foundation and the W. K. Kellogg Foundation that we previously mentioned, that have a special interest in health care have provided funding for studies and focused efforts. Many of these projects were centered on defining and implementing differentiated practice based on an educational model in an effort to ensure that the size and educational mix of the nursing workforce would be sufficient to meet nursing care needs across all settings.

The Robert Wood Johnson Foundation also sponsored the Nursing Practice and Education Consortium (N-PEC), a group formed in 1997 comprising 10 major national nursing organizations that collaborated to address vital concerns about the future of nursing. The specific purpose of the consortium was to create a comprehensive plan for nursing practice and education that would distinguish the specific competencies needed for nursing to meet its social mandate. A product of this group was the publication of a paper titled "Vision 2020 for Nursing" (Nursing Practice and Education Consortium, 2001). This paper advocates discrete scopes of practice and differentiated licensure tied to educational preparation and includes a strategic plan objective and outcome. The vision for the future would "have a nursing education system that is based in institutions of higher education and prepares nursing clinicians for clearly differentiated roles." It goes on to envision "a practice environment in which nurses practice in distinct and clearly differentiated roles" (Nursing Practice and Education Consortium, 2001). In November 2002, the members agreed to dissolve the consortium, with the recommendation that the Vision 2020 document be transferred to Nursing's Agenda for the Future (NAF) initiatives.

NURSING'S AGENDA FOR THE FUTURE

In mid 2001, the ANA appointed a steering committee comprising representatives from 19 national nursing organizations to develop a comprehensive strategic and tactical plan for nursing. This began with a Call to the Nursing Profession summit meeting held in September 2001, funded by a grant of $100,000 from the American Nurses Foundation. Participants representing 60-plus national nursing organizations were instructed to envision what nursing should look like and where it should be by the year 2010. *Nursing's Agenda for the Future* is the result of this work.

Nursing's Agenda for the Future (available through American Nurses publishing at www.NursesBooks.org or www.NursingWorld.org) identifies 10 domains or areas of concern demanding action: leadership and planning, delivery systems, legislation/regulation/policy, professional/nursing culture, recruitment/retention, economic value, work environment, public relations/communication, education, and diversity.

Work groups were assigned to each domain to identify strategies, objectives, and plans for implementation. Co-champions that represent organizations that will monitor the implementation and results of the plans guide the work of each domain (ANA, 2002).

IMPACT ON THE NEW GRADUATE

As you read through the preceding material you may have asked yourself, "So what does all this have to do with me? As a new graduate, how will I be affected?" Let's begin with the area of economics, because most new graduates are concerned about the dollars they will earn. One of the objectives of the *Nursing's Agenda for the Future* is the design of a model for reimbursement for nursing services. This will involve much data collection, accountability, and unification by nurses. As a new graduate you could be involved in all of these. As nurses work to establish the economic value of nursing, the need for quantified nursing data is critical. If you are working on a unit in which data are being collected, it is important that you take the extra time and effort needed to complete required reports. Nurses will be working together as a united whole to achieve established goals. Thus, supporting others and providing encouragement and assistance takes on new meaning. You will want to work in an environment in which nurses respect and care for one another and collaboration is of the essence.

You may seek employment in a health care facility that has implemented an integrated practice model. Perhaps this model will employ evidence-based practice. You will need to be flexible with regard to change. You may want to attend additional workshops or classes to gain more information on evidence-based practice. If these are not activities in which you want to be involved, you will want to be selective about seeking employment. If these activities are ones that excite you, you will want to learn as much about them as you can. As you seek employment, you may want to discover which hospitals in your area are committed to futuristic plans. Most interviews provide an opportunity for the person being interviewed to ask questions. You may want to prepare some well-thought-out questions that will provide such information to you.

If the facility in which you are hoping to gain employment is implementing a differentiated practice model, how will that affect what you will be doing as a nurse? Does this model result in a broader sharing of accountability among the nurses on the unit? How does this model affect staffing? How does it affect the quality of nursing care that staff can provide? Is shared governance a part of the model? Are collaborative work relationships promoted and supported? You can seek answers to these questions by talking with others employed in the facility or by discussing them during the interview. If you are thinking about seeking employment in a health care facility to which you were assigned for clinical experience, you can be exploring some of these areas as a student.

If you are interested in a leadership role in nursing, you will be interested in the professional development programs that are available to the new graduate. If a differentiated practice model is being used in a hospital in which you wish to work that bases that differentiation on education, do you need to consider additional formal education?

How can you remain informed about changes in nursing once you leave school? Participating in a professional nursing organization is one place to begin. Another activity that will allow you to remain informed is to subscribe to and read a professional nursing journal. Attending workshops and conferences that focus on current topics represents another avenue to remaining current.

Critical Thinking Exercise

Select one of the facilities in which you have had experience as a student. Discover what model of care delivery is being used in that hospital at the present time. Have any efforts been made to differentiate practice? Is it based on education, experience, or both? Is it related to salary benefits? Does it affect the role of the supervisors or managers? Are patients involved in assessing the quality of patient care? Compare your findings with those of a classmate who completed this assessment at a different facility.

Nursing Practice Models

A variety of new approaches to nursing practice models also have a major focus on differentiated practice. A nursing practice model may be defined as "operational models for redesigning nursing practice for the provision of patient care in organizational settings, primarily hospitals and long-term care facilities" (Weisman, 1992). Two of the factors that made the practice models reported by Weisman (1992) innovative as compared with traditional models were the degree to which the practice of individual nurses was differentiated according to education level or performance competencies and the degree to which nursing practice at the unit level was self-managed rather than being managed by traditional supervisors.

Some of the models were initiated primarily to address nursing shortages whereas others were motivated primarily to contain costs. Many of the models included consumer input regarding the quality of care in the data that was collected and most included patient outcomes. Often several elements were included in the same model.

EXAMPLE *Community Hospital's Clinical Ladder Program*

Community Hospital designated three categories of registered nurse roles as Clinical Nurse 1, Clinical Nurse 2, and Clinical Nurse 3. Each role had different educational and experience requirements. Clinical Nurse 1 required the completion of a probationary period and registered nurse's licensure. Clinical Nurse 1 was assigned to direct patient care on standard medical surgical nursing units. Susan James decided to apply for promotion to the Clinical Nurse 2 role. As part of the application process, she prepared a portfolio with information on both her education and experience. This promotion required that she have either a bachelor's degree in nursing or significant continuing education as well as three years of practice. She obtained the required peer reviews of practice and the administrative evaluation that was required. After she was promoted to the new role, Susan received a salary increase, but she also had increased responsibilities. She now worked as charge nurse, served on at least one practice-related committee for the hospital, and acted as a preceptor for new nurses.

A unit-based Differentiated Group Professional Practice Model at the University of Arizona College of Nursing includes three components: group governance (including participative management, staff by-laws, peer review, and professional salary structure); differentiated care delivery (including differentiated practice for RNs, use of nurse extenders, and primary case management); and shared values (including a culture-building process that valued quality of care, entrepreneurship, and recognition of practice excellence) (Weisman, 1992). The goal of this project was to create an opportunity for professional practice that would retain nurses and create a desirable work environment.

Another example is the research demonstration project at the University of Rochester School of Nursing, which was designed to increase nurses' control over practice at the unit level and to provide professional compensation. The project included five hospitals, experimental and control units, as well as pre- and posttest design. Patients' perceptions of the hospital experience, morbidity and mortality, and any unplanned hospital readmission up to 30 days after discharge were included in the patient outcomes that were studied.

Like the projects mentioned earlier, these projects were often funded by outside organizations such as the National Center for Nursing Research (NCNR) and the Division of Nursing. Through a program entitled "Strengthening Hospital Nursing: A Program to Improve Patient Care," 20 projects have been funded by the Robert Wood Johnson Foundation and the Pew Charitable Trust.

It is beyond the scope of this chapter to mention all the studies that are currently being conducted to implement and evaluate the effect of differentiated practice on quality care. We leave this topic by assuring you that as a new graduate you will encounter many opportunities to be involved in such study.

Just as you may have wondered how all the discussion of differentiated practice will affect you are a new graduate, you may also wonder about the various practice models. Many of the same suggestions apply here that we discussed earlier. It is always wise to gain as much information about prospective employers as possible before submitting applications to them (see Chapter 10).

EXAMPLE   *Surveying Employers*

Mark Morris was preparing to graduate from a nursing program in a large urban area. There existed a number of different health care facilities that were planning to hire new graduates. Mark wanted to be certain that he selected hospitals that embraced shared governance, were futuristic in their approach, and supported differentiated practice. To begin gathering this information, Mark went to the Web site of each hospital. He researched their mission statement and reviewed their values. He then clicked on the link titled "Governance Structure" to learn more about how they were structured. Following this, he gathered information on the history of each facility and explored links addressing legislative advocacy and classes that were offered. He concluded his Web search by going to the Web site of the local newspaper and searching the name of each facility for articles that had appeared in recent editions of the paper. He then ranked the facilities as first choice, second choice, and third choice and prepared to send his resumé to each.

Critical Thinking Exercise

You have been assigned to gather information about differentiated practice to be used in developing a project on the unit on which you work. From what you have read here, would you be more inclined toward a model differentiated on the basis on education or one based on competency? What factors have influenced your choice? What information would you gather to share with others? How would you go about gathering it? What resources are available to you?

■ ORGANIZATIONAL ADVISORY GROUPS IMPACTING NURSING

When an organization such as the Joint Commission on Accreditation of Healthcare Organizations (JCAHO), the Secretary of Health, or Congress what expert advise regarding issues with which they must deal, it is not unusual that an advisory group will be appointed to address specific concerns. Your career in nursing will be affected by the input several of these groups make. Therefore, we believe it is to your advantage to be able to recognize these groups and know their focus.

National Advisory Council on Nurse Education and Practice (NACNEP)

Authorized under Title VIII of the Public Health Service Act, the National Advisory Council on Nurse Education and Practice (NACNEP) provides advice and recommendations to the Secretary of Health and to Congress covering a wide range of topics. This group which is comprised of nursing leaders appointed by the Secretary of Health and Human Service addresses issues such as the nurse workforce, nursing education, and nursing practice improvement. For example, in its 1996 *Report to the Secretary on the Basic Nursing Workforce* this council identified the need to increase the racial/ethnic diversity of the registered nurse workforce (Bureau of Health Professions, 1996). They emphasized that a culturally diverse workforce is essential to meeting the health care needs of the Nation's population, citing increases in minority populations, that these populations have higher rates of certain diseases, lower rates of successful treatment, and sometimes shorter life expectancies.

As a result of NACNEP's recognition of the need for additional expertise to identify the issues related to workforce diversity, the Division of Nursing convened the Expert Workgroup on Diversity. The 18 members of the Workgroup are recognized for their nursing expertise and knowledge of workforce diversity issues represent a variety of organizations including national minority nurse organizations, schools of nursing, national nursing associations, national health care associations, national medical school associations, and private organizations. This group provided advice to NACNEP in the development of a national agenda to address this concern. They developed recommendations that covered four broad themes: education, practice, leadership, and cultural competency. The goals and actions were accepted by NACNEP who then issued the following goals.

- Enhance efforts to increase the recruitment, retention, and graduation of minority students
- Promote minority nurse leadership development
- Develop practice environments that promote diversity
- Promote the preparation of all nurses to provide culturally competent care.

As a result of these goals educational programs, regulatory agencies, and health care organizations are taking actions to assure that racial/ethnic diversity is increased in nursing. This includes, among other features, special programs for members of minority groups in both education and leadership, increasing the number and percentage of baccalaureate-prepared minority nurses, increasing the number of minority faculty, increasing the use of mentors for students and nurses young in their careers, and establishing cultural competence standards in education and practice. Diversity in nursing is discussed later in this chapter.

As you have progressed through your nursing program you may have recognized some of these goals in action. As you move into a work environment you will have additional opportunity to assist the profession to achieve these purposes.

Critical Thinking Exercise

You have been employed on a medical unit of an urban hospital for 6 months. A newly licensed minority nurse has been hired to work on this unit. What things can you do to facilitate this nurse's transition to the work environment? How will these things help? Are there others you need to involve in these activities? How will you know that your goals have been realized?

The Nursing Advisory Council of Joint Commission on Accreditation of Healthcare Organizations (JCAHO)

Throughout this textbook we have discussed the JCAHO. This group, that surveys health care facilities and measures their performance against a set of established standards, relies on a variety of **advisory groups** to assure that the public is provided with safe and quality care. These groups provide JCAHO leaders with feedback that assists them to develop and revise standards, policies and procedures. One such group is the Nursing Advisory Council.

The Nursing Advisory Council was established in the first quarter of 2003 to address issues in nursing such as the nurse shortage. The 30-member council composed of representatives from leading nursing organizations, the Federation of American Hospitals, researchers, labor representatives, and public members, is charged with addressing recommendations set forth in a white paper published in August 2002 entitled *Health Care at the Crossroads: Strategies for Addressing the Evolving Nursing Crisis.* The council meets several times a year to counsel the Joint Commission of nursing issues that affect health care quality and patient safety, provide a nursing perspective on new initiatives and identify way to optimize the effects of nursing-related changes to JCAHO's standards and accreditation processes (JCAHO, 2003).

Public Advisory Group

The Public Advisory Group is another council that was formed in 1999 to advise the JCAHO on current and evolving care issues that are of concern to the public. The 25 individual members and organization representatives come from public advocacy groups, prevention associations and consumer groups. They define public expectations for quality in health care and offer suggestions for improving the accreditation process. This represents just one more instance of consumer input to expectations regarding the quality of health care and the standards that ensure it (Facts About Advisory Groups, 2003.)

As a new graduate you will soon become aware of the role of the JCAHO in accreditation of health care facilities. You will want to learn which of your nursing activities fall under one of the standards this group assesses. More information regarding the JCAHO and its role of assuring quality care is discussed in Chapter 4.

■ REGULATORY AGENCIES IMPACTING NURSING

Several regulatory agencies impact nursing practice in agencies and institutions.

State Board of Nursing

The most significant regulatory agency impacting nursing is the state board of nursing or its equivalent. This agency administers the nurse practice act. Nurse practice acts are the policing power of the state and exist to protect the public safety, specifically against negligence, **malpractice,** or other torts committed by nurses. Most states have similar nurse practice acts that define nursing and establish the scope of practice, mandate and set standards for licensure and examination, regulate and set the standards for nursing education programs, and investigate reports of violation of nursing practice with ensuing discipline when violation has occurred. Some states also stipulate the requirements for continuing education; however, continuing education is not required for continued licensure in all states. Once you have completed your nursing program, you will be eligible to write the licensing examination in your state that, when passed, will result in a license that will permit you to practice nursing as defined by that state. Therefore, nurses must remain informed about the legal ramifications of nursing practice and stay abreast of any changes in the language of the nurse practice act in the state in which they are practicing in order to protect themselves from disciplinary action by the state.

As nurses have moved into roles with greater responsibility and accountability for professional practice, the nurse's liability or legal accountability has also increased. Patients who believe they have been harmed by improper actions on the part of professional nurses may seek compensation or redress through civil courts.

Although the root of many errors committed by nurses is found in system problems rather than personal incompetence, the nurses remain liable for their action. Negligence is a broad term that refers to conduct that does not show due care. Malpractice refers to the negligence of a specially trained or educated person in the performance of his or her job that results in harm to the patient (Ellis & Hartley, 2004).

Major areas in which nurses are involved in malpractice litigation include situations involving patient falls, failure to identify and document pertinent information, failure to perform treatments or nursing care correctly, failure to communicate significant data and errors in medications (Swansburg & Swansburg, 2002). For example, it has been reported from an observational study of nurses administering medications, that 19% of the doses were erroneous with 43% given at the wrong time, 30% omitted, 17% being the wrong dose, and 4% being an unauthorized drug. Seven percent of the errors were considered clinically significant (ASN Reports: Using Technology to Address Medication Errors, 2003).

Because of the increase in suits brought against nurses, many nurses choose to purchase personal malpractice insurance. This is a wise practice. Most professional liability insurance policies provide support for legal counsel in both suits against the nurse and for disciplinary actions by the board of nursing as well as paying for any judgment against the nurse. However, the best action any nurse can take to protect against malpractice claims in to maintain a high standard of care. Nurses should perform only those nursing skills they are competent to perform that are allowed within the scope of practice outlined in the nurse practice act of the state.

Health Care Agency Certification and Accreditation

If you choose to work in a hospital after graduation, it is important that you have a basic understanding of the standards against which that facility is accredited. This occurs in the form of certification and accreditation. When the standards of a governmental agency are met it is referred to as **certification;** when the standards of a non-governments agency are met it is referred to as **accreditation.** Health care facilities may be surveyed by the state Department of Health and then certified. Medicare/Medicaid funding requires that specific federal standards be met to qualify for those funds. The agency that meets those standards is termed Medicare certified. The major organization responsible for the accreditation of hospitals is the Joint Commission on Accreditation of Healthcare Organizations (JCAHO). This organization also accredits home care agencies associated with hospitals. The Community Health Accreditation Program (CHAP) accredits community health and home health agencies.

Both certification and accreditation require site visits by evaluators who examine all aspects of an institution's functioning. These evaluative visits are stressful for everyone involved because of the serious consequences of failure to meet the standards. If you are employed at a health care agency, you will usually be expected to participate in education to prepare you to respond appropriately when the agency is expecting a site evaluation. As these visits move to the process of being unscheduled, you will want to have a general understanding of the criteria that affect your practice. In particular, you will want to assure that standards are being followed for nursing-related processes, such as documentation, discharge planning, and medication administration.

EXAMPLE ***Learning About Standards of the Joint Commission on Accreditation of Healthcare Organizations (JCAHO)***

Jacob Justice had accepted a position as an RN in a community hospital in the area in which he lived with his family. Shortly after he began work on the surgical unit to which he was assigned, he learned that members of the accrediting team of JCAHO had recently visited and had cited the facility on several standards. Jacob had learned little about JCAHO standards in his nursing education program and felt the need to develop a better understanding of the accreditation process. He began by visiting the JCAHO Web site, where he learned that he could sign up for e-mail newsletters and additional information. He explored links to frequently asked questions and pursued areas in which JCAHO was placing increased emphasis, such as safety and infection control. He learned that effective January 2004, all hospitals are required to avoid the use of "dangerous" abbreviations in clinical documentation. He had never thought of some of the abbreviations as causing concern. Included among the examples he found was the requirement that QD and QOD be written out, because one can be confused with the other. Similarly, he learned that International Units (IU) needed to be written out because it was to frequently misread as IV (intravenous). Jacob decided to set aside an hour each day after he had completed his shift at the hospital to learn more about the JCAHO standards. In addition, he decided to talk with his unit manager about finding a way in which he could share his new knowledge with fellow employees.

 ■ **LEGISLATION IMPACTING NURSING**

The activities of nurses increasingly are being affected by enacted legislation. This legislation may come from federal, state, or local groups. For example, the federal government legislated the Health Insurance Portability and Accountability Act (HIPAA) of 1996 that is currently being implemented in health care facilities. Aimed at protecting patient privacy, one section places severe limitations on the information that can be released regarding patients. All nurses must be informed about such legislation and the restrictions that it imposes. In many instances, the legislation requires changes in the way or the type of services are delivered to patients. Many of the recent legislative mandates have been directed at providing patients a greater role in decision making regarding their care. Being aware of these requirements is a part of providing competent care.

The Public Health Security and Bioterrorism Response Act of 2002 authorizes funding to train health care professions, including nurses, to prepare for and respond to bioterrorism. Nurses should be aware that they are eligible for such funds. The Smallpox Emergency Personnel Protection Act of 2003 (PL 108-20) addressed the role of the federal government in assuring the proper administration of smallpox vaccinations and established a compensation program for individuals injured by the vaccine (McKean, 2003). As informed health care workers, nurses should know of this legislation.

In California, legislation has been enacted that stipulates maximum nurse:patient ratios. This will affect nursing practice in that state. Thus, it is essential that nurses be informed about state legislative mandates. Nurses are often involved in the process of developing the language of the legislation and encouraging its passage.

■ A NURSING NOMENCLATURE

Another fairly recent development in the nursing profession that promises to grow and flourish is the development of a unique language that would describe the clinical judgments made by nurses that are not in medical language systems. As long ago as 1909, nurses with a strong eye to the future and professionalism recognized that nursing would someday need a language of its own However, throughout the development of nursing as a profession, nursing had relied on disease entities from medical classifications as the basis for thinking, speaking and writing. The first steps toward the goal of systematic nursing terminology were the development and exploration of nursing theories and the introduction and implementation of the nursing process problem solving approach to care in the mid-twentieth century. The terminology established in these efforts proved to be the first steps toward a broader nursing terminology that emerged in the 1970s.

Defining a language for nursing primarily involves the development and refinement of **nursing nomenclatures** and **classification systems** that communicate information and guide data collection about nursing activities. The term nursing nomenclature refers to the words by which we name or describe phenomena in nursing. A classification is the systematic arrangement or a structural framework of these phenomena. Establishing a specialized language for nursing has evolved from a need for objective, science-based information to use in decision making. These data also provide the basis for accountability and the documentation supporting processes and outcomes of care. The data can be used further to answer research questions about nursing and nursing actions.

In December 1995, the ANA Board of Directors approved the establishment of the Nursing Information & Data Set Evaluation Center. The group's purpose is to review, evaluate against defined criteria, and recognize information systems that support documentation of nursing care. Groups wanting to have their information system included among those approved by the ANA complete necessary application packets and pay established fees. Depending on the number of applications, the review process occurs twice a year. The recognition is granted for a period of 3 years, after which another application must be completed and another review conducted.

At present, the language of nursing primarily addresses nursing diagnoses, nursing interventions, and nursing outcomes. Four systems that currently are the most widely used are discussed in the following.

North American Nursing Diagnosis Association (NANDA)

The first steps toward a common language for nursing started in 1973 at the First National Conference on Classification of Nursing Diagnosis. National Conferences have been held on a regular basis since that time. The National Group for the Classification of Nursing Diagnosis became a formal organization after the fifth conference and was renamed the North American Nursing Diagnosis Association **(NANDA).**

The association addresses two main purposes: to develop a diagnostic classification system (also known as a **taxonomy**) and to identify and approve nursing diagnoses.

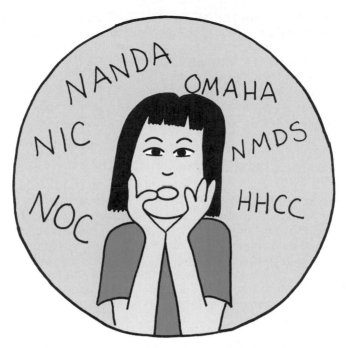

The language of nursing can be overwhelming at first.

McCormick and Jones (1998) define taxonomy as a hierarchical system that includes vocabulary and terms. After the first meeting of NANDA participants, 29 conceptual areas were identified with approximately 100 terms. The current classification system contains 71 conceptual areas and 143 terms (Gordon, 1998).

The following is the definition of a nursing diagnosis accepted by the NANDA (1997): "Nursing diagnosis is a clinical judgment about individual, family, or community response to actual or potential health problems/life processes. Nursing diagnoses provide the basis for selection of nursing interventions to achieve outcomes for which the nurse is accountable."

The list of nursing diagnoses (concepts that are given word labels) continues to grow as nurses encounter diagnoses in clinical practice that have not been included and submit these to NANDA for consideration. As a student, you have some familiarity with nursing diagnoses from the nursing care plans you develop for patient care and in the case studies you discuss in your classes.

Nursing Interventions Classification (NIC)

The University of Iowa began work on the classification of nursing interventions in 1996. The Nursing Interventions Classification **(NIC)** represents a comprehensive, standardized language describing treatments that nurses perform in all settings and in all specialties and includes both physiological and psychosocial interventions. To facilitate computerization, the interventions are numbered. There are 486 interventions organized into 30 classes and 7 domains. Each intervention listed contains a definition and a set of detailed activities that describe nursing actions. The interventions have been linked with NANDA, the Nursing Outcomes Classification (NOC), Patient Outcomes, Omaha System problems, long-term resident assessment protocols (RAPS), and the OASIS outcome measures mandated by home health care. They facilitate the implementation of a Nursing Minimum Data Set (University of Iowa, 2003a). The use of NIC to plan and document care will assist in the collection of large databases, which will allow the study of the effectiveness and cost of nursing treatments. Ultimately, it is hoped that this information will help to establish the importance of the nurse's role in delivery of health care.

Nursing Outcomes Classification (NOC)

Also developed at the University of Iowa, the Nursing Outcomes Classification (**NOC**) was published in 1997. Listed in alphabetical order, the classification includes 247 individual level outcomes, 7 family outcomes, and 6 community outcomes. An outcome is defined as a "measurable individual, family, or community state, behavior or perception that is measured along a continuum and is responsive to nursing interventions" (University of Iowa, 2003b). Each outcome has a definition and a list of indicators that assist in evaluation of patient status.

The outcomes are organized into 29 categories, called classes. Classes are grouped in seven domains: functional health, physiologic health, psychosocial health, health knowledge and behavior, perceived health, and family health and community health. Each outcome has a unique code number to facilitate its use in computerized clinical information systems that will allow manipulation of data to respond to questions about the quality and effectiveness of nursing care. In 1997, the first joint international NANDA, NIC, and NOC Conference was held in St. Charles, Illinois (University of Iowa, 2003c).

The Omaha System

The **Omaha System,** another example of early classification efforts, is based on federally funded research conducted by the Visiting Nurse Association of Omaha from 1975 to 1993. It was designed as a three-part, comprehensive yet brief approach to documentation and information management for multidisciplinary health care professionals who practice in community settings. The goal was "to provide a useful guide for practice, and method for documentation, and a framework for information management" (The Omaha System, 2003). The system includes an assessment component (Problem Classification Scheme), and intervention component (Intervention Scheme) and an outcomes component (Problem Rating Scale for Outcomes). It offers terms and codes to classify the client's health-related concerns or problems, the interventions that nurses and other health care professionals use, and the client's outcomes. Client problems can be identified for individuals, families, and groups of all ages, locations, medical diagnoses, socioeconomic ranges, spiritual beliefs, and culture. The interventions describe both plans and interventions for specific client concerns. The outcome scales evaluate a client's health-related changes through the use of problem-specific knowledge, behavior, and status ratings. The Omaha System is recognized by the ANA and is used by an international community (Omaha System, 2003).

DISPLAY 14-2 **Classification Systems Recognized by the ANA**

- North American Nursing Diagnosis Association (NANDA)
- Nursing Interventions Classification System (NIC)
- Nursing Outcomes Classification System (NOC)
- Nursing Management Minimum Data Set (NMMDS)
- Home Health Care Classifications (HHCC)
- Omaha System
- Patient Care Data Set (PCDS)
- Perioperative Nursing Dataset (PNDS)
- SNOMED RT
- Nursing Minimum Data Set (NMDS)
- International Classification for Nursing (ICNP)
- ABC codes
- Logical Observation Identifiers Names & Codes (LOINC)

Other Classification Systems

Several other classification systems have emerged. In some instances, they were developed for a particular specialty. It is not within the purview of this textbook to discuss each, but data identifying those systems recognized by the ANA are found in Display 14-2.

Critical Thinking Exercise

Review the listing of nursing classifications presented in Display 14-2. What do you perceive as the future for such endeavors? How do you believe nursing will benefit? What resources are necessary for the full development of such systems? What experience have you had using the systems thus far in your nursing education? What long-term benefits can be anticipated?

■ INCREASING DIVERSITY REPRESENTATION IN NURSING

Disparities in health and health care are not new occurrences and they continue to be problematic. In 2000, the U.S. Census Bureau reported that 25% of the U.S. population is composed of ethnic minority groups, with African Americans comprising the largest number. At the present growth rate, the Hispanic population is expected to increase by 21% by the year 2040 (U.S. Bureau of the Census, 2000). The history of the United States reveals a disparity in the health care services received by members of minority groups, which has resulted in increased disease morbidity and mortality rates experienced by minority ethnic/racial groups.

Disparities are considered differences in the quality of health care that are not due to access-related factors or clinical needs, preferences, and interventions. Included among the causes of the disparities are provider–patient relationships, provider bias and discrimination, and patient variables such as mistrust of the health care system and refusal of treatment (Baldwin, 2003). Thus, we see increased incidence of such conditions as cardiovascular disease, cancer, and diabetes among members of minority groups.

Key to correcting this disparity is the education of physicians, nurses, and allied health professions. Physicians and nurses represent the largest group of health care providers. At the present time, 12.3% of RNs have been documented as racial and ethnic minorities (Smedley et al., 2002). This does not represent a large enough group to effectively meet the nation's future health care needs. A culturally diverse workforce is essential to meeting the health care needs of the nation's population.

Why is it important that there be a sufficient number of racial and ethnic minorities in the health care workforce? First, many believe that insensitivity to patients resulting from racial bias and discrimination exists in the current managed care system. In addition, many minority patients do not trust the health care system and as a result refuse treatments (Baldwin, 1996). Another concern is that cultural differences often result in problems in communications (see Chapter 5). All these point to the need for health care systems to create programs that will help their staff to become culturally competent and sensitive to the needs and values of a more diverse clientele (see Chapter 11).

Another solution that will help resolve this problem is organized around recruiting and retaining more racial and ethnic minorities in the health care professions. It has been reported that minority nurses tend to practice in their own communities once they have completed their education (Smedley et al., 2002). Minority nurses contribute significantly to the development of models of care and provision of care that address the special needs of racial/ethnic minority populations.

A number of projects have been launched to support and increase the number of minorities in nursing. *Nursing's Agenda for the Future* (2002) sets forth several objectives that address diversity issues, including obtaining funding to support an increase in minority enrollment, identifying a specific mobility track for nurses of diverse cultures throughout their careers, creating a specific curriculum to address diversity, and developing and distributing promotional and recruitment materials to attract individuals from diverse backgrounds into nursing.

You have probably noted that the curriculum for your nursing program has included content that will assist you to become culturally competent. As you move into a position in nursing, you may notice that some of the more experienced nurses have not had the advantage of this content. You can do much teaching by example. You can help create and maintain a workplace environment that is sensitive to the needs of all people.

■ KEY CONCEPTS

- The first nursing programs in the United States were apprenticeship in nature with students learning by working along side a more experienced individual.
- The first nursing programs were established in the late 1800s and were typically 18–24 months long.
- As the country moved from an agricultural to an industrialized nation, hospitals were constructed, medical advances occurred, and many hospitals established educational programs to prepare nurses with little attention to standards. By the 1950s, this was a concern for the profession.

- In 1965 the ANA published its first position on nursing education that promoted the requirement of a baccalaureate degree for entry into professional nursing. Hotly debated at the time, the position continues to be a contentious issue in nursing.
- Differentiated practice is the practice of structuring nursing roles on the basis of education, experience, and competence. By the mid 1980s, several projects, often funded by foundations, were implemented to differentiated practice based on nursing education.
- Differentiated practice can also be put into practice by recognizing individual competencies. This approach has been implemented in some health care organizations and may be encountered by the new graduate seeking employment.
- The term *competency* has become very popular in nursing and health care and a number of organizations have identified needed competencies for nursing practice. Among these organizations are the Pew Health Professions Commission and the IOM.
- In 2001, the ANA published *Nursing's Agenda for the Future* that looked at where nursing should be by 2010. Ten areas of concern were identified.
- In an effort to recognize and implement differentiated roles in nursing, a number of hospitals have participated in projects, which have resulted in the development of practice models that are based on the education and experience of nurses. Foundations that have an interest in health care often fund these projects.
- A number of organizational advisory groups also impact the practice of nursing. Some of these groups are legislative in origin, such as the National Advisory Council on Nurse Education and Practice; others are regulatory, such as the state boards of nursing; whereas still others represent special councils of groups responsible for the accreditation and approval of health care organizations.
- Since the 1970s, nursing has been developing a nomenclature unique to the practice of nursing. The NANDA was the first of these.
- Other nursing classifications commonly used in nursing include the NIC, the NOC, and the Omaha System. Currently, the ANA recognizes 13 different language systems, some of which are focused on specialties in nursing practice.
- Nursing continues to recognize and support an increase in the number of racial and ethnic minorities in the profession. The recruitment and retention of minorities in nursing is critical to correcting racial and ethnic disparities that occur in health care.

REFERENCES

American Association of Colleges of Nursing. (1995). *A Model for Differentiated Nursing Practice.* Washington, DC: Author.

American Nurses Association's First Position on Nursing Education. (1965). *American Journal of Nursing, 65*(12), 106–111.

American Nurses Association (ANA). (2002). *Nursing's Agenda for the Future* [Online]. Available at www.nursingworld.org/naf. Accessed November 1, 2003.

ASN reports: "Using Technology to Address Medication Errors." (2003). *American Journal of Nursing, 103*(4):25.

Baldwin, D. M. (1996). A model for describing low-income African American women's participation in breast and cervical cancer early detection and screening. *Advances in Nursing Science, 19*, 27–42.

Bellack, J. P., & O'Neil, E. H. (2000). Recreating nursing practice for a new century. *Nursing and Health Care Perspectives, 21*(1), 14–21.

Benner, P. (1984). *From Novice to Expert: Excellence and Power in Clinical Nursing Practice.* Menlo Park, CA: Addison-Wesley.

Boston, C. (Ed.) (1990). Differentiated practice: an introduction. In *Current Issues and Perspective on Differentiated Practice* (pp. 1-3). Chicago: American Organization of Nurse Executives.

Bureau of Health Professions. (1996). Executive Summary [Online]. Available at http://bhpr.hrsa.gov/nursing/nacnep/divrepex.htm. Accessed May 21, 2004.

Cadmus, E., Dickson, G. L., Tuella C., et al. (2004). An integrated competency-based nursing practice model [Online]. Available at http://www.njccn.org/pdf/Competency_Model.pdf. Accessed May 17, 2004.

Ellis, J. R., & Hartley, C. L. (2004). *Nursing in Today's World: Trends, Issues, & Management* (4th ed.). Philadelphia: Lippincott Williams & Wilkins.

Gordon, M. (September 30, 1998). Nursing nomenclature and classification system development. *Online Journal of Issues in Nursing.* Available at http://www.nursingworld.org/ojin/tpc7/tpc7_1.htm. Accessed October 4, 1999.

Institute of Medicine. (2003). *Health Professions Education: A Bridge to Quality.* Greiner, A. C. & Knebel, E. [Eds.], Committee on the Health Professions Education Summit. Washington, DC: The National Academics Press.

Joint Commission on Accreditation of Healthcare Organizations (JCAHO). (2003). *Facts About Advisory Groups* [Online]. Available at http://www.jcaho.org/about+us/advisory+groups/. Accessed on September 20, 2003.

McCormick, K. A., & Jones, C. B. (1998). Is one taxonomy needed for health care vocabularies and classifications? *Online Journal of Issues in Nursing.* Available at http://www.nursingworld.org/ojin/tpc7/tpc7_2.htm. Accessed on October 4, 1999.

McKean, E. (2003). Smallpox compensation legislation passes. *American Journal of Nursing, 103*(6), 29.

North American Nursing Diagnosis Association (1997). *1997–1998 NANDA Nursing Diagnoses: Definitions and Classifications (1997–1998).* Philadelphia, PA: Author.

Nursing Practice and Education Consortium (N-PEC). (2001). *Vision 2020 for Nursing* [Online]. Available at http://www.nursingsociety.org/programs/vision2020.rtf. Accessed on September 14, 2003.

Rick, C. (2003). AONE's leadership exchange: differentiated practice—get beyond the fear factor. *Nursing Management, 34*(1), 11.

Smedley, B. D., Stith, A. Y., & Nelson, A. R. (2002). Unequal treatment: confronting racial and ethnic disparities in health care. *Institute of Medicine Report.* Washington, DC: National Academy Press.

Swansburg, R. C., & Swansburg, R. J. (2002) *Introduction to Management and Leadership for Nurse Managers* (3rd ed.). Boston: Jones and Bartlett Publishers.

The Omaha System: Omaha System Overview [Online] Available at http://www.omahasystem.org/systemo.htm. Accessed September 28, 2003.

University of Iowa. (2003a). *Nursing Interventions Classification: Overview* [Online]. Available at http://www.nursing.uiowa.edu/centers/cncce/nic/nicoverview.htm. Accessed September 28, 2003.

University of Iowa. (2003b). *Nursing Outcomes Classification: Overview* [Online]. Available at http://www.nursing.uiowa.edu/centers/cncce/noc/nocoverview.htm. Accessed September 28, 2003.

University of Iowa. (2003c). *Center for Nursing Classification & Clinical Effectiveness: History Timeline and Highlights* [Online]. Available at http://www.nursing.uiowa.edu/centers/cncce/history.htm. Accessed September 28, 2003.

U.S. Bureau of the Census. (2000). *Statistical Abstract of the United States.* Washington, DC: U.S. Government Printing Office.

"Using Technology to Address Medication Errors." (2003). *American Journal of Nursing, 103*(4):25.

Weisman, C. S. (1992). Nursing practice models: research on patient outcomes In *Patient Outcomes Research: Examining the Effectiveness of Nursing Practice* (pp.112–120), DHHS.NIH Publication No. 93-3411. Washington, DC: National Academy Press.

Glossary

Absenteeism. The pattern of being absent from work or an assignment.

Abstract. A brief summary of a scientific article or work.

Acceptance theory. A view of authority that proposes that authority is earned by a leader from the subordinate.

Accommodating. A strategy for dealing with conflict in which the individual gives in to the wishes of another to preserve harmony or build up social credits.

Accountability. As associated with responsibility, often viewed as the liability associated with actions.

Accountable. The situation of being answerable in a legal sense for particular actions or activities.

Accreditation. An acknowledgment given to a school or organization to certify that it has met a certain set of standards.

Achievement. Accomplishments.

Achievement motivation. According to McClelland, motivation that is based on the accomplishment itself and not on external rewards.

Achievement-oriented leadership. A part of the path–goal theory developed by House, a type of leadership behavior that concentrates on identifying challenging goals that capable subordinates are expected to achieve.

Active listening. Communication strategies designed to encourage another person to communicate his or her thoughts, feelings, or perceptions.

Adhocracy. A type of structure that employs the use of teams of specialists who are organized to complete a particular project or task. Members of the team may come from a variety of disciplines and the role of the leader is to create the process for effective problem solving.

Adult learning. An approach to teaching and learning that acknowledges the unique needs of adults.

Adversarial model. A method of approaching advocacy that assumes that the other individual does not have the same goals.

Advisory groups. Groups composed of individuals with certain expertise who come together to offer advise to an organization or institution.

Advocacy. Helping clients to be autonomous and informed decision makers and to accomplish their own goals and objectives.

Advocate. An individual who helps clients to be autonomous and informed decision makers and to accomplish their own goals and objectives.

Affective learning. Changes that encompass attitudes, values, and feelings.

Affiliation. According to McClelland, motivation that is based on the desire to feel related to other people.

Affirmation. A statement of positive regard for another individual.

Agency shop. A condition in collective bargaining in which all employees are required to pay dues for membership. If because of religious or philosophical beliefs, employees are unwilling to pay dues to the bargaining group, provisions may be made to pay the same sum to a nonprofit group.

Aggressive. Behavior that infringes on the rights of another person.

Algorithm. A systematic method of solving a certain kind of problem; a set of actions to be followed in a given situation.

Anger. A feeling of displeasure resulting from injury, mistreatment, opposition, and the like that typically shows itself in a desire to fight back or "get even."

Apprenticeship. A method of learning in which a student works for a given period of time with a master craftsman to learn the skills of that trade.

Assertiveness. Behavior that clearly outlines one's own boundaries and rights.

Assessment. Gathering information to determine whether an unmet need, problem, or concern is present.

Assignment. A specific set of duties given to an individual to accomplish as part of the job.

Assistive personnel. Persons, usually unlicensed, to whom nursing tasks are delegated.

Audit. A formal and often periodic examination and checking of accounts, financial records, or operations to verify their correctness.

Authoritarian or autocratic leadership/management style. A leadership style that is characterized by strong control by the manager over the workgroup.

Authority. The official power an individual has to approve an action, to command an action, or to enforce a decision. Power held by virtue of the position an individual holds within the organization; the right to act and make decisions.

Autonomy. An ethical principle that refers to the right to make one's own decisions.

Avoiding. An approach to dealing with conflict in which the individual chooses not to address the issue at hand.

Behavioral theory. Also referred to as the humanist approach, it represents a theory of leadership that looks at the behaviors in which the leaders engaged.

Benchmark. A specific quantitative standard to which one compares one's own accomplishment.

Beneficence. An ethical principle that refers to the commitment to do or bring about good.

Bioethics. Ethical issues that result from technological and scientific advances, especially in biology and medicine.

Boundary violation. A situation in which a professional infringes on the space that exists between the professional's power and the client's vulnerability.

Brain sheet. An informal written organizational tool.

Brainstorming. A type of decision making in which a group of people gather and suggest all possible alternatives that they can envision to a problem.

Budget. A formal plan for managing financial resources.

Budget hearings. Meetings in which proposals for the new budget are presented.

Budget processes. The method of determining a budget for an organization.

Budget variance. The difference between the planned and the actual expenditures or income.

Bureaucracy. A type of administration in which the organization operates through a complex structure of departments and subdivisions, usually following an inflexible routine.

Capital budget. The funds assigned to purchases of a relatively permanent nature, often defined as a specific budget amount.

Capitation. A method of health care reimbursement based on a fixed payment per individual in the plan.

Career. A profession or occupation for which one trains and which one pursues as a life work.

Career counselor. An individual schooled in assisting others in the development of their careers.

Career development. The process of establishing or planning one's career or life work.

Career mapping. The process by which one develops a master plan for career advancement.

Career styles. The form, manner, or stages of career development.

Case management. A type of care delivery in which a case manager monitors a patient's health care for purposes of maximizing positive outcomes and containing costs.

Case method. A type of nursing care delivery in which a nurse provides all the care a patient needs and often assumes other household responsibilities, often living in the home.

Centralized. To gather together or to make central; to organize under one control.

Certification. A written statement or specified process attesting to the accomplishment of certain goals or standards.

Chain of command. The path of authority and accountability from one individual with top administrative authority to the individuals at the very base of the organization.

Champion. Another term applied to the change agent.

Change. To alter or to become different; to transform.

Change agent. The person who seeks to cause or create change.

Channels of communication. The patterns of message-giving within an organization.

Charisma. The power that attracts one person to another and relates to the way the leader looks, acts, talks, walks, and associations to which he or she belongs.

Checklists. A type of evaluation form that describes the standard of performance, and the rater indicates whether the employee demonstrates that behavior by placing a check mark in a column.

Chemical dependence. The physical need of the body for a particular substance.

Chemically impaired/chemical impairment. A term used to describe the condition that exists when an individual's professional practice has deteriorated because of chemical abuse, specifically the use of alcohol and drugs.

CINAHL. Cumulative Index to Nursing and Allied Health Literature. A comprehensive index of journal articles, books, computer programs, and videos that relate to all areas of nursing and allied health professions.

Classification systems. In nursing, a term applied to nursing language that communicates information and guides data collection about nursing activities.

Clinical career ladder. A system of advancing nurses developed around specific criteria that are used to evaluate and promote nurses who wish to remain at the beside as opposed to pursuing different jobs in nursing, such as administration, teaching, or research.

Clinical incompetence. When an individual fails to perform clinical skills in a manner that meets established standards.

Clinical pathways/critical paths. In nursing care, a series of spelled-out interventions and activities to be taken with specific outcomes along a given timeline.

Coach. To instruct or train; to develop potential.

Coaching. A process of using feedback to assist others to achieve their own personal bests and to support the entire team in achieving desired outcomes.

Coaching role. The position one occupies when instructing or training.

Coerce/coercion. The act or power of restraining or constraining by force or threats.

Coercive power. Power that is achieved from verbal threats of punishment and that is based on fear of punishment.

Cognitive learning. Changes that encompass thoughts, ideas, and intellectual understanding.

Collaborate. To work in a cooperative manner with others.

Collaborating. An approach to conflict in which the individuals involved in the conflict work toward common goals.

Collective bargaining. A process of negotiation between organized workers and their employer for reaching an agreement on wages, fringe benefits, hours, working conditions, and the like.

Communication. The giving or exchanging of information, either verbal or nonverbal, between individuals.

Competence/competencies. A demonstrated ability or skill.

Competing. An approach to conflict in which the individual works for his or her particular desired solution exclusively.

Complaints. In organizations, a formal charge or accusation.

Compromise. An approach to conflict that involves give and take on the part of all persons involved.

Concurrent audit. A review of patient records while the patient is still hospitalized.

Confidentiality. The act of keeping information confidential, that is, not sharing it with others.

Conflict. The situation that occurs when people with different values, interest, goals, or needs view things from a different perspective.

Confrontation. Addressing a problem directly with the person involved.

Connection power. Power based on having connections (or associations) with others who are powerful.

Consensus. In decision making, an agreement among all participants to accept the proposed solution.

Constraints on advocacy. Factors that tend to restrict an individual from successfully acting as an advocate.

Consultant. A knowledgeable individual from outside the organization who has specialized expertise and skills and who is called in to help rectify a situation.

Contingency theory of leadership. A theory of leadership developed by Fiedler, which included the leader–member relationship, the structure of the task to be performed, and the position power wielded by the leader.

Continuing education. Learning activities designed to maintain or expand competence in a chosen field.

Continuous quality improvement (CQI). A formal process in which ongoing analysis and improvement lay the foundation for change.

Control group. In a research study, the group that does not receive any treatment or intervention.

Control procedures. Processes used to monitor expenditures.

Convenience sample. In research, a sample of the population that is composed of those whose participation may be easily (conveniently) obtained.

Co-optation. Enlisting key people from the opposition onto your side by giving them desirable roles in the process and thereby ensuring their commitment.

Cost containment. Efforts to diminish the rate of increase in the cost of health care.

Cost standards. The ratio of the cost in resources when compared with a given health care outcome.

Cost–benefit ratio. A comparison between the economic cost of any plan and the benefits to be derived from it. Also termed *cost-effectiveness.*

Cost-effectiveness. The relationship between the cost of some aspect of health care and its effects on health care outcomes. A comparison between the economic cost of any plan and its effectiveness in accomplishing its goals. Also termed *cost–benefit.*

Cost-shifting. The process used by hospitals of charging more to those who can pay to cover the costs of care delivered to those who have no source of payment.

Cover letter. A letter sent to an organization along with a resumé to inquire about available positions.

Critical thinking. According to Paul, the intellectually disciplined process of actively and skillfully conceptualizing, applying, analyzing, synthesizing, or evaluating information gathered from observation, experience, reflection, reasoning, or communication.

Critical-incident technique. An evaluation method in which specific instances of the employee carrying out responsibilities critical to the job are documented.

Cross-functional. A process used in health care organizations to train an individual to carry out the responsibilities of another worker or area of work.

Cultural competence. Demonstrating knowledge and understanding of the client's culture; accepting and respecting cultural differences.

Cultural desire. A term defined by Campinha-Bacote as the nurse's motivation to want to engage in the process of becoming culturally aware, knowledgeable, and skillful, and seeking cultural experiences.

Culturally appropriate. Patient care that takes into consideration all aspects of cultural differences.

Damage control. A technique of management in which the manager distributes assignments so that a single individual who fails to meet expectations will cause minimal disruption to the unit.

Decision. A judgment or choice between two or more alternatives.

Decision grid. Also referred to as a matrix; a visual grid that allows comparison of alternative strategies for dealing with a problem.

Decision making. A systematic cognitive process in which alternatives are identified and evaluated, a conclusion is reached, and an action is selected.

Decision-making competence. The ability to make good decisions.

Decision tree. A graphic tool that provides a means of organizing the key elements that go into a decision.

Delegate. When individuals authorize a competent person to act for them or in their stead.

Delegatee. The individual to whom tasks are assigned.

Delegation. The process of transferring specific job responsibilities to another person.

Delegator. The person who is doing the delegating.

Delphi method. A decision making process in which a group of individuals propose, analyze, and rate alternatives, and in which the members work independently and the membership of the group is known only to the manager.

Democratic leadership/management style. A leadership style in which the manager focuses on involving subordinates in decision making; sees himself or herself a as coworker; and stresses communication, consensus, and team work.

Dependent variable. That which changes as a result of the independent variable.

Descriptive research. A type of nonexperimental research that has as its purpose a more accurate and more precise description of the population.

Diagnostic related groups (DRGs). A category to which a medical diagnosis is assigned based on the average number of days of hospitalization and costs for care. Used to determine reimbursement under Medicare and Medicaid.

Differentiated nursing practice. The practice of structuring nursing roles on the basis of education, experience, and competence.

Directive leadership. A part of the path–goal theory of leadership developed by House in which the leader focuses on rules and policies and gives specific direction to expectations and task accomplishment.

Disciplinary procedures. A set of steps or actions to be taken when an employee's performance is consistently unacceptable.

Discoverable. Information that must be made available to a legal counsel of a plaintiff bringing suit.

Dissatisfiers. According to Herzberg, a category of job attributes that can cause dissatisfaction in their absence but are not sufficient to cause satisfaction when present. Also termed *hygiene factors.*

Divided loyalties. The feelings that exist when one finds oneself wanting to be supportive of two groups that may have differing values and goals.

Documentation. The act of recording all activities or actions that have taken place.

Dominance power. Control, authority, or influence over others.

Driving forces. Forces that call for change.

Due process. In employment, problems; includes the employee being notified of the problem, being told what must be done to correct the problem, receiving help (coaching and/or teaching) in remedying the problem, and being given time for this to occur.

Effectively. Performing in such a manner as to accomplish the desired outcomes.

Efficiently. Performing in such a manner as to accomplish the desired outcomes within a designated time framework.

Embarrassment. A emotion that exists when one is caused to feel self-conscious, confused, ill-at-ease, or flustered.

Empirical-rational strategy. An approach to change that says change will be accepted by a person, group, or organization when it is seen as desirable and is aligned with the interest of those affected.

Employee assistance program. A program designed to help employees who have problems.

Employee performance evaluation. Another term used for performance evaluation. A formal evaluation process for employees.

Empower. To assist others to take action to achieve their desired outcomes.

Empowerment. The process by which a leader shares power with others or enables them to act.

Entrepreneur. A person who organizes and manages a business undertaking.

Entry into practice. The point at which one enters a career after completing the education preparation for that particular discipline.

Ethnocentrism. The emotional attitude that one's own culture, ethnic group, or nation is superior to others.

Ethnography. A type of research in which the researcher becomes involved in the culture being studied and tries to describe it as completely as possible.

Evaluation. The process of determining the effectiveness of an individual's performance. The process of determining the outcomes and effectiveness of any action taken.

Evaluation standards. A set of criteria that can be used in the evaluation process.

Evidence-based practice (EBP). The process of applying to patient care approaches to that care that have been demonstrated as effective through research.

Exit interview. An interview conducted at the termination of employment or other final activity.

Experimental group. The group in a research study that receives the treatment or intervention.

Experimental research. A research strategy in which the researcher is determining the effect of an independent variable controlled by the researcher.

Expert power. Power that is gained through the possession of special knowledge, skill, or ability.

External forces. Factors encouraging change that originate outside the person or organization.

Extraneous variable. Variable other than the independent variable that might also affect the dependent variable and could confuse the relationship between the independent and dependent variables.

Extrinsic motivator. Something outside of the person that tends to support behavior.

Feedback. Information given to an individual regarding his or her performance.

Fee-for-service. Reimbursement for health care based on the specific services performed.

Fidelity. An ethical principle referring to the responsibility to carry out the agreements and responsibilities one has undertaken.

Field review. An evaluation method that allows comparison of the ratings of several supervisors for the same employee to be compared.

Findings. The information disclosed by the research study.

First reprimand. Informing the employee about the problem behavior, identifying acceptable behavior and officially reprimanding the employee for the poor performance; may be a verbal reprimand.

Fiscal year. A 12-month period chosen as the budgeting year, commonly from January 1 through December 31 or July 1 through June 30.

Flat or decentralized organization. A type of organizational structure with few levels and a broad span of control.

Force field analysis. A theory of change developed by Lewin, which describes the forces that push toward change balanced against the forces that restrain change.

Forcing. An action taken during a conflict that involves working for one's particular desired solution exclusively.

Formal education. A planned program of learning usually occurring in a school or other educational institution.

Functional method. A type of care delivery characterized by having nurses assigned to various tasks, for example, a treatment nurse or a medication nurse.

Generalization. The application of findings from a research sample to the entire population.

Goals. The broad statements of overall intent of an organization, department, unit, or individual; an object or end that one strives to attain or accomplish.

Great Man theory. An early theory of leadership which contends that some people are born to lead and others are born to be led.

Grievance process. The steps or process that spells out an orderly method to be used in mediating the grievance between parties.

Health maintenance organizations (HMOs). Health provider organizations founded on the principles of keeping the subscribers healthy and avoiding high cost care.

Hierarchy of needs. According to Maslow, the order of primacy of the various human needs.

History. Events other than the experimental variable that can affect a research outcome.

Humiliation. The emotion one feels when one's pride or dignity is wounded or when one is caused to seem foolish or contemptible.

Hygiene factors. According to Herzberg, a category of job attributes that can cause dissatisfaction in their absence but are not sufficient to cause satisfaction when present. Also termed *dissatisfiers.*

Hypothesis. The reasoned prediction of the outcome of a research study that is based on the theoretical framework and previous research.

Independent variable. The variable that is manipulated by the researcher.

Index Medicus. The print form of a comprehensive index of medical and biomedical literature compiled by the National Library of Medicine.

Informal organization. The group of individuals within an organization that is responsible for much of the socialization of employees.

Informational power. Described by Heineken and McCloskey, the power that exists when individuals have information that others must have to accomplish particular goals.

Integrative decision making. An approach to decision making or conflict resolution that involves problem solving and collaboration among those involved.

Internal forces. Factors encouraging change that come from within the organization or person.

Internet service provider (ISP). A company that provides a link from individual computers into the Internet system.

Interpersonal competence. Refers to having the ability to relate effectively with coworkers, clients, family members, and members of the community.

Interview. Typically, a meeting of people face to face during which each learns about the other, or a time during which the evaluator meets with the employee to discuss the evaluation.

Intrapersonal conflict. Occurs within an individual in situations in which he or she must choose between two alternatives.

Intrinsic motivator. Something within the person that tends to support behavior.

Job. A specific task or work that one has agreed to do for pay.

Job descriptions. Written statements that describe the duties and functions of the various jobs within the organization.

Journal. A periodical publication aimed at a specific professional or technical field.

Justice. An ethical principle that relates to the obligation to be fair to all people.

Key indicator. Selected data, monitored on an ongoing basis, that reveal the need for more extensive data collection or remedial action.

Laissez-faire leadership/management style. A style of leadership that provides the least structure and control; little or no direction is provided by the leader.

Leadership. The process of guiding, teaching, motivating, and directing activities of others toward attaining goals.

Leadership style. The manner in which one goes about planning, organizing directing, and controlling the actions of others.

Learning style. The manner of presentation in which an individual most effectively learns.

Legitimate power. Often termed *authority,* the power granted by an official position.

Letter of inquiry. A letter written to inquire about available positions in an organization.

Level of significance. The probability at which the changes in the dependent variable would be identified as being due to the action of the independent variable rather than chance.

Lines of authority. The pattern of responsibility and accountability that is passed from one level to the next within the organization.

Linguistically appropriate. Services that are provided in ways that meet the language needs of the client and family. This includes translation services if needed, signs in various commonly used languages, and the use of language seen as respectful by the client.

Listserv. A type of group discussion conducted by e-mail messages.

Lose–lose. An outcome of conflict in which neither party wins or achieves the desired outcome.

Majority rule. Acceptance of a ruling, decision, or outcome that is favored by the greatest number of the participants.

Malpractice. Negligence on the part of a professional in the performance of his or her job; may be inappropriate actions taken or failure to take appropriate actions.

Managed care. Any health plan system in which care is actively managed by the third-party payer who sets the ground rules for care and determines where, how, and by whom care will be provided.

Management. The coordination and integration of resources through planning, organizing, directing, and controlling in order to accomplish specific goals and objectives within an organization.

Management by objectives. A method of managing through developing specific, predetermined outcomes or goals. When applied to performance evaluation, a method of basing evaluation on the evaluator's observations of the employee's performance as measured against very specific, predetermined objectives or goals that have been jointly agreed on by the employee and the evaluator.

Marginal employee. An employee whose work meets only the minimum standards considered acceptable.

Matrix structure. A type of organizational structure in which a second structure overlies the first, creating two directions for lines of authority, accountability, and communication.

Maturation. The fact that differences measured from one point in time to another may be due to changes in the subject over time rather than to the independent variable.

Mediate. To bring about resolution of a conflict or dispute through friendly or diplomatic intervention, sometimes involving a third party who serves as a go-between.

Mediation. The process of resolving differences through having a third party as a go-between for others.

Mediator. A person who helps the involved parties to negotiate toward a solution.

Medicaid. A program supported by the federal and state governments and administered by the states that is designed to provide health care to those meeting specific low income standards.

Medicare. A federal program to provide health care to those over 65 years of age, the disabled, and others on Social Security.

MEDLINE. A computerized index to biomedical and health literature compiled by the National Library of Medicine.

Mentor. An individual who serves as a role model, guide, and support to a novice.

Mentoring. Assisting a selected individual to prepare for advancement and greater opportunities; support offered to those with promise and potential.

MeSH. Medical subject heading used for subject category indexing by the National Library of Medicine.

Meta-analysis. Combining through statistical techniques the results of several different research studies to determine the overall findings of the studies collectively.

Minimal disruption of the unit. A situation in which the action chosen is the one that causes the very least disruption or harm to a unit.

Mission statement. A statement that outlines what the organization plans to accomplish, its aims or function, and the group to whom services are directed.

Modular care. A type of care delivery system similar to team nursing, in which patient care units are divided into modules and the same team of care providers is consistently assigned to each module.

Mortality. The loss of participants in a research study. Also termed *attrition*.

Motivation. The drive to accomplish or engage in specific behaviors.

Motive/motivator. A factor that drives behavior.

Movement. The second stage in the change process identified by Lewin in which the change agent identifies, plans, and implements appropriate strategies to bring about the change.

Multicratic style. A leadership style that requires the leader to employ the style the particular situation calls for, using structure when needed and providing maximum group participation in other instances.

Multidisciplinary team. A group of individuals with differing professional skills and abilities who collaborate to support the client in achieving desired outcomes.

Multitasking. Working on several tasks simultaneously.

NANDA. Acronym for North American Nursing Diagnosis Association, one of the classification systems in nursing.

Narrative or essay technique. An evaluation technique in which the evaluator writes a paragraph or more (usually more) outlining an employee's strengths, weaknesses (or areas for improvement), and potential.

Negative feedback. Information provided to an individual about performance that does not meet the standard.

Negotiating. Reaching an agreement through conferring, bargaining, or discussing the issues.

Negotiation. The process of finding areas in which both parties may give something and then both parties gain.

Newsgroup. A type of online group discussion in which messages are posted at one site and individuals can access that site to read the posted messages.

NIC. Acronym for Nursing Implementation Classifications, one of the nursing classification systems.

NOC. Acronym for Nursing Outcomes Classifications, one of the nursing classification systems.

Nominal group technique. A decision-making process in which a group of individuals selected by the manager write down alternatives, which are then shared, analyzed, and ranked.

Nonmaleficence. An ethical principle that means to do no harm.

Nonproductive employee behaviors. Actions taken by an employee that do not benefit the organization or its clientele.

Nonverbal communication. The communication of meaning through body movement and position and facial expressions.

Normative reeducative strategy. An approach to change that maintains that change will take place only after changes in attitudes, values, skills, and significant relationships have occurred.

Null hypothesis. The statement that no relationship exists between the independent and dependent variables. Used as a statistical tool.

Nursing informatics. The use of technology to retrieve and manage information relevant to nursing practice.

Nursing nomenclature. Another term for nursing language usually found in nursing classifications.

Objectives. The specific accomplishments that help achieve the goal.

Ombudsman. A person with the official role of advocate for individuals in a specific setting or in relationship to a specific organization.

Omaha System. A classification of nursing focused on community nursing.

Operating budget. Funds designated to be used for the day-to-day operating expenses.

Organization. A group of people that come together for some specific purpose.

Organizational chart. A graphic, pictorial means of portraying various roles and patterns of interaction among parts of the system.

Organizational climate. The prevailing feelings and values experienced by individuals who work in an organization.

Organizational culture. The sum total of organization values, formal and informal communication patterns, and historical patterns that influence how an organization operates.

Organizational effectiveness. The degree to which and the ease with which an organization achieves it purpose.

Organizational function. The way interactions actually occur within the organization.

Organizational hierarchy. The path of authority and accountability within an organization.

Organizational structure. The way in which a group is formed, its chains of command, its lines of communication, and the process by which decision making occurs.

Outcome standards. A statement of the expected results of care for the patient that can be used for evaluation.

Participant. In a research study, each member of the sample, also termed a subject.

Participative. An approach to activities that allows all involved individuals to have a part or the share in the decisions.

Participative decision making. A process of decision making that allows a group of individuals to make the decision rather than a single individual.

Partnership models. A type of nursing care delivery in which patients are cared for by a pair of caregivers, often a registered nurse and a nursing assistant.

Paternalism. The restricting of an individual's liberty by making decisions for the person, in the manner of a father making decisions for his children. It usually involves withholding information and is justified because the decision maker "knows what is best" for the person.

Patient classification systems. Methods used to separate patients into groups based on acuity or resource utilization.

Peer evaluation. In nursing, staff nurses are asked to evaluate other staff nurses as a contribution to their growth and development in nursing.

Peer reviewed. Something that has been reviewed and evaluated by a group of peers.

Performance appraisal. A formal evaluation process for employees.

Performance feedback. Providing the individual with information on his or her own behavior in relationship to expectations and standards.

Performance improvement. Another term for quality improvement.

Performance standards. Criteria for performance, usually found in writing.

Permissive (leadership). Another term used for the laissez-faire leadership style.

Phenomenology. A type of research designed to describe experience as it is lived by people.

Philosophy. Provides a statement of beliefs and values that are basic to the operation of the organization, service, or unit.

Physiological needs. One of the levels of needs described by Maslow that is essential for one's physical existence.

Policy(ies). Designated plans or courses of action for a specific situation.

Policy manuals. A written document that contains all the policies for a given organization.

Population. The entire group of people in whom a phenomenon is of interest.

Positive feedback. Information provided to an individual about performance that meets or exceeds the standard.

Positive performance. Performance that meets standards and expectations for the role.

Power. The ability to influence others; or the ability to act or accomplish objectives.

Power-coercive strategy. An approach to change that is employed when the leader orders change and those with less power comply.

Preferred providers. Health care providers that have contracted with a health care plan to provide care at a predetermined lower price.

Primary nursing. A type of nursing care delivery in which one nurse is assigned the responsibility for the care of a patient from the time the patient is admitted to the hospital until discharge.

Prioritize. To determine the order of importance for accomplishing a set of tasks.

Proactive. To take action to prevent problems.

Probability. The statistical likelihood of an event occurring.

Problem employees. Those individuals who, for various reasons, are unable to perform as fully contributing team members.

Problem solving. A method of conflict resolution in which the individuals involved work toward common goals. Also referred to as the *collaborative approach.*

Procedures. A document that spells out how a particular nursing activity is to be completed.

Process standards. A statement of the processes intended to accomplish the desired outcomes that should be in place and that can be used for evaluation.

Process theories. Theories of leadership that look at leadership as it relates to group interaction.

Procrastination. To put off action.

Progressive discipline. A series of steps or actions to be taken with an employee when that employee's work consistently fails to meet expectations.

Project structure. An organizational structure that is centered around a group of specialists who come together to accomplish a certain project or task.

Promotion. Advancement in rank, position, grade, or salary.

Pros and cons. A listing of the advantages or favorable consequences of an action and the disadvantages of unfavorable consequences.

Prospective reimbursement. A predetermined payment schedule for a given surgery or episode of illness based on some type of statistical average.

Protocols. A term applied to special unit policies.

Proximal cause. The individual action that created the error.

Psychomotor (technical) competence. Those abilities that are related to "doing" or "performing" a skill.

Psychomotor learning. A type of learning related to the acquisition of motor skills.

Punishment power. The authority to discipline or reprimand others for wrong-doings.

Qualitative. A type of research concerned with the subjective and contextual; that is, it looks at phenomena in their environment instead of attempting to isolate them.

Quality assessment and improvement (QAI). The ongoing activities designed to objectively and systematically evaluate the quality of patient/resident care and services, pursue opportunities to improve patient/resident care and services, and resolve identified problems.

Quality assurance (QA). Activities that are used to monitor, evaluate, and control services provided to consumers.

Quality assurance reports. A written statement describing a situation in which standards were not met or an error occurred. May also be referred to as an incident report.

Quality circles. Groups of first line workers who meet to develop strategies for improvement.

Quality improvement (QI)/quality improvement movement. The emphasis within all types of organizations on continuing to improve all aspects of the organization.

Quality indicators. Data that indicate that high standards of care are being maintained.

Quantitative. A type of research that emphasizes experimentation and statistical analysis.

Random sample. A method of assigning participants (subjects) into groups through a method that would allow every participant the same chance of being in any group.

Rapid process improvement. A strategy of quality improvement in which the problem is identified, the team assembled, and plans for change made and implemented in very short time frame such as ten days to two weeks.

Rater bias. The tendency to make judgments based on factors other than the official standards of performance.

Rating scales. An evaluation tool that consists of a set of behaviors or characteristics along with a method to indicate the degree to which the person being evaluated demonstrates each behavior.

Reactive change. Change that occurs in response to some event or problem as it arises.

Recruitment. The process of actively searching for qualified personnel.

Referent power. Identified by French and Raven, the power a leader has because others identify with that leader or what that leader symbolizes.

Refreezing. The final stage of change identified by Lewin in which changes that have been made are integrated and stabilized.

Reinforcement. A reward given to a learner for making the desired response.

Relational model of leadership. A theory of leadership in which leadership is viewed as a relational process designed to accomplish a common goal to benefit all.

Reliability. The degree of consistency or dependability with which an assessment tool measures something.

Reprimand. A serious or formal rebuke, especially by a person in authority.

Research. A systematic approach to the study of a phenomenon.

Research design. A plan for carrying out a research study.

Resistance. A force that retards, hinders, or opposes motion or change, or the act of opposing or withstanding a concept or change.

Responsible model. An approach to advocacy that uses negotiation, compromise, and persuasion and involves interaction with other persons associated with the situation.

Restraining forces. Forces that are opposed to change.

Resumé. A brief written overview of one's qualifications for a position.

Retrospective audits. Reviewing charts after the patients have been discharged.

Reward power. Identified by French and Raven, the power that is achieved by having the ability to grant favors to others or the promise of reward that they value.

Risk management. Taking actions that minimize the risk to the institution or agency of an error or problem that could result in legal action or liability.

Role ambiguity. Occurs when employees do not know what to do, how to do it, or what the outcomes must be.

Role conflict. Occurs when two or more individuals in different positions within the organization believe that certain actions or responsibilities belong exclusively to them.

Root cause analysis. A comprehensive, often complex, process that seeks to identify all the contributory factors to an error and identify their share of causation.

Safety needs. A level of needs described by Maslow that deal with being secure or safe.

Samples. Portions of the population chosen for study.

Satisfiers or motivators. According to Herzberg, those attributes of an employment situation that make people feel satisfied with their job.

Scarcity of resources. Exists when there is an inadequate amount of supplies, equipment, funds, space, employees, or other elements critical to the operation of an organization.

Scope of practice. The activities, procedures, and treatments that a licensed individual may do as specified by the licensing act governing that profession.

Second reprimand. The second serious or formal rebuke, especially by a person in authority, usually in writing.

Selection. Refers to choosing subjects and sorting them into control and experimental groups. If the choice of subjects and the assignment to groups are not random, there may be significant undetected differences between the two groups.

Self-actualization. The highest level of needs described by Maslow, which relate to reaching one's full potential.

Self-determination. Making one's own decisions.

Self-esteem. A person's self-evaluation of worth.

Self-evaluation. Examining oneself and determining to what extent one meets the standards one has set.

Servant leadership theory. A theory of leadership in which the successful leader is pictured as being able to influence others as a result of dedicating his or her life to serving others.

Shared governance. A form of administration in an organization in which the running of the organization (governance) is shared among all levels of employees. The aim is the empowerment of individuals within the decision-making system.

Situational theory of leadership. A theory of leadership that focuses on the context or the situations in which the leader functions.

Smoothing. An approach to dealing with conflict in which the individual tries to eliminate anger and expressions of difference without addressing the issue itself.

Social change model of leadership. A leadership theory in which individuals and groups work toward a common goal and improve the quality of life for all by promoting basic values.

Socializing. Engaging in personal conversation and activities.

Span of control. The number of individuals one person is responsible for managing.

Stakeholders. Those affected by a change or action; the client system.

Standards for critical thinking. Criteria for the measurement of the quantity, extent, value, or quality of an individual's thinking process.

Standards of care. Authoritative statements that describe a common or acceptable level of client care.

Standards of nursing practice. Expected behaviors of the registered nurse that can be used as a basis for measuring performance.

Story board. A report of the changes that are implemented from start to finish of a project that serves as a report and identifies progress along the way.

Strategies. In the world of management, alternative actions.

Structural standards. A statement of the organizational structures that are intended to accomplish the desired outcomes, should be in place, and that can be used for evaluation.

Subject. Individual chosen to participate in a research study. Also termed *participant.*

Subject headings. Categories used for indexing.

Substance abuse. A term applied to the overuse of chemicals or alcohol.

Supervisor. One responsible for overseeing and directing the activities of others.

Supervisory role. The role one occupies when he or she oversees and directs the activities of others.

Suspension. An official period of time, usually without pay, during which an individual is not to return to work because of unacceptable behavior.

Tall organization. A type of organizational structure in which most of the decision-making authority and power is held by a few persons.

Task force. A group of individuals appointed by the manager to work on a specific problem.

Taxonomy. In nursing, another term for classification system.

Teaching. The process of instructing others.

Team building. An activity that has as its goal the generation of a type of synergy, in which the outcomes of people working together toward common goals have a greater effect that can be realized by the sum efforts of people working individually.

Team nursing. A type of nursing care delivery in which care providers on a unit are organized into groups comprising individuals with various levels of education.

Termination. The formal ending of employment, either voluntarily or involuntarily.

Testing. Refers to the fact that a testing procedure can itself pose a threat to research integrity, because it can produce changes in a patient.

Theory X. A theory of leadership developed by McGregor that viewed workers as basically lazy, in need of constant supervision, unwilling to assume responsibility, indifferent to organizational goals and purposes, and seeking rewards in money and fringe benefits.

Theory Y. A theory of leadership developed by McGregor that viewed workers as reliable, self-motivated, and willing to work hard to achieve personal and organizational goals.

Theory Z. Developed by Ouchi, an expansion of McGregor's Theory Y to include consensus decision making, job security, quality circles, and strong bonds between superiors and subordinates.

Thesaurus. A listing of the categories used for indexing along with an explanation of the attributes of that category.

"Thinking hats." A strategy that encourages looking at a situation from multiple perspectives.

Third-party payers. Those health plan or government entities that pay for health care provided to the client by a separate health care provider.

Time management. A planned approach to organizing activities to maximize the amount that can be accomplished in the time available.

Total patient care. A nursing care delivery system in which a registered nurse or licensed practical (vocational) nurse is assigned to all care needs of a group of four to six patients.

Total quality management (TQM). An overall management program to implement continuous quality improvement.

Trait or attribute theory of leadership. A theory of leadership that attributes ability to lead to particular traits of an individual, such as intelligence, decisiveness, or creativity.

Transactional leadership. A leader who functions in a caretaker role and is focused on day-to-day operations.

Transformational leadership theory. A leader who motivates followers to perform at their full potential by influencing changes in perceptions and by providing a sense of direction to the group.

Trust. The first belief or confidence in the honesty, integrity, or reliability of another person.

Unfreezing. The first stage of change identified by Lewin in which the change agent loosens or unfreezes the factors or forces that are maintaining the status quo.

Unlicensed assistive personnel (UAP). Unlicensed personnel to whom tasks are assigned.

Validity. The degree to which an assessment tool actually measures what it is supposed to measure.

Value analysis. A systematic approach to the evaluation of products, including supplies, equipment, pharmaceuticals, and new technology, that are used in providing patient care.

Variance. A difference between the planned expenditure and the actual expenditure.

Veracity. An ethical principle that refers to the obligation to tell the truth.

Verbal communication. Words exchanged in an interaction.

Win–lose. An outcome of conflict in which one of the parties wins (dominates) and the other loses (submits).

Win–win. An outcome of conflict in which both parties win.

Withdrawing. A strategy for dealing with conflict in which the individual retreats from the situation or ignores it.

Written reprimand. A written warning regarding the effects of behavior that are unacceptable.

Zero-base budgeting. A budgeting plan in which every department starts from zero and must justify all budget requests, not just new or increased requests.

Index

Page numbers followed by an "f" denote figures; those followed by a "b" denote boxes; those followed by a "t" denote tables; those followed by a "d" denote displays.